Field and Laboratory Methods for Grassland and Animal Production Research

Field and Laboratory Methods for Grassland and Animal Production Research

Edited by

L. 't Mannetje
Department of Plant Sciences
Wageningen University
Wageningen
The Netherlands

and

R.M. Jones
CSIRO
Tropical Agriculture
St Lucia
Australia

CABI *Publishing*

CABI *Publishing* is a division of CAB *International*

CABI Publishing
CAB International
Wallingford
Oxon OX10 8DE
UK

Tel: +44 (0)1491 832111
Fax: +44 (0)1491 833508
Email: cabi@cabi.org
Web site: http://www.cabi.org

CABI Publishing
10 E 40th Street
Suite 3203
New York, NY 10016
USA

Tel: +1 212 481 7018
Fax: +1 212 686 7993
Email: cabi-nao@cabi.org

A catalogue record for this book is available from the British Library, London, UK.

Library of Congress Cataloging-in-Publication Data
Field and laboratory methods for grassland and animal production research / edited by L.
't Mannetje and R.M. Jones.
    p.   cm.
   Replaces Measurement of grassland vegetation and animal production. 1978.
   Includes bibliographical references.
   ISBN 0-85199-351-6 (alk. paper)
   1. Pastures--Research. 2. Feed utilization efficiency. I. Mannetje, L. 't II. Jones, R. M.
(Richard M.)

  SB199 .F44 2000
  633.2'02--dc21

00-037816

ISBN 0 85199 351 6

Typeset by AMA DataSet Ltd, UK.
Printed and bound in the UK by the University Press, Cambridge.

Contents

Contributors

A.T. Adesogan, *Welsh Institute of Rural Studies, Llanbadarn Campus, University of Wales, Aberystwyth SY23 3AL, UK.* Email: ata@aber.ac.uk

K.E. Basford, *Department of Agriculture, University of Queensland, St Lucia 4067, Australia.* Email: K.E.Basford@mailbox.uq.edu.au

G.N. Bastin, *CSIRO, Department of Wildlife and Ecology, PO Box 2111, Alice Springs 0871, Australia.* Email: Gary.Bastin@dwe.csiro.au

W. Bayer, *Rohnsweg 56, D-37085 Göttingen, Germany.* Email: wb.waters@link-goe.de

J. Bouma, *Department of Environmental Sciences, Laboratory for Soil Science and Geology, Wageningen University, PO Box 37, 6700 AA Wageningen, The Netherlands.* Email: Johan.Bouma@BodLan.BenG.WAU.NL

D.I. Bransby, *Department of Agronomy and Soils, 202 Funchess Hall, Auburn University, Auburn, AL 36849, USA.* Email: dbransby@acesag.auburn.edu

V. Chewings, *Centre for Arid Zone Research, CSIRO, Division of Wildlife and Ecology, PO Box 2111, Alice Springs 0871, Australia.* Email: Vanessa.Chewings@dwe.csiro.au

D.B. Coates, *CSIRO, Davies Laboratory, Private Mailbag, PO Aitkenvale 4814, Australia.* Email: David.Coates@tag.csiro.au

J.P. Curry, *Department of Environmental Resource Management, Faculty of Agriculture, University College, Belfield, Dublin 4, Ireland.* Email: james.curry@ucd.ie

M.H. Friedel, *CSIRO, Division of Wildlife and Ecology, PO Box 2111, Alice Springs 0871, Australia.* Email: Margaret.Friedel@dwe.csiro.au

D.I. Givens, *ADAS, Nutritional Sciences Research Unit, Drayton Manor Drive, Alcester Road, Stratford-upon-Avon, Warwickshire CV37 9RQ, UK.* Email: Ian.Givens@adas.co.uk

M.B. Hardy, *Crop Development, Department of Agriculture, Western Cape, Private Bag X1, Elsenburg 7607, South Africa.* Email: markh@wcape.agric.za

M.J.M. Hay, *AgResearch, Private Bag 11008, Palmerston North, New Zealand.* Email: HayM@agresearch.cri.nz

V.J.G. Houba, *Department of Environmental Sciences, Wageningen University, PO Box 8005, 6700 EC Wageningen, The Netherlands.* Email: Victor. Houba@BodGenG.BenP.WAU.NL

S.C. Jarvis, *Institute of Grassland and Environmental Research, North Wyke Research Station, North Wyke, Okehampton, Devon EX20 25B, UK.* Email: steve.jarvis@bbsrc.ac.uk

R.M. Jones, *CSIRO Tropical Agriculture, 306 Carmody Road, St Lucia 4067, Australia.* Email: dick.jones@tag.csiro.au

A.M. Kelly, *Queensland Department of Primary Industries, Toowoomba, 4352, Australia.* Email: Kellya@dpi.qld.gov.au

E.A. Laca, *Department of Agronomy and Range Science, One Shields Avenue, 249 Hunt Hall, University of California, Davis CA 95616-8515, USA.* Email: ealaca@ucdavis.edu

W.A. Laycock, *Department of Rangeland Ecology and Watershed Management, College of Agriculture, University of Wyoming, Box 3354, Laramie WY 82071, USA.* Email: KBrewer@UWyo.Edu

G. Lemaire, *INRA, Station d'Écophysiologie des Plantes Fourragères, 86600 Lusignan, France.* Email: lemaire@lusignan.inra.fr

A.R. Maclaurin, *University of Zimbabwe, PO Box 167, Mount Pleasant, Harare, Zimbabwe.* Email: maclauri@cropsci.uz.zw

L. 't Mannetje, *Department of Plant Sciences, Wageningen University, Haarweg 333, 6709 RZ Wageningen, The Netherlands.* Email: ltmannet@bos.nl

G.M. McKeon, *Queensland Centre for Climate Applications, Department of Natural Resources, Indooroopilly 4068, Australia.* Email: greg.mckeon@dnr.qld.gov.au

O. Oenema, *Wageningen University and Research Centre, Alterra, PO Box 47, NL-6700 AA Wageningen, The Netherlands.* Email: o.oenema@alterra.wag-ur.nl

D.M. Orr, *Queensland Department of Primary Industries, PO Box 5545, Rockhampton 4702, Australia.* Email: Orrd@dpi.qld.gov.au

E. Owen, *Department of Agriculture, University of Reading, Earley Gate, PO Box 236, Reading RG6 2AT, UK.* Email: E.Owen@reading.ac.uk

P. Penning, *Institute of Grassland and Environmental Research, North Wyke, Okehampton, Devon EX20 2SB, UK.* Email: Peter.penning@bbsrc.ac.uk

K.G. Rickert, *School of Natural and Rural Systems Management, University of Queensland, Gatton Campus, Gatton Q4343, Australia.* Email: krickert@uqg.uq.edu.au

M.L. Roderick, *Ecosystem Dynamics, Research School of Biological Sciences, Australian National University, Canberra 0200, Australia.* Email: Michael. Roderick@anu.edu.au

R. Schultze-Kraft, *Institute of Plant Production and Agroecology in the Tropics and Subtropics, University of Hohenheim (380), PO Box 700562, D-70593 Stuttgart, Germany.* Email: rsk@Uni-Hohenheim.de

R.C.G. Smith, *Remote Sensing Services, Department of Land Administration, PO Box 471, Perth 6014, Australia.* Email: Richard_Smith@notes.dola.wa. gov.au

J.W. Stuth, *Department of Rangeland Ecology and Management, Texas A&M University, College Station, TX 77843-2126, USA.* Email: jwstuth@ rasc-sparc.tamu.edu

A. Waters-Bayer, *Rohnsweg 56, D-37085 Göttingen, Germany.* Email: wb.waters@link-goe.de

R.D.B. Whalley, *Botany Department, University of New England, Armidale 2531, Australia.* Email: rwhalley@metz.une.edu.au

Preface

This book presents a critical review of methods used for measuring properties of grassland ecosystems in terms of plants, animals, soils and environment. It is a replacement for *Measurement of Grassland Vegetation and Animal Production*, edited by L. 't Mannetje, first published in 1978 and reprinted in 1982 and 1987 by the Commonwealth Bureau of Pastures and Field Crops and its successors (now incorporated into CAB *International*). This, in turn, replaced Dorothy Brown's *Methods of Surveying and Measuring Vegetation* published in 1954. The 1978 publication has been out of print for several years and since then there have been many developments in grassland research and methodology. Aspects of grassland ecosystems other than vegetation and animal production were not considered at all in the 1978 publication. Thus, we have included chapters on soils and nutrients, remote sensing and sociology. In addition there is a separate chapter on rangeland monitoring, because rangelands require a different approach than more intensive grasslands. Some changes in methodology, such as in measuring botanical composition and yield of pastures, have been developments of existing methods rather than new ones.

Each chapter is essentially self-contained, hence there is some overlap in the sense that some topics are mentioned in more than one chapter. However, to avoid unnecessary duplication, we have encouraged cross-referencing between chapters. For example, nitrogen fixation by legumes is mentioned in Chapters 12 and 13, but the description of the methodology for measuring it is in Chapter 13.

As in the 1978 publication, this is not a book of recipes but rather an introduction to grassland ecosystem and animal production research methodology and a guide to the available techniques. Contributors were asked to adopt a critical approach to the description of methods and their application. In most cases it will be necessary for readers to refer to the original publication or some other references for details of the methods described. For this reason, considerable thought has been given to the provision of suitable references.

The book of 16 chapters is the joint effort of 34 authors from ten countries, each author having wide experience in research methodology in her or his own field. In many chapters the joint authors come from different countries. This was encouraged as a way of ensuring that the topics were dealt with from a broad perspective.

The chapters fall into seven groups. There are those concerned with analysis and modelling (Chapters 2 and 3), measurements of grassland vegetation at the plant or quadrat level (Chapters 4 to 8), measurements on vegetation at a larger scale (Chapters 9 and 10), laboratory methods (Chapter 11 and part of Chapter 12), soils and nutrients in grasslands (part of Chapter 12 and Chapter 13), animal studies (Chapters 14 and 15) and sociological research (Chapter 16).

The predecessor of this book found many satisfied users and we trust that the present volume will fill a need for a critical presentation and appraisal of field and laboratory methods used in research in grasslands and animal production.

L. 't Mannetje
R.M. Jones

Grassland Vegetation and its Measurement

L. 't Mannetje[1] and R.M. Jones[2]

[1]Department of Plant Sciences, Wageningen University, Wageningen, The Netherlands; [2]CSIRO Tropical Agriculture, St Lucia, Australia

What is Grassland?

The term 'grassland' has several meanings. It can refer to a plant community, contrasting with 'forest', to an ecosystem comprising vegetation, soil, domestic and/or wild animals and management, and also to a ruminant production system. These three entities have in common that grasses (species of the family *Gramineae*) play a major part in their botanical composition. However, the strict definition, 'land covered only by grasses', is adequate only in a minority of cases. It usually applies only to areas newly sown to grasses, or areas that are maintained as such (e.g. sports fields and lawns), because species from other families will almost always invade and become part of grassland communities. Such species are commonly present in well-established sown and natural grasslands and include other monocotyledons (e.g. rushes and sedges) and both herbaceous and woody dicotyledons. Moore (1964) and Spedding (1971), amongst others, have defined grassland as a plant community in which grasses are dominant, shrubs rare and trees absent. However, on a global scale, most areas in which grasses are dominant in the ground cover, whether used for domestic ruminant production or as game reserves, contain woody species. Therefore, the definition of grassland as a 'plant community in which woody species do not exceed 40% of the total cover' (UNESCO-UNEP-FAO, 1979), is much more appropriate. As detailed discussions about definitions are usually not very fruitful, we shall consider grassland as 'ecosystems in which grasses play a dominant role in the (ground) vegetation, in which woody species do not exceed 40% of the total cover, whether or not they are used for animal production'.

It is sometimes useful to distinguish between treeless (pure) and wooded grasslands, because they require, in part, a different approach to sampling. The latter are sometimes referred to as grazing lands, or open woodlands, savannas or steppe, notwithstanding the fact that the terms savanna and steppe originally referred to treeless grassy plains. Tothill and Mott (1985) have edited a useful collection of papers on the savanna ecosystems of the world.

Another distinction can be made between 'rangeland' and 'improved/sown grasslands'. Rangelands are grasslands that consist of native and/or naturalized species, on which management is usually limited to grazing, burning and the control of woody species. Improved or sown grasslands may consist of or be oversown with selected/improved species and management may be extended to fertilization, irrigation, drainage and weed and pest control. Grasslands as part of a crop rotation system are usually referred to as 'leys' and play an important role in maintaining soil fertility and in reducing soil borne pests and diseases.

Grassland vegetation used for feeding animals is commonly referred to as 'forage' or 'herbage', although a distinction could be made between these two terms. 'Herbage' can be regarded as herbaceous biomass in general, e.g. as used in ecological studies of grassland vegetation, whereas 'forage' refers to animal feed in keeping with the term 'foraging': the animal's actions of selecting and ingesting herbaceous feed. The term 'pasture' is sometimes used for feed, but this is confusing, as 'pasture' also stands for a grazed grassland field.

Origin of Grasslands

Grasslands (including savannas and open forests) form the second greatest terrestrial biome, in terms of biomass, after tropical forest (Long and Jones, 1992).

Grasslands may be 'natural' or 'induced'. Ecologically, natural grasslands are pure or wooded vegetation types controlled by a combination of climate, soil, topography, biotic factors and fire (Moore, 1964). Natural grasslands generally occur in climates that are either too dry or too cold for forest to persist – for example, arid or semi-arid areas, monsoonal tropics with a long dry season, mountainous areas above the tree line (alps) or tundras in the arctic regions. Therefore, there are generally no natural grasslands in equatorial or temperate lowlands with humid or subhumid climates. Grasslands are also more likely to occur on heavy-textured soils or in areas that are regularly burnt.

In humid and subhumid climates most grasslands are induced (man-made), because the climate lacks the conditions needed for natural grasslands. Generally speaking, land is used for animal production from grassland only when other, more profitable land use systems are not possible. Thus, even natural grasslands, such as the prairies in North America, pampas in Argentina, llanos in Colombia, cerrados in Brazil, downs in Australia, steppe in Russia and pusta in eastern Europe, have been converted to croplands when soil conditions and rainfall were sufficiently favourable for cereal production. Figure 1.1 gives a schematic view of the origin of grasslands based on rainfall, soil fertility, economics and management choice. Apart from climatic considerations, economic reality plays an important role in the choice of grassland or cropland as the most suitable form of land use. Not all land that is cultivable will be cropland, because there may not be ready markets for the products, or animal production may be more profitable.

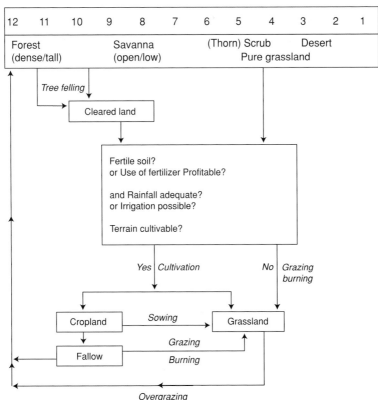

Fig. 1.1. The origin of grasslands on the basis of rainfall, soil fertility and management options.

Grassland and Animal Production Research

Since the publication of the predecessor of this book (Mannetje, 1978) the emphasis of grassland research has shifted from pure vegetational and animal production aspects to more multidisciplinary research on all parts of the ecosystem. Soil-related, environmental and sociological issues are also being studied. Thus, we are interested not only in forage yield, forage quality and botanical composition of the vegetation, but also in the persistence of both abundant and rare grassland species, in the characteristics of the soils and in flows and losses of major nutrients. Modelling has developed to such an extent that it has become a necessary tool in research, akin to statistics and pattern analysis. It is being recognized that for research to be more effective, the people who live on and manage grasslands also need to be involved in and often are a subject of the research. Underlying all these aspects are the interests in sustainability, in maintaining biodiversity and avoiding accelerated soil erosion and nutrient losses.

Research requires measurements and the main objective of this book is to present modern methodology to meet the needs of the grassland and ruminant animal production student and scientist.

Vegetation is measured for a wide range of purposes, including: (i) description in terms of its floristics, ground cover, amount of dry matter, quality of dry matter; (ii) assessing changes in vegetation brought about by changes in management (e.g. fertilizer, grazing pressure and grazing system) or by changes in climate; and (iii) determining the ability of the vegetation to provide feed for different types of livestock.

The methods used for measuring vegetation will vary with the objective. For example, the contribution of a species to botanical composition can be measured in terms of yield, basal cover, density or frequency of occurrence (Chapters 7 and 4). If vegetation measurements are to be related to concurrent animal production, then botanical composition would be assessed in terms of weight of dry matter contribution to the pasture. If the emphasis is on long-term botanical change, then measurements of basal cover, density and frequency may provide information that is less dependent on short-term changes due to differences in rainfall and grazing pressure.

Similarly, measurements of grassland soils (Chapters 12 and 13) can be made to: (i) describe soil chemical, physical and biological properties; (ii) assess changes in soil brought about by management; and (iii) determine the impact of soils on grassland productivity.

Grassland vegetation, by its very nature, is well adapted to the prevention of soil erosion and this is important no matter whether the grassland is used for animal production, recreation or environmental conservation. In every case well-managed grassland offers stability to the environment and protects the soil – which is one of the key resources of the earth for continuing terrestrial life of all kinds, including humans.

The importance of grassland soils for carbon sequestration, comparable to forest soils, is not generally recognized but is an undisputed fact, well supported by research findings (e.g. Goudriaan, 1992; Long and Jones, 1992; Fisher *et al.*, 1994).

Increasingly in some areas, the main purpose of grasslands is for conservation of biodiversity in terms of plant species and communities, and as wildlife reserves. The sustainability of these rangelands depends on the stocking rate of the wild animals in relation to the carrying capacity of the rangeland. Thus the measurement of non-agricultural attributes of grasslands may be as important as those of immediate agricultural relevance. Most of the methods discussed in this book are directly applicable to these situations.

Perhaps the greatest difficulty in measuring grasslands occurs when measurements of vegetation are to be related to consumable animal products. Many plant factors, such as the ability of the vegetation to provide energy, protein and minerals over time, are involved. Superimposed over this is the ability of a grazing animal to select from the available forage. Furthermore, direct measurement of animal performance is expensive and often not possible due to lack of resources.

More research is now being carried out off-station than before, either on-farm or in communally used rangelands. Under the latter circumstances, strict orthogonal-type experimental designs are often not applicable. In the case of animal production research on communally grazed rangelands, the investigator may not even be sure that the same animals will be involved. Observational (e.g. condition scoring) and indirect measurements (e.g. girth circumference) may be the only methods possible to investigate the performance of the animals. It is particularly under these conditions that the herders or owners of the animals can be directly involved in the research, and sociological research (Chapter 16) should be combined with the biological.

Choosing the Right Measurements to Take

No matter what the topic is, the key requirement is to define clearly the purpose of the study and then decide on what needs to be measured to meet these objectives. It is all too easy to collect a lot of data that turns out to be very site specific and of little value either in explaining the outcomes of that particular study or in the development of general principles. Once it has been decided what to measure, the next step is to determine the intensity of measurements that is needed and the methods that will be used. For example, sometimes only a general description of yield and botanical composition may be required to describe broadly the grassland in which a study was carried out. To undertake regular and very detailed measurements of botanical composition in this situation would be a waste of time and resources. Likewise the methods used must be appropriate to the desired outcome. There is no point in using a highly elaborate and time-consuming method if a simpler and quicker yet less accurate method will be adequate.

In keeping with the role of grassland as the main supplier of feed for herbivores, the measurements of greatest interest are usually those concerning the plant community, rather than the individual plant. However, it is sometimes necessary to measure individual plants as, for example, in demographic studies (Chapter 6), to understand the community. Botanical composition is important because it gives information on the basic elements of the pasture that provide energy, protein and minerals to feed animals. Furthermore, plant species differ in their adaptability to climatic and edaphic conditions and have different growth rates, chemical composition and digestibilities. Pasture yield can be expressed as dry matter produced over a certain period or available at a certain time, but to be really useful in terms of animal performance it needs to be qualified as green material on a dry matter basis or as metabolizable or net energy. For the calculation of rations for stall-fed or feedlot animals or the need for supplements to grazing animals, accurate knowledge about the energy value, crude protein and mineral concentrations of the feed on offer are necessary.

A very important consideration is whether or not a particular measurement is necessary. Dry matter yields and chemical analyses of pasture plots or liveweight of animals are often measured (or measured too frequently) merely because the methods are available and they give results, whereas simple observations and common sense, or less frequent measurements, would suffice for the purpose of the investigation. Many of the countless analyses of nitrogen that have been made on plant samples from grazed pastures are of questionable benefit because they were 'whole plant' samples bearing little relation to what animals were eating.

We also believe that in many situations grassland scientists have not taken advantage of the unique opportunities offered in long-term species evaluation and grazing trials. Species evaluation trials are too often destroyed after the formal investigation period has expired. Much valuable information on persistence can be obtained by simply leaving the area intact, particularly when it can be grazed. The long-term persistence of species that may have been discarded because of low dry matter yields or poor initial establishment may become evident without any further measurement or special management. Such events, for example, led to the release of the tropical forage legume *Vigna parkeri* cv. Shaw in Queensland (Cook and Jones 1987).

Grazing experiments are expensive to establish and run, but there are few of them and, if the experiments have been adequately designed, they offer unique opportunities to examine how variables such as fertilizer and grazing pressure affect many aspects of grasslands vegetation and soils. With the increasing interest in whole systems these trials offer many opportunities. For example, there is currently increased interest in sustainability and biodiversity of grassland systems. Most experiments with stocking rate as a variable do not include biodiversity in their experimental objectives, yet such trials provide unique opportunities to ascertain how this is affected by stocking rate. Similarly, it is possible to examine the long-term effects of stocking rate on soil properties such as infiltration rate and bulk density. Jones *et al.* (1995) considered the value of long-term trials in more detail.

Variability

Readers will note that there is no chapter on conventional statistics in this book. This is partly because some of the chapters deal with statistics as it relates to their particular topic (e.g. Chapter 14). Furthermore, the subject of statistics is usually adequately covered at university level; and there are many books on statistical methods and many statistical computer programs are available. Particular emphasis on the role of statistics in grassland research was given in the chapter by McIntyre in Mannetje (1978) and a more detailed discussion of statistical analysis of plant communities was given in Digby and Kempton (1987).

Most use of statistics in grassland research has been and is directed towards reducing 'errors' and optimizing the opportunity for differences between treatments to be 'significantly' different. However, one feature that is highlighted in many chapters in this book is that variability in grassland is a 'real' and important feature and that its importance has often been overlooked. This variability can occur at the individual plant or plant-part scale (as discussed in the case of soil biology in Chapter 12), at the 'patch' scale (Chapter 5), or at a large scale of kilometres in rangelands (Chapters 9 and 10). If we are to make continued progress in understanding and modelling how grasslands function, grassland scientists will sometimes have to put more effort into describing variability and understanding its effects, instead of regarding variability as a somewhat embarrassing error term around a mean value.

References

Cook, B.G. and Jones, R.M. (1987) Persistent new legumes for intensive grazing. 1. Shaw creeping vigna. *Queensland Agricultural Journal* 113, 89–91.

Digby, P.G.N. and Kempton, R.A. (1987) *Multivariate Analysis of Ecological Communities.* Chapman & Hall, London, 206 pp.

Fisher, M.J., Rao, I.M., Ayarza, M.A., Lascano, C.E., Sanz, J.I., Thomas, R.J. and Vera, R.R. (1994) Carbon storage by introduced deep-rooted grasses in the South American savannas. *Nature* 371, 236–238.

Goudriaan, J. (1992) Biosphere structure, carbon sequestering potential and the atmospheric ^{14}C carbon record. *Journal of Experimental Botany* 43, 1111–1119.

Jones, R.M., Jones, R.J. and McDonald, C.K. (1995) Some advantages of long-term grazing trials with particular reference to changes in botanical composition. *Australian Journal of Experimental Agriculture* 35, 1029–1038.

Long, S.P. and Jones, M.B. (1992) Introduction, aims, goals and general methods. In: Long, S.P., Jones, M.B. and Roberts, M.J. (eds) *Primary Productivity of Grass Ecosystems of the Tropics and Sub-tropics*. Chapman & Hall, London, pp. 1–24.

Mannetje, L. 't (1978) (ed.) *Measurement of Grassland Vegetation and Animal Production*. Bulletin No. 52, Commonwealth Bureau of Pastures and Field Crops, Hurley, UK, 260 pp.

Moore, C.W.E. (1964) Distribution of grasslands. In: Barnard, C. (ed.) *Grasses and Grasslands*. Macmillan, Melbourne, pp. 182–205.

Spedding, C.R.W. (1971) *Grassland Ecology*. Clarendon Press, Oxford, 221 pp.

Tothill, J.C. and Mott, J.J. (1985) (eds) *Ecology and Management of the World's Savannas*. Australian Academy of Science, Canberra, and CAB International, Farnham Royal, UK, 340 pp.

UNESCO-UNEP-FAO (1979) *Tropical Grazing Land Ecosystems*. A State-of-the-Art report. United Nations Educational, Scientific and Cultural Organization, United Nations Environmental Programme, Food and Agriculture Organization, Paris, 655 pp.

Pattern Analysis in Grassland and Animal Production Systems

A.M. Kelly[1] and K.E. Basford[2]

[1] Queensland Department of Primary Industries, Toowoomba, Australia; [2]Department of Agriculture, University of Queensland, St Lucia, Australia

Introduction

The aim of this chapter is to provide research workers in grassland and animal production systems with an overview of pattern analysis procedures. These techniques are commonly used for the exploratory analysis of complex multivariate data as they determine and display the underlying patterns in such data. Although some information is sacrificed in this process, the aim is to discard only noise. The detail of how this is achieved will not be discussed, but rather guidance given on where and how pattern analysis could be useful. We illustrate its application to data from grassland and animal production systems, discussing some of the inherent problems and outlining the main advantages and disadvantages of different techniques. We also discuss some procedures that assist with the interpretation of results and ways to compare trends over time.

Background

It is important to distinguish pattern analysis techniques, which aim to detect and summarize underlying patterns in data, from those used in testing hypotheses. Consider, for instance, analysis of variance and regression techniques, with which most readers will be familiar. The former are used to test whether there are differences between treatments of some sort while the latter test whether the variation in one attribute can be explained by a particular (perhaps linear) relationship on other attributes. Pattern

©CAB *International* 2000. *Field and Laboratory Methods for Grassland and Animal Production Research* (eds L. 't Mannetje and R.M. Jones)

analysis techniques are exploratory in the sense that they are not testing hypotheses that have been formed before data collection. However, they may help to generate hypotheses about the relationship between the individuals on which the multivariate data are recorded and the underlying influential factors. Belbin and McDonald (1993) also recommended that such pattern-finding techniques can be usefully employed at an early stage of analysis to detect errors and identify outliers.

A single analytical procedure will not usually provide complete insight into any reasonably sized multivariate data set. Ordination and classification techniques can both be used to summarize and extract information and it is their combined use which is referred to as pattern analysis (Williams, 1976). These two approaches are complementary as they explore different aspects of the data. Classification or clustering most commonly divides the set of individuals into distinct groups, so that individuals within a group are more similar to each other than to individuals in other groups. Strictly, we should use the term 'clustering' rather than 'classification' for this process. Clustering refers to the situation when the categorization is into groups that are determined from the data, whereas classification is most often used when individuals are being assigned to (or classified as belonging to) one of several pre-specified groups (Gnanadesikan, 1977). Ordination gives a geometrical (or spatial) representation of the individuals in a low (usually two- or three-) dimensional space, such that the distance between points (individuals) represents their dissimilarity. Ordination methods are also useful for determining whether natural groupings of the individuals exist. By combining these approaches, scientists can deal with and 'interpret' a graphical display across a small number of dimensions or make comparisons between a few groups.

To illustrate this complementarity, consider how Miles (1979) summarized the nature of vegetation by stating that it 'can be viewed as a mosaic of distinct patches or types, or as a pattern of intergrading populations. All patches are different and unique, yet some are more similar than others.' Emphasis on these opposing properties has governed the types of methods employed to describe vegetation. Clustering can be used to distinguish between the different types of vegetation that may be of practical importance. Because it is acknowledged that these types usually intergrade, the division into discrete units may be arbitrary, or may meld intermediate types. Ordination is better used to describe continuous change because the individuals are preserved in the summary graphics. The choice of group level in a clustering or number of dimensions in an ordination is analogous to looking through a microscope: with greater magnification we see more detail, while with less magnification we see the bigger picture. Belbin and McDonald (1993) stated that ordination could be considered to be more powerful than clustering when applied to ecological data because it can better detect gradients and the nature of clusters, but it is computationally more demanding and more likely to mislead, e.g. through the presence of outliers. Although clustering is less influenced by outliers, it will allocate individuals into groups whether or not they reflect an underlying group structure and this can also be misleading.

Pattern analysis techniques are appropriate for a variety of grassland and animal production systems as they make minimal assumptions about the underlying structure of the data. They are particularly suitable for large-scale survey information where little is known about the response of species to ecological gradients and the variation in response is large. The acceptance of such descriptive methodology was initially hampered by the belief that any correct or meaningful type of analysis should be based on classical techniques for hypothesis testing which assumed some form for the underlying distribution of the data. In practice, the sampling methods applied may not be appropriate for more conventional forms of statistical analysis and/or explicit hypotheses may not have been formulated. In addition, recent advances in computer technology have allowed more straightforward implementation of these descriptive techniques.

To end this section, we briefly illustrate the scope and breadth of applications. Foran *et al.* (1986) claimed that using such multivariate methods can produce 'objective and repeatable results, and reduce the subjectivity inherent in most range assessment procedures'. Their analysis involved three stages. Firstly, sites were classified into distinct range types using data on soil type, trees, shrub and long-lived plants in the herbage layer. In the second stage, they applied both clustering and ordination methods to species composition data to determine condition states within each range type, and then superimposed the influence of climate, grazing, soil type and fire on to these states. The third stage involved monitoring change in condition over time by comparing the position of sites between different ordination outputs. Other applications in rangeland assessment in arid climates include Bosch (1989), Friedel (1990) and Stuart-Hill and Hobson (1991). Books dealing with applications to data from the ecological arena include Williams (1976), Gauch (1982), Greig-Smith (1983), Pielou (1984), Digby and Kempton (1987), Legendre and Legendre (1987) and Manly (1994). This methodology has been used in finding patterns in data from experiments with conventional statistical design and layouts (Annicchiarico, 1992; DeLacy *et al.*, 1996; McDonald *et al.*, 1996), for the analysis of succession along an environmental gradient (Austin and Belbin, 1981; Burrows *et al.*, 1984) and for the construction of state and transition models (Westoby *et al.*, 1989). It has also been used to summarize diversity in a collection of accessions (Pengelly and Eagles, 1995, 1996) and in rainfall events (Taylor and Tulloch, 1985; Stone and Auliciems, 1992).

Data Form and Type

Multivariate data from grassland and animal production systems often consist of measurements of various attributes (or variables) on the same set of individuals (or objects). For instance, if n individuals are assessed on the basis of p attributes then the data might be recorded in an $n \times p$ matrix. An example common to many ecological studies is the site by species matrix, where at each site a measurement is made for each of the species. The type of data to be collected depends on both the aims of the study and the available resources. These data types include binary, nominal, ordinal, interval and ratio scales of measurement. Binary data are recorded as simply presence/absence of a species, or on/off information such as hairy or glabrous leaves. The nominal scale describes data classified into one of a number of categories, e.g. the accumulation of surface material at a site can be defined as belonging to one of the following classes: tree litter, silt, gravel, rock, or debris. An ordinal scale involves logical sequencing of the categories of each variable; for example, compactness of the soil surface can be assessed as an ordinal variable with three categories: loose, moderate, or hard. Quantitative variables (which use ratio or interval scales, depending on whether or not there is a true zero) provide a greater level of detail for each of the individuals, e.g. frequency or basal area of each species. For large-scale studies across heterogeneous individuals (or sites), it may be cost effective to record only binary data, yet still retain an adequate level of detail. Conversely, when individuals have more in common, the gain in information from measuring quantitative variables will be substantial (Digby and Kempton, 1987).

Sometimes data are presented in the form of an association matrix with entries corresponding to some measure of association between each pair of individuals; for example, the number of times two species appear together at a site may be used as an indication of their similarity. Although not central to all clustering and ordination techniques, the concept of 'likeness' between individuals across several measured attributes is required in some of the methods under consideration. Different terms used for the measure of 'likeness' include association measure, similarity, and proximity, while the converse (or opposite) is a dissimilarity or distance measure. Regardless of which is recorded, it is a relatively straightforward transformation between dissimilarity and similarity, given certain assumptions and standardizations (Gordon, 1981).

The procedure for combining information across attributes or calculating association for a real data set can be complicated by many factors. Firstly, it is necessary to consider the types of attributes (e.g. always observed or conditionally present) and the scales upon which they are measured (e.g. binary to numeric). Are the units of measurement consistent and comparable? Should all attributes be converted to the same scale or combined in some way? If they are to be combined, e.g. with the Gower (1971) general similarity coefficient, should there be equal or unequal weighting of the various attributes – for example, because some attributes are known to be better discriminators than others or because unimportant or 'noisy' attributes might swamp the important information? If not directly applied, the weight is implicitly dependent on the scale of measurement of the attributes or the data values themselves. This implicit weighting can be removed by standardizing (centring and/or scaling) the attributes, but there are different views on the usefulness of this process (Greig-Smith, 1983; Pielou, 1984; Digby and Kempton, 1987). Lastly, the data should be examined for missing values and a decision made as to how these will be handled (Gordon, 1981; Little and Rubin, 1987). None of these issues will be covered in detail here and readers are referred to the literature for more information.

Clustering

Suppose that several attributes have been measured on a set of individuals. Methods of clustering can be used to group these individuals in such a way that members within a group have similar characteristics, and this distinguishes them from the members of other groups. These procedures seek some sort of internal cohesion and external isolation of groups or clusters. However, the clustering should not impose some inappropriate dissection where members in different clusters possess as many common characteristics as members in the same cluster (Gordon, 1981). Thus the question may be asked as to whether the individuals fall naturally into these distinct groups (assuming that overlapping groups are not allowed) or whether they interrelate in a continuous way. If distinct groups do emerge, then a summary of group properties is an efficient account of the main information in the data. A lack of distinct grouping is information in itself, and other methods, which deal with change on a more continuous basis, can be employed.

Hierarchical and non-hierarchical procedures

Available methods of seeking clusters can be categorized broadly as being hierarchical or non-hierarchical. The former class is one in which every cluster is a merger or split of the clusters at a previous stage. Thus it is possible to visualize not only the two extremes of clustering, i.e. each cluster contains only one individual (very weak clustering) and one cluster which contains all individuals (very strong clustering), but also a monotonically increasing strength of clustering going from one level to another. Hierarchical strategies always optimize a route between these two extremes (Williams, 1976). The route may be defined by progressive fusions, beginning with single individual groups and ending with a single group of all individuals (agglomerative hierarchy), or by progressive divisions, beginning with a single group and decomposing it into individuals (divisive hierarchy).

If we consider data in the form of a matrix of association measures between each pair of individuals, it can be useful to understand how clustering procedures affect this space of all possible associations. As individuals merge, the original properties of the space may be distorted in some way, unless the strategy employs rules that are space conserving. Space-contracting strategies tend to obscure boundaries between groups because of the chaining process. Conversely, dilating strategies tend to sharpen boundaries by increasing the intensity of the clustering. However, they tend to form groups in which the members of a group can be quite different from one other. For this reason, some authors, such as Greig-Smith (1983), preferred to adopt a space-conserving strategy.

With a non-hierarchical strategy, it is the structure of the individual groups which is optimized, since these are made as homogeneous as possible for a particular number of groups (Williams, 1976). No route is defined between the groups and their constituent elements, and so the infrastructure of groups (how they relate to one another) cannot be examined. For those applications for which homogeneity of groups is of prime importance, the non-hierarchical strategies are very attractive. Then, a crucial question is the computational feasibility of any specific algorithm. An examination of all possible partitions of the data, to determine a clustering that is optimal with respect to some criterion, is prohibitively expensive and may be impossible.

In general, non-hierarchical methods have a distinct advantage when classifying large data sets (Belbin, 1992). This is because they do not require the calculation and storage of the full set of associations between pairs of individuals and are not restrained by an inefficient early partition or combination. Hawkins *et al.* (1982) commented that most writers on cluster analysis 'lay more stress on algorithm and criteria in the belief that intuitively reasonable criteria should produce good results over a wide range of possible (and generally unstated) models'. They strongly supported the increasing emphasis on a model-based approach to clustering. For instance, the mixture approach to clustering (McLachlan and Basford, 1988) assumes that the data consist of samples from a mixture of underlying populations in various proportions. The aim is to estimate the parameters of the specified distributions for these populations and assign the individuals to their unknown population of origin. The probability that each individual comes from each of these populations (or groups) can be estimated. An outright allocation is only obtained when the individuals are assigned to the group to which they have the largest probability of belonging.

Both hierarchical and non-hierarchical procedures do have problems in their implementation. In the former case, a distance measure and grouping strategy must be specified and the level (number of groups) at which the dendrogram (graphical representation of the hierarchy) is to be truncated must also be determined. This decision is often subjective and based on a 'satisfactory' amount of variation being accounted for among the groups. Equivalently, the number of underlying populations (groups) must be specified in a non-hierarchical model. The latter procedures are usually iterative and some initial allocation of the individuals into groups or estimates of the parameters of the underlying distributions must be specified. In addition, most algorithms do not guarantee convergence to the global maximum of whatever criterion is being considered; see McLachlan and Basford (1988) for more detail.

There is no generally accepted 'best' method and different clustering procedures will often produce different results on a given set of data (Manly, 1994). As would be expected, the identification of clusters of individuals will depend on the attributes measured on them. If another set of attributes were measured, then different results could be expected from the same clustering procedure.

An example of cluster analysis

To illustrate the application of a clustering procedure on data from a production system, consider the paper by Pengelly and Eagles (1995) on genetic diversity (the variation among individuals within the same species). A collection of 53 accessions of the tropical legume *Macroptilium gracile* from a wide range of sites was grown and data on 24 attributes (including the ability to set both aerial and subterranean seed and a small set of morphological and phenological attributes) were recorded. The 24 attributes (Table 2.1) included underground tubers, although this was missing from the original table in Pengelly and Eagles (1995), and they are coded here as attributes A to X. They used the Gower (1971) metric to establish a similarity matrix among accessions and then a hierarchical clustering procedure with the incremental sum of squares fusion strategy to group the accessions. The dendrogram for the clustering (down to the ten-group level) is displayed in Fig. 2.1. Pengelly and Eagles (1995) discussed the characterization of the groups via their mean responses for each attribute and concluded that 'the resulting classification has provided a framework for the selection of representative accessions from the collection for evaluation studies'. Not only did the analysis enable the rational selection of germplasm from the collection for plant improvement programmes, but it would also assist in the placement of further germplasm acquisitions into this framework. Thus the clustering procedure provided a useful summary of the variation among the accessions with respect to the measured attributes.

One of the interpretation issues with dendrograms (particularly for the novice user) is the 'closeness' or similarity of the groups. In this example,

Table 2.1. Attributes used in the cluster analysis of 53 accessions of *Macroptilium gracile* and their code for later displays. (Adapted from Pengelly and Eagles, 1995.)

Attributes	Code	Attributes	Code
Days to 50% emergence	A	No. branches at 45 DAS	M
Cotyledonary node height (mm)	B	Days to first flower	N
Juvenile leaf length (mm)	C	Days to first ripe seed	O
Juvenile leaflet width (mm)	D	Pod length (mm)	P
Juvenile leaf height (mm)	E	No. seeds per pod	Q
No. nodes at 30 DAS	F	Amphicarpy (present or absent)	R
No. branches at 30 DAS	G	Canopy density (1–4)	S
Node no. at first branch	H	Pod width (mm)	T
Terminal leaflet length (mm)	I	Seed weight (g per 100 seeds)	U
Terminal leaflet width (mm)	J	Density leaf hairs (adaxial) (1–4)	V
Internode length (mm)	K	Density leaf hairs (abaxial) (1–4)	W
No. nodes at 45 DAS	L	Underground tubers (1–4)	X

DAS = days after sowing.

Groups 6 and 7 are the most similar of the ten groups, but it is not apparent which of these is more like Group 5, for example. This is because the horizontal axis in Fig. 2.1 does not correspond to any response variable; rather, it is a somewhat arbitrary numbering of the groups which have been equally spaced along this axis.

In interpreting the groups obtained from the clustering, Pengelly and Eagles (1995) took advantage of further information about the origin of the accessions. For instance, the non-amphicarpic groups (Groups 1 to 5) were generally from the northern regions of South America or Brazil while the geographical distribution of plants with amphicarpy (Groups 6 to 10) encompassed almost the full latitudinal range of the species. Accessions in Groups 6 and 7 were from South America, those in Group 8 from southern Mexico and northern Guatemala together with one accession collected from a semiarid region of southern Baja California; those in Group 9 mainly originated from alkaline soils of the Yucatan Peninsula, while those in Group 10 (distinguished from Group 9 largely on the basis of internode length) were from a region with similar rainfall and similar latitude, but from acid soils.

Ordination

Ordination techniques aim to display the information from a multivariate data set in a reduced dimensional space. To achieve this, they attempt to condense the information on the individuals as ordered scores on a few new attributes (usually two or three) which define the dimensions of this new space. Individuals can then be plotted as points in this space, such that

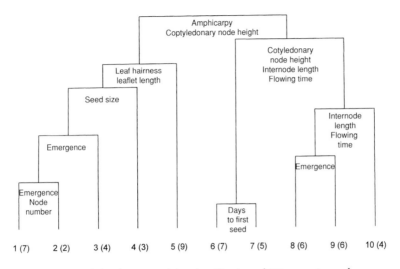

Fig. 2.1. Truncated dendrogram of the classification of 53 accessions of *Macroptilium gracile* using 24 attributes, although only those attributes which contributed most at each level of the dendrogram are shown. The number in brackets following the group number indicates the number of accessions within the group. (Adapted from Pengelly and Eagles, 1995.)

the distance between any pair of points approximates the original dissimilarity measure between the individuals. In this attempt at dimension reduction, 'all ordinations distort the original multivariate data set and information is inevitably lost. There is a trade off between loss of information and the simplification of data in order to detect pattern' (Beals, 1984). The success of the technique lies in retaining the bulk of relevant information and discarding noise, but various ways of measuring the amount of lost information can be considered. Some techniques, such as multidimensional scaling, are based on 'stress' minimization, where stress measures the difference between the original dissimilarity of the individual pairs, and the way in which this is represented as distances between points on the ordination diagram. An analysis with low stress gives a meaningful representation of the data in which most of the relevant information is retained. Many other techniques measure the amount of information retained by calculating the percentage of variation explained by each of the new attributes, as in principal components analysis. This is analogous to linear regression where the square of the correlation coefficient indicates the amount of variation in the dependent variable accounted for by the regression.

The most meaningful interpretation of the graphical output of an ordination can be made when data are superimposed onto it. Data internal to the ordination analysis (i.e. used in it) can be displayed on the diagram to highlight the influential attributes. On the other hand, data external to the analysis (i.e. not used in it) can be superimposed on the diagram to determine which other factors discriminate between individuals.

Detecting trends and gradients

The first and simplest application of gradient analysis was an ordering of sites along a known environmental gradient – direct gradient analysis (Whittaker, 1967). These gradients were typically formed from elevation and topographic lines. However, when no obvious environmental index exists, a more indirect method of ordering sites (or individuals) is needed. Multivariate ordination techniques used for this purpose include principal components analysis (Hotelling, 1933), principal coordinates analysis (Gower, 1966) and correspondence analysis (Hirschfeld, 1935), which was applied in the ecological field as reciprocal averaging (Hill, 1973, 1974). Modifications to the classical methodology resulted in canonical correspondence analysis (Braak, 1986, 1994) which may be viewed as a form of principal components analysis applied to categorical rather than quantitative variables. Yet another approach is semi-strong hybrid scaling (Belbin, 1991) which follows the methodology of multidimensional scaling (Kruskal and Wish, 1978). All these methods arrange the sites along axes of variation that may or may not represent environmental factors. In principal components analysis, the first axis represents the direction of maximum variation in the data, the second axis displays the largest amount of independent variation, and so on. In other methods, such as multidimensional scaling, the axes are arbitrary and major trends can be revealed across any rotation of the axes.

To illustrate this process, a principal components analysis was applied to the data of Pengelly and Eagles (1995) to represent the major variation among the accessions, as measured by the 24 attributes, in a reduced space of two or three dimensions. However, the output will not be displayed until the next section, where we discuss the combined presentation of the results of ordination and clustering procedures.

Interpreting and Extending the Information from a Pattern Analysis

Once the clustering and ordination techniques have been undertaken, a number of devices can be employed to complement and assist with interpretation of the output.

Biplots

Biplots can be considered to be the multivariate analogue of scatter plots (Gower and Hand, 1996). They are used to represent simultaneously the variation among the individuals and the attributes (hence the name) on the same diagram. Usually only the first two or three dimensions of the new ordination space are used. As well as displaying patterns in the individuals, such a representation displays the interrelationships among the attributes and the way in which they discriminate among the individuals. Thus, biplots can be used to detect patterns in the data, and to display the results of more formal methods of analysis.

Biplots of the output from the principal component analysis (using the singular value decomposition algorithm) of the data from Pengelly and Eagles (1995) are presented in Figs 2.2 and 2.3. Here, all 53 accessions and 24 attributes are plotted using the first three components, which accounted for 65% of the total variation in the data. As recommended by Kroonenberg (1995), the accessions are represented by points (here symbols coinciding with membership at the ten-group level determined from the clustering procedure and displayed in Fig. 2.1) while the attributes (coded A to X, as in Table 2.1) are displayed as vectors from the origin. In these displays, the origin represents the average response. Plotting accessions as points and attributes as vectors has the advantage that the two types of points on the graphs (accessions and attributes) are clearly distinguished from each other.

We now briefly discuss how these biplots may be interpreted; for a more detailed discussion see Kroonenberg (1995). To interpret the response of

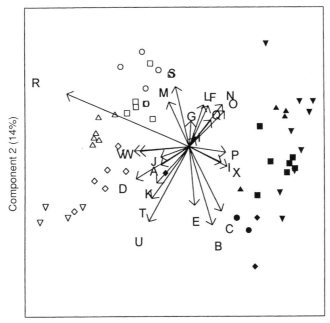

Component 1 (41%)

Fig. 2.2. Biplot of principal components 1 and 2 from the ordination of 53 accessions using 24 attributes. Accessions are plotted with symbols (■ Group 1, ● Group 2, ▲ Group 3, ◆ Group 4, ▼ Group 5, □ Group 6, ○ Group 7, △ Group 8, ◇ Group 9, ▽ Group 10) and attributes are plotted as vectors (see Table 2.1 for attribute code).

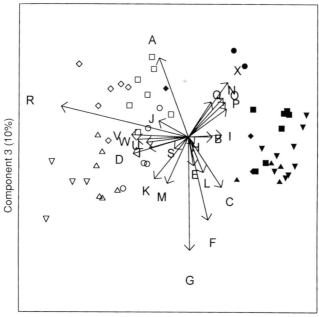

Fig. 2.3. Biplot of principal components 1 and 3 from the ordination of 53 accessions using 24 attributes. Accessions are plotted with symbols (■ Group 1, ● Group 2, ▲ Group 3, ◆ Group 4, ▼ Group 5, □ Group 6, ○ Group 7, △ Group 8, ◇ Group 9, ▽ Group 10) and attributes are plotted as vectors (see Table 2.1 for attribute code).

any particular accession with respect to any particular attribute, a pendicular line is dropped from the accession point on to the attribute vector. In this process, the vector may need to be extended in the positive or negative direction from the origin. If this projection is far from the origin in the positive direction, then the accession has a considerably above-average response, while if it is far from the origin in the negative direction, then the accession has a considerably below-average response. These statements are comparative in that all responses are compared with the origin which corresponds to the average response in each of the environments. If attribute vectors are parallel to each other then there is a positive correlation in their response, while if they are in opposite directions, they are negatively correlated. If attribute vectors are at right angles to each other, their responses are independent of each other. If all attributes were equally well represented in these displays, then we would expect the vectors to be of equal length.

From Figs 2.2 and 2.3, we see that accessions within each of the ten groups tend to be relatively close together. However, accessions within Groups 4 and 5 tend to be less similar to each other as they are more widely spread. Accessions in Groups 1 to 5, apart from one accession in Group 4, have a negative score (projection) on the vector corresponding to attribute R (Amphicarpy), while those in Groups 6 to 10 have a positive score on this vector. This attribute is particularly well described in the reduced three-dimensional space, as the vector representing it is quite long in comparison with the others and was used by Pengelly and Eagles (1995) to interpret the major dichotomy between Groups 1 to 5 and Groups 6 to 10 (Fig. 2.1).

From Fig. 2.2, we can see that component 2 has attributes B, C, E and U (cotyledonary node height, juvenile leaf length, juvenile leaf height and seed weight) in one direction and attributes S and M (canopy density and number of branches at 45 days after sowing) in the other. Thus this component could be considered to be mainly a contrast between these attributes. Component 3 has attributes F and G (the number of nodes and branches at 30 days after sowing) in one direction and attribute A (the number of days to 50% emergence) in the other. Thus component 3 mainly represents a contrast in the response to these attributes.

Networks

Yet another perspective of the data may be revealed by exploring networks or interrelationships between individuals (Belbin, 1992). Network methods focus on the localized neighbourhood of an individual and form links between these. The methods are a useful adjunct to clustering and ordination, as the individual linkages can be superimposed on either output and aid in interpretation. Minimum spanning trees (Gower and Ross, 1969) concentrate on an accurate representation of close neighbours, but will distort the overall spatial configuration of individuals. They yield a set of lines that link all individuals, where the length of the line represents the dissimilarity between the individuals. The tree is formed so that the length of this network of lines is a minimum. In this way, they reveal information about the local neighbourhood of each individual by the way in which it is interconnected with other individuals.

Pengelly and Eagles (1995) also used a minimum spanning tree, constructed from the same similarity matrix used in the clustering and ordination procedures, to display the diversity within the groups and the relationships among them (Fig. 2.4). They commented on the close agreement between the results of this analysis and those of the clustering and the ability for this graphic to display the variation within groups. For instance, those groups that were relatively homogeneous did not have links to members of other groups before linking all members of that group. In Fig. 2.4, only Groups 4, 5 and 6 were not continuous and Group 5 was the most heterogeneous. This is consistent with the spread of accessions within these groups in Figs 2.2 and 2.3. The minimum spanning tree can also be thought of as a simpler summary of the low dimensional representation from the

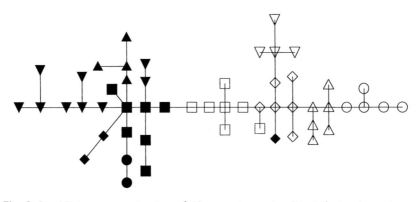

Fig. 2.4. Minimum spanning tree of 53 accessions using 24 attributes. Accessions are plotted with symbols (■ Group 1, ● Group 2, ▲ Group 3, ◆ Group 4, ▼ Group 5, □ Group 6, ○ Group 7, △ Group 8, ◇ Group 9, ▽ Group 10). (Adapted from Pengelly and Eagles, 1995.)

ordination analysis displayed in Figs 2.2 and 2.3. In particular, variation along the tree is consistent with variation along principal component 1.

Both ordination displays (biplots and minimum spanning trees) allow better interpretation of 'closeness' and 'compactness' of the groups than the dendrogram used to display the hierarchical clustering. This has been demonstrated in the above discussions and is, in some sense, a consequence of the presentation of the individual accessions in the ordination displays, rather than simply the group structure (which groups join or split from which other groups) presented in the dendrogram.

Comparing ordinations

To illustrate a situation where ordination diagrams may need to be compared, consider a field survey of the botanical composition of sites conducted over a number of growing seasons. Botanical composition may change in response to short-term effects of climate and management but also may exhibit slower changes or long-term effects. The former are usually reversible while the latter may not be. Comparison of ordination patterns over time can assist in differentiating between short-term and long-term fluctuations. The comparison of two different ordinations on the same set of individuals can be achieved using standard procrustes analysis (Gower, 1975). When more ordinations are involved, generalized or multiple procrustes analysis may be applied, depending on the purpose of the comparison.

Procrustes analysis involves matching the ordination diagrams through the processes of translation, rotation and dilation. Once matched, a measure of stress indicates the magnitude of change in the position of the individual across the two ordinations. In addition to magnitude of change, direction of change is also important and is measured by the angles between vectors joining the same individuals across the two ordinations. In terms of botanical composition, these vectors indicate whether all sites are moving in the same direction, maybe due to a more favourable season. Sites with divergent trajectories may be tagged as those subject to some atypical influence that is affecting botanical composition.

Different ordinations on the same set of individuals can arise in a number of ways. Various ordination techniques can be applied to the same data with the aim of comparing the outcome from each method. If the same sites are observed over time, it may be desirable to measure the consistency of ordinations across years or seasons. Alternatively, individuals can be ordered separately across a number of different data sets based on different types of attributes. Then the similarity of relationships across the different types of data may be of interest.

Full Example

The following example illustrates how classification and ordination procedures can complement each other.

Mullen *et al.* (1998) collected data on 25 accessions of *Leucaena* spp. planted in experiments at 19 sites over a 2.5 year period to identify agronomic adaptation to environmental challenges and to gain an understanding of limitations to *Leucaena* growth. Because different experimental conditions could be imposed at each site (such as high and low psyllid pressure, fertile and acid-infertile soils, high and low temperatures and wet and dry seasons), the individual combination of experimental condition and site was called an environment. Hence data on 25 accessions grown in 61 environments were actually recorded. Pattern analysis of dry matter yield showed an F_1 hybrid (*L. pallida* K748 × *L. leucocephala* K636) to be distinctly different from all other accessions in that it was comparatively very high yielding in all environments and displayed excellent broad adaptation. Because it was so different, it was subsequently excluded and dry matter yields on the remaining 24 accessions grown in the 61 environments were reanalysed using pattern analysis methodology. In both cases, the data were standardized within environments before accessions and environments were separately classified into groups using a hierarchical, agglomerative procedure with incremental sums of squares as the fusion strategy and squared Euclidean distance as the dissimilarity measure. The dendrograms were truncated at the nine-accession group level and the 11-environment group level. The first two components of a principal component analysis (using the singular value decomposition algorithm) explained an adequate amount of the variation and these were used in a biplot (Fig. 2.5) to display the variability among the individual accessions and environment groups. As

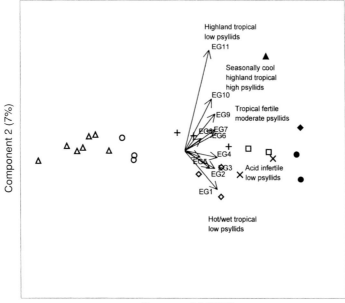

Fig. 2.5. Biplot of principal components 1 and 2 from the ordination of 24 accessions using 61 environments. Accessions are plotted with symbols (◆ Group 1, ● Group 2, ▲ Group 3, □ Group 4, × Group 5, ◇ Group 6, + Group 7, ○ Group 8, △ Group 9) and vectors for the individual environments have been replaced by those for environment groups (EG1 to EG11) identified by the cluster analysis. (Adapted from Mullen et al., 1999.)

before, the accession group composition is displayed on the biplot using a different symbol for each group.

Mullen et al. (1998) reported that the accession scores on principal component 1 were highly correlated with accession mean yields, while those on component 2 were correlated with severity of psyllid damage. Thus the accession points on the biplot (Fig. 2.5) were reasonably interpreted in terms of dry matter yield potential on principal component 1 and psyllid resistance and other unknown factors on component 2.

The environment groups were an effective summary of the 61 environments and environment group vectors have replaced the individual environment vectors in the biplot (Fig. 2.5). General descriptors of environmental types have also been added on the biplot to aid interpretation. In particular, Mullen et al. (1998) noted that no exclusive acid-infertile environment groups were identified, with acid-infertile environments in several environment groups. As all environment groups tended to score similarly on principal component 1 (Fig. 2.5), this component did not discriminate between them. The environment scores on principal component

2 were correlated with maximum and minimum temperatures and psyllid damage ratings, but not with acidity, infertility indices or rainfall. Thus the biplot environment scores on this component were interpreted in terms of accession response to temperature and psyllids.

Overall, pattern analysis methodology enabled clear identification of broad and specific adaptation in the genus *Leucaena*. For example, accession Group 1 displayed broad adaptation with high yields, while accession Groups 8 and 9 were very low yielding in all environments. On the other hand, accession Group 3 was identified as being specifically adapted to seasonally cool highland tropical and high psyllid pressure environments, while accession Group 2 was less productive in these types of environments but more productive in humid tropical, low psyllid pressure environments.

The results indicated that specific adaptation to temperature and psyllids existed, but not to acid or infertile soils or to low rainfall. The best performing accessions in acid infertile soils were broadly adapted accessions which produced comparatively high yields in all environments. However, even the highest yields in strongly acid infertile environments were unlikely to provide sufficient dry matter to recommend accessions confidently to farmers. In addition, the summarization of growth of *Leucaena* accessions at experimental sites into seasonal 'environment groups' allowed growth to be matched to relatively specific environmental factors.

Conclusions

Pattern analysis techniques are very powerful in determining and displaying the underlying response patterns, especially in large data sets for which conventional statistical analysis is inappropriate.

One of the strengths of pattern analysis is that it involves multiple facets, each of which reveals differing aspects of the data. Clustering will impose group boundaries, whether these are clearly defined or not. Ordination has the power to reveal overall trends, and will give insight into whether distinct clusters exist. Network methods deal purely with links between individuals within their local neighbourhood, and can be useful to clarify the interpretation of the previous two approaches.

A weakness of the current methodology is that many methods, either for clustering or ordination, are not based on an underlying ecological or statistical model. Future applications can benefit from the adoption of model-based methodology, although this will not be appropriate for all data sets.

It must be realized that pattern analysis may sometimes impose a pattern of its own on the data. This is not a problem if the user understands the methods, but it can be hazardous for the inexperienced user. To some extent, this concept provides an answer to the questions from sceptics: 'How can I get four different answers by applying four different clustering techniques?' and 'Which one is correct?' There is no correct answer. Different methods may give somewhat different answers and it is necessary to interact with experienced users and experts in the field of study to ensure that the method being applied is appropriate for the data under consideration.

Acknowledgements

We thank Bruce Pengelly and David Eagles for the use of their data to illustrate some of the procedures of pattern analysis, and also the *Australian Journal of Agricultural Research* for permission to reprint tables and figures from Pengelly and Eagles (1995). We also thank The Australian Centre for International Agricultural Research (ACIAR) for permission to reprint figures from Mullen *et al.* (1998).

References

Annicchiarico, P. (1992) Cultivar adaptation and recommendation from alfalfa trials in Northern Italy. *Journal of Genetics and Breeding* 46, 269–278.
Austin, M.P. and Belbin, L. (1981) An analysis of succession along an environmental gradient using data from a lawn. *Vegetatio* 49, 19–30.
Beals, E.W. (1984) Bray–Curtis ordination: an effective strategy for analysis of multivariate ecological data. *Advanced Journal of Ecological Research* 14, 1–55.
Belbin, L. (1991) Semi-strong hybrid scaling, a new ordination algorithm. *Journal of Vegetation Science* 2, 491–496.
Belbin, L. (1992) *PATN Technical Reference Manual.* CSIRO Division of Wildlife and Ecology, Canberra, 220 pp.
Belbin, L. and McDonald, C. (1993) Comparing three classification strategies for use in ecology. *Journal of Vegetation Science* 4, 341–348.
Bosch, O.J.H. (1989) Degradation of the semi-arid grasslands of Southern Africa. *Journal of Arid Environments* 16, 143–147.
Braak, C.J.F. ter (1986) Canonical correspondence analysis: a new eigenvector technique for multivariate direct gradient analysis. *Ecology* 67, 1167–1169.
Braak, C.J.F. ter (1994) Canonical community ordination. Part 1: Basic theory and linear methods. *Ecoscience* 1, 127–140.
Burrows, W.H., Beale, I.F., Silcock, R.G. and Pressland, A.J. (1984) Prediction of tree and shrub population changes in a semi-arid woodland. In: Tothill, J.C. and Mott, J.J. (eds) *Ecology and Management of the World's Savannas.* Australian Academy of Science, Canberra, pp. 207–211.
DeLacy, I.H., Basford, K.E., Cooper, M., Bull, J.K. and McLaren, C.G. (1996) Analysis of multi-environment trials – an historical perspective. In: Cooper, M. and Hammer, G.L. (eds) *Plant Adaptation and Crop Improvement.* CAB International, Wallingford, UK, pp. 39–124.
Digby, P.G.N. and Kempton, R.A. (1987) *Multivariate Analysis of Ecological Communities.* Population and Community Ecology Series. Chapman & Hall, London, 206 pp.

Foran, B.D., Bastin, G. and Shaw, K.A. (1986) Range assessment and monitoring in arid lands: the use of classification and ordination in range survey. *Journal of Environmental Management* 22, 67–84.

Friedel, M.H. (1990) Some key concepts for monitoring Australia's arid and semi-arid rangelands. *Australian Rangelands Journal* 12, 21–24.

Gnanadesikan, R. (1977) *Methods for Statistical Data Analysis of Multivariate Observations.* Wiley, New York, 311 pp.

Gauch, H.G. Jr (1982) *Multivariate Analysis in Community Ecology.* Cambridge University Press, New York, 298 pp.

Gordon, A.D. (1981) *Classification.* Chapman & Hall, London, 193 pp.

Gower, J.C. (1966) Some distance properties of latent root and vector methods use in multivariate analysis. *Biometrika* 53, 325–338.

Gower, J.C. (1971) A general coefficient of similarity and some of its properties. *Biometrics* 27, 857–874.

Gower, J.C. (1975) Generalised procrustes analysis. *Psychometrika* 40, 33–51.

Gower, J.C. and Hand, D.J. (1996) *Biplots.* Chapman & Hall, London, 277 pp.

Gower, J.C. and Ross, G.J.S. (1969) Minimum spanning trees and single linkage cluster analysis. *Applied Statistics* 18, 54–64.

Greig-Smith, P. (1983) *Quantitative Plant Ecology.* Blackwell Scientific Publications, Oxford, 359 pp.

Hawkins, D.M., Muller, M.W. and Kroonden, J.A. ten (1982) Cluster analysis. In: Hawkins, D.M. (ed.) *Topics in Applied Multivariate Analysis.* Cambridge University Press, Cambridge, pp. 303–356.

Hill, M.O. (1973) Reciprocal averaging: an eigenvector method of ordination. *Journal of Ecology* 61, 237–249.

Hill, M.O. (1974) Correspondence analysis: a neglected multivariate method. *Applied Statistics* 23, 340–354.

Hirschfeld, H.O. (1935) A connection between correlation and contingency. *Proceedings of the Cambridge Philosophical Society* 31, 520–524.

Hotelling, H. (1933) Analysis of a complex of variables into principal components. *Journal of Educational Psychology* 24, 417–441, 498–520.

Kroonenberg, P.M. (1995) *Introduction to Biplots for G×E Tables.* Centre for Statistics Research Report 51, The University of Queensland, Brisbane, 22 pp.

Kruskal, J.B. and Wish, M. (1978) *Multidimensional Scaling.* Sage University Paper Series on Quantitative Applications in the Social Sciences. Sage Publications, Beverly Hills, California, 93 pp.

Legendre, L. and Legendre, P. (eds) (1987) *Developments in Numerical Ecology.* Springer Verlag, New York, 585 pp.

Little, R.J.A. and Rubin, D.B. (1987) *Statistical Analysis with Missing Data.* Wiley, New York, 278 pp.

Manly, B.F.J. (1994) *Multivariate Statistical Methods*, 2nd edn. Chapman & Hall, New York, 215 pp.

McDonald, C.K., Jones, R.M. and Silvey, M.W. (1996) Effect of seasonal soil moisture, nitrogen fertiliser and stocking rate on unsown species in a sown subtropical pasture. *Tropical Grasslands* 30, 319–329.

McLachlan, G.J. and Basford, K.E. (1988) *Mixture Models: Inference and Applications to Clustering.* Marcel Dekker, New York, 253 pp.

Miles, J. (1979) *Vegetation Dynamics.* Chapman & Hall, London, 80 pp.

Mullen, B.F., Shelton, H.M., Basford, K.E., Castillo, A.C., Bino, B., Victorio, E.E., Acasio, R.N., Tarabu, J., Komolong, M.K., Galgal, K.K., Khoa, L.V., Co, H.X., Wandera, F.P., Ibrahim, T.M., Clem, R.L., Jones, R.J., Middleton, C.H., Bolam, M.J.M., Gabunada, F., Stur, W.W., Horne, P.M., Utachak, K. and Khanh, T.T. (1998) Agronomic adaptation to environmental challenges in the genus, *Leucaena*. In: *ACIAR Proceedings No. 86, Leucaena – Adaptation, Quality and Farming Systems*, ACIAR, Canberra, Australia, pp. 39–50.

Pengelly, B.C. and Eagles, D.A. (1995) Geographical distribution and diversity in a collection of the tropical legume *Macroptilium gracile* (Poeppiga ex Bentham) urban. *Australian Journal of Agricultural Research* 46, 569–580.

Pengelly, B.C. and Eagles, D.A. (1996) Diversity in the tropical legume *Teramnus*. *Tropical Grasslands* 30, 298–307.

Pielou, E.C. (1984) *The Interpretation of Ecological Data*. Wiley, New York, 263 pp.

Stone, R. and Auliciems, A. (1992) SOI phase relationships with rainfall in eastern Australia. *International Journal of Climatology* 12, 625–636.

Stuart-Hill, G.C. and Hobson, F.O. (1991) An alternative approach to veld condition assessment in the non-grassveld regions of South Africa. *Journal of the Grassland Society of South Africa* 8, 179–185.

Taylor, J.A. and Tulloch, D. (1985) Rainfall in the wet-dry tropics: extreme events at Darwin and similarities between years during the period 1870–1983 inclusive. *Australian Journal of Ecology* 10, 281–295.

Westoby, M., Walker, B. and Noy-Meir, I. (1989) Opportunistic management for rangelands not at equilibrium. *Journal of Range Management* 42, 266–274.

Whittaker, R.H. (1967) Gradient analysis of vegetation. *Biological Reviews* 42, 207–264.

Williams, W.T. (1976) *Pattern Analysis in Agricultural Science*. Elsevier, Amsterdam, 331 pp.

Modelling Pasture and Animal Production

3

K.G. Rickert[1], J.W. Stuth[2] and G.M. McKeon[3]

[1]*School of Natural and Rural Systems Management, University of Queensland, Gatton Campus, Gatton, Queensland, Australia;* [2]*Department of Rangeland Ecology and Management, Texas A&M University, College Station, Texas, USA;* [3]*Queensland Centre for Climate Applications, Department of Natural Resources, Indooroopilly, Australia*

Introduction

This chapter refers to the prediction of pasture and animal production by a series of mathematical equations that are based on various biophysical inputs, which influence or control production. The mathematical equations are arranged in a computer program to mimic 'real-life' processes that determine pasture and animal production. The computer program is called a model, and modelling is a term that refers to model building as well as using a model to study pasture and animal production. This chapter reviews the structure, applications and steps in building models of pasture and animal production. It provides an overview of principles and approaches, points to appropriate literature, and gives an example of a simple model of pasture and animal production. It is a preliminary guide for persons who are considering the development or use of such models.

Model builders and model users have distinct responsibilities. Model builders are responsible for the integrity of the model. They must ensure that the mathematical expressions in the model are a true representation of the underlying biophysical processes, within specified limits. On the other hand, model users must ensure that the input data are accurate and within the design specifications of the model. Both groups are subject to a basic law of modelling – the GIGO law (garbage in, garbage out), since the validity of predictions from a model depend on the validity of the mathematical descriptions and on the validity of the user's application (Rickert and McKeon, 1991). The degree to which users were involved in model development, and to what extent a model is supported in its application by the

©CAB *International* 2000. *Field and Laboratory Methods for Grassland and Animal Production Research* (eds L. 't Mannetje and R.M. Jones)

model developer or experienced users, all greatly impact on the success of a model.

Modelling pasture and animal production first emerged in the 1960s as computers became available for research. Many pasture scientists were first introduced to the topic by two notable papers at the XI International Grasslands Congress. One described a simple empirical model of sheep production (Spedding, 1970), and the other a complex mechanistic model of production on a short-grass prairie (Dyne, 1970), thereby illustrating two basic approaches to modelling that persist today. A rapid expansion in the range, scope and role of models followed, in response to the even more rapid expansions in the power and accessibility of computers, and because the models proved to be a valuable aid to research, extension and management (Bouman *et al.*, 1996). A rapid expansion in modelling crop production also occurred during this period and models of pastures and crops each have a common focus on plant production. The history and evolution of scope and expectations of modelling can be traced through many books on the topic, such as Dent and Anderson (1971), Dent *et al.* (1979), France and Thornley (1984), Keulen and Wolf (1986), Muchow and Bellamy (1991) and Peart and Curry (1998). Additional insight into the progress and philosophy of modelling pasture and animal production is obtained from reviews by Seligman and Baker (1993), Stuth *et al.* (1993) and Sorensen (1998).

Terminology and Concepts

Since modelling pasture and animal production involves biology, mathematics and computers, the appearance of jargon and new terminology is not surprising. Some key terms and concepts are explained below to avoid confusion in the following sections.

Pasture and animal production can be regarded as a *system* – a group of interacting components that operate together for the common purpose of converting specific inputs into outputs (Fig. 3.1). Two implications follow from this definition. Firstly, because the components of a system interact, the whole system is conceptually greater than the sum of the individual components. This concept justifies the use of modelling as an integrative tool, since a change in one component affects other components in a system. Secondly, the components are contained within a *boundary*, which varies across models and is specified by the model builder. The model boundary is a concept that may coincide with the physical boundary, such as a field or farm, although it often includes factors that impact on production but are not within a physical boundary. For example, depending on the scope of a model, the boundary might include options for managing pastures and animals, markets, costs and prices, or taxation policy (Fig. 3.1). Thus the boundary reflects the role of a model and is a vital concept,

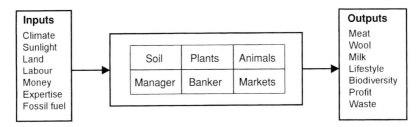

Inputs		Outputs
Climate		Meat
Sunlight		Wool
Land	Soil | Plants | Animals	Milk
Labour		Lifestyle
Money	Manager | Banker | Markets	Biodiversity
Expertise		Profit
Fossil fuel		Waste

Fig. 3.1. A schematic representation of an animal production system on a farm where the boundary includes the attitudes of consumers (markets) and the banking fraternity outside the farm. If appropriate, the boundary could be expanded to include social attitudes expressed through government policies on pollution, land clearing, animal welfare, etc. Note that outputs may be expressed in both quantitative and qualitative terms.

which is specified by the model builder and needs to be appreciated by a model user.

The process of running a model to mimic or simulate a system is called *simulation*, and a series of simulations, which are conducted in response to a systematic change in one or more inputs, is called a *simulation experiment*. Simulation experiments answer 'what if?' questions posed by a user, lead to better understanding of the system and indicate ways to improve or repair a system. All simulations are a form of *systems analysis*, a general term which refers to any study of the interactions between components in a system. Systems analyses need not involve modelling, since modelling is one of several techniques available (Morley, 1981). However, simulation experiments with a model are a popular method of systems analysis.

Output from computer models usually includes variables that reflect the status of a system and, depending on the purpose of the model, these may estimate the productivity, stability and sustainability of a system. These are three key but often conflicting criteria for evaluating performance of farming systems (Conway, 1985). *Productivity* within a production period refers to familiar terms such as kilograms of wool, milk or liveweight gain. Rather than absolute units, productivity is commonly expressed as a ratio of output to animal or land inputs (e.g. kg per animal or kg ha^{-1}), but many other convenient ratios can be used. For example, profit per unit of forage allows the efficiency of using forage resources to be compared across different animal management systems (James *et al.*, 1996). *Stability* or reliability refers to the variation in productivity in response to natural variation in inputs such as rainfall or prices. It is reflected in the coefficient of variation for average production, or if there is a long history of productivity, by probability distributions of productivity (Rickert and McKeon, 1985). *Sustainability* refers to the ability of a system to withstand stress without becoming irreversibly damaged from factors such as low prices, high stocking rates, climate change, or a sudden shock such as fire, flood or out-of-season frost. Models are particularly useful tools for estimating temporal trends in productivity and other impacts of stress on a system (McKeon et al., 1990; Parton and Ojima, 1994; Hall et al., 1998; Landsberg et al., 1998).

Computer models that are aids to managing complex, ill-structured problems are often called *decision support systems* (DSS). However, this definition is too narrow. Contemporary DSS may also include databases that store input data, the interface and operating instructions for users, utilities for generating and interpreting reports of output, mechanisms to maintain the computer software, and procedures for communicating with users (Stuth et al., 1993). This expanded description recognizes that a DSS may not consist of a model; instead it might consist of a database or an expert system with utilities for extracting and interpreting information (e.g. Gillard, 1993; Clarkson et al., 1997).

Purposes and Approaches to Modelling

Benefits

A model is a collection of mathematical equations that mimic biophysical processes. Each equation can be regarded as a hypothesis pertaining to a specific process or component of the system, and a model can be regarded as a collection of hypotheses, derived from past research, that can be further modified and developed through new research. Indeed, model building tends to identify gaps in our knowledge that point to future research. Thus, a model becomes a repository for past research and a precursor for future research (Ebersohn, 1976; Dent et al., 1979) and model construction is a common and legitimate research activity (Seligman and Baker, 1993; Sorensen, 1998).

However, decision support models for 'real-life' managers exist because of two other attributes. Firstly, good computer models provide a quantitative description of complex systems consisting of many interacting components, some of which may have opposing or conflicting responses (Black et al., 1993). This is a powerful and unique attribute that greatly exceeds the analytical capacity of the human mind. A simple example of conflicting responses is provided by the familiar relationships between stocking rate and liveweight gain (Jones and Sandland, 1974). In regard to beef cattle, as stocking rate increases the liveweight and value per animal decrease, variable costs increase and production per hectare first increases and then decreases. A manager must balance the trade-offs between profit, risk, pasture degradation and premium prices (Rickert, 1996). Similar trade-offs between productivity, stability and sustainability are common in farming systems (Conway, 1994) and a model can be a tool for teaching how to avoid 'real-life' errors in managing grazing systems.

Secondly, a good model provides an objective and quantitative extrapolation in space and time of information derived from past research and experiences. This is another powerful and unique attribute that reduces the need to repeat research across environments. If the input files contain a long history of daily weather data, then the year-by-year output can be expressed as probability distributions, an indication of system stability as mentioned above. By repeating the process for different management options (a simulation experiment), the reliability of different options can be compared in respect to the long-term variability in climate (Rickert and McKeon, 1985). Similarly, by applying a model and processing the historical weather for each land unit in a region, a large-scale evaluation of past management is possible (McKeon *et al.*, 1990). Further, if the spatial model uses current weather data as input, the output is a near real-time display at a regional or national level of pasture and/or animal production (Hall, 1997). All of these applications rely on a model's ability to extrapolate information in temporal and spatial dimensions, and this attribute is fundamental to the role of models in information transfer (Stuth *et al.*, 1993).

A wide range of models dealing with different aspects of plant and animal production can be arranged in a hierarchy of increasing scale of operation (Table 3.1). Commonly, elements from lower-level models are used in the large-scale higher-level models. As the level increases the roles of models change from being tools for research through management aids for farmers to aids for making industry or government policy, and there is a parallel increase in interest by the wider community in the predictions and policies arising from the models. As a result, both the model and the model builders who influence government policy are exposed to a high level of public scrutiny and the validity of the model and its predictions need to be sound and transparent. Notably, the models in Table 3.1 focus on the biophysical and economic components of pasture and animal production, and tend to ignore the social attitudes and aspirations of managers or the community. Because social attitudes influence a manager's acceptance of new technology, the role and effectiveness of models in fostering new technology has been questioned (Jiggins and Baker, 1993; Cox, 1996; Rickert, 1998).

Categories

Models of plant and animal production can be classified into the following broad categories (Loewer, 1989; Rickert and McKeon, 1991): (i) word and diagrammatic models; (ii) deterministic or probabilistic (stochastic); (iii) static or dynamic; and (iv) mechanistic (theoretical) or empirical.

Word and diagrammatic models describe the context and boundary of a system using common language and/or convenient diagrams (e.g.

Table 3.1. A short selection of models that involve pasture and animal production arranged in hierarchy of scale of operation.

Level	Scope	Purpose	Examples
1	Organs within a plant or animal, or individual plants or animals	Research into processes and a basis for higher-level models	Intake and rumen models (Fisher and Baumont, 1994; Poppi, 1996)
2	Plants in a community or field; animals in a mob	Basis for higher-level models and on-farm DSS	Pasture growth and quality (Gustavsson et al., 1995); animal production (White et al., 1983; Freer et al., 1997); feeding a dairy herd (Hulme et al. 1986)
3	Farm forage supply and herd structure and management	Evaluation of new technology and strategic and tactical decisions	Management strategies (Stafford Smith and Foran, 1988; Bowman et al., 1989; Cobon and Clewett, 1999)
4	Whole-farm enterprise mix and management	Selection of preferred management strategies	Crops and livestock (Morrison et al., 1986; Kreuter et al., 1996; Rickert and Sinclair, 2000)
5	Regional or national assessment of industry or land condition	Advice on policy to industry or government agencies	Safe stocking rate and land condition (McKeon et al., 1990; Scanlan et al., 1994); land clearing and hydrology (Lemberg et al., 1998)
6	Assessment of impact of climate change on plants and/or animals	Advice to governments and negotiations on global policy	(Howden et al., 1994; Parton and Ojima, 1994; Eckert et al., 1995; Day et al., 1997; McKeon et al., 1998)

Fig. 3.2). Such descriptions should occur early in the process of building a model as they guide the process of model development.

Deterministic models do not reflect the natural or random variation in inputs, whereas inputs or decision rules in *probabilistic models* display natural variation. Typically, models that use average values of input variables are deterministic, while the output from stochastic models reflects natural variation. In practice, models of grazing systems often combine deterministic and probabilistic elements to simulate the day-by-day variation in, for example, pasture yield and animal liveweight by keeping all inputs constant (deterministic) with the exception of day-by-day variation (stochastic) in climate.

Static models determine the new status of the system for given inputs and a single production period, whereas a dynamic model repeats the calculations for a number of production cycles specified by the user. Static models have been used to estimate herd or flock structure (Holmes, 1988), ration formulations (Hulme *et al.*, 1986) and supplementation programmes (Stuth *et al.*, 1999). After inputs are changed, static models calculate the new status of a system in a manner similar to recalculation of a spreadsheet.

Dynamic models operate on a standard time step, commonly one day, and the arrangement of data in input and output files reflects the standard time step. Dynamic models are particularly useful for analysing grazing systems since the temporal trends in predictions of state variables can be displayed in response to variations in inputs of climate or management (McKeon *et al.*, 1990).

Empirical models usually estimate the underlying processes by equations developed from experimental data which display a relationship between the process and one or more influencing variables. For example, several empirical equations are available for the calculation of intake as a function of forage digestibility and animal liveweight (Poppi, 1996). On the other hand, *mechanistic models* use equations that reflect a theoretical understanding of the factors that control the process. For example, in a mechanistic model, intake becomes a function of rumen size, rate of digestion and energy metabolism (Poppi, 1996; Weston, 1996). The relative merits of mechanistic and empirical approaches have been hotly debated (France and Thornley, 1984; Black *et al.*, 1993; Seligman and Baker, 1993; Passioura, 1996). Mechanistic models, because of their stronger theoretical base, tend to be more versatile and robust than empirical models, but, since they often contain parameters that are difficult to determine in practical situations, they tend to be used as research models. Furthermore, the components of a mechanistic model at one level are often derived from an empirical relationship at a lower level. For example, the rumen size used in a mechanistic estimation of intake might be derived from an empirical function based on animal liveweight (Herrero *et al.*, 1998). Mechanistic models may not be more accurate than empirical models, but because of the theoretical base they are more likely to explain why observations occur. Conversely, the

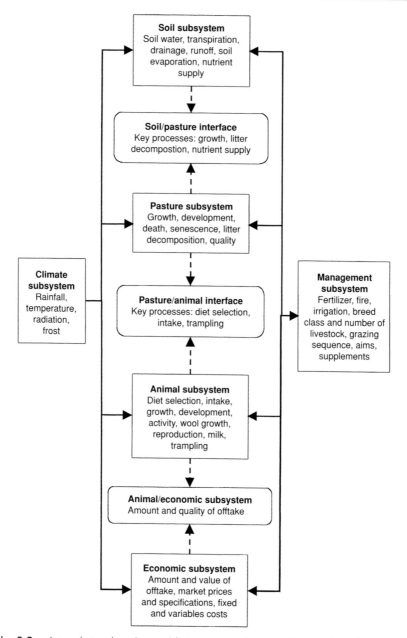

Fig. 3.2. Interrelationships (arrows) between six subsystems (rectangles) often found in models of pasture and animal production. Each subsystem consists of processes that control the state variables in the subsystems. The interface between two subsystems (rounded rectangles) is expressed through key processes, which are influenced by factors in two or more adjoining subsystems. The climate and management subsystems impact on the soil, pasture, animal and economic subsystems, but influence is two-way for management and one-way for climate.

robustness of an empirical function is a reflection of the accuracy and range of experimental data used in its derivation. The danger with an empirical equation is that spurious results might occur if it operates outside of the range in the data used to derive the equation. To avoid this problem, a model user should be familiar with the derivation of functions that describe key processes in a model, and model output should be treated with caution when the input data contains extreme values. Because of convenience, empirical relationships are widely used in practical decision-support models of pasture and animal production. As a variation on the above distinction, some DSS actually process and interpret the results previously stored from many simulation experiments with a mechanistic model.

The above plethora of pasture and animal production models suggests a lack of convergence in the representation of the biophysical processes of Fig. 3.2. McCown *et al.* (1996) developed a modelling approach whereby a special software shell or 'engine' allows different submodels of the same biophysical process to be compared while other components are held constant. Whilst this approach has facilitated a convergence in describing crop models, it has not been used with models of complex pasture–animal-management systems and an understandable lack of convergence remains.

Types of models

It is convenient to group the models in Table 3.1 into three broad types: (i) research models used by a few interested persons; (ii) commercial models which are sold as DSS to farmers or advisors who display a wide range in computer and managerial skills; and (iii) policy models which have wide implications for government or industry and are used and maintained by teams of skilled operators. Commercial models are considered separately later because their development involves more steps than developing a research or policy model.

Research models are particularly useful for analysing the complex interactions in pasture and animal production (Fig. 3.2). Research models do not need a sophisticated presentation, particularly if the model builders and model users are one and the same. A spreadsheet is a useful medium for a research model because the equations are visible, results can be readily displayed in figures or tables, and inputs can be easily changed. Indeed, spreadsheet models have made a useful contribution to science and management (Holmes, 1988; Rickert and McKeon, 1988; McIvor and Moneypenny, 1995). Sometimes a research model evolves into a commercial or policy model. Many of the existing commercial packages originated in this manner, thereby reducing development costs. Conversion from a research to a commercial product is obviously beneficial, provided the ongoing need for the model is justified and the commercialization process is handled properly.

Policy models serve policy makers by estimating trends in key components such as the economy, and environment (Table 3.1). With regard to pasture and animal production, policy models range from those that target a specific question to those that provide a regular ongoing service. An example of a specific analysis that influenced policy was the acceptance, at the 1997 Kyoto conference on climate change, of shrub encroachment in rangelands as a sink for reducing greenhouse gases. An example of a regular ongoing service is the monthly maps of relative pasture yield, adjusted for prevailing stocking rates, which are derived from a pasture production model operating on 5×5 km grid for the State of Queensland (Brook and Carter, 1994). The maps provide an objective assessment of drought status for government and industry. Constructing and maintaining a policy model of this scope is a demanding task that requires an integrated team of scientists, programmers and support staff. A policy model gains credibility through demonstrating its scientific base and validity.

The compilation of data at the proper scale is critical for policy models, and linking economic and environmental analyses is a big challenge (Hall, 1997). Most economic data are collected along political boundaries (e.g. province, county) while environmental data are normally stratified by ecosystems (e.g. river basin, soil association, ecological sites). To partition economic data properly within districts requires synchronization between the response and the environmental conditions associated with that response. For instance, a district might span several precipitation zones, whereas only one zone might grow a given forage species. Therefore, policy that impacts on that species is only applicable to one zone and regional economic data must be properly partitioned to reflect interzonal economic responses and environments.

Getting Started as a Model User

Getting started as a model user requires an appropriate model and computer, some prior understanding of pasture and animal production and some basic computing skills. A good portion of patience and tenacity of purpose is also needed, as a model, like other computer software, demands a commitment in time and effort to develop skill and experience with the package.

Table 3.2 lists a selection of models that have useful attributes for model users who are novices. Also, each is readily available, can be set up without difficulty on IBM-type personal computers, and has a contact for after-sale advice. Before acquiring one of these models (or any other one, for that matter), users should ensure that the computer requirements for the model match the specifications of their computer. The more advanced the computer, the better it is for modelling. Running big models on old computers is a slow and frustrating exercise that is best avoided.

Getting Started as a Model Builder

Models of pasture and animal production are usually complex as they involve parallel flows of mass (soil, water, carbon, nitrogen), energy (solar radiation, metabolic energy), information (management decisions) and money (Fig. 3.2). Because of this complexity it is not surprising that many different models of grazing systems exist, but the following protocol has underpinned the development of many of the successful models:

1.   Clear objectives based on the issues being addressed are essential and a model should not be built unless these are specified.
2.   Word and diagrammatic models give the 'big picture' by defining boundaries to the system and the information required for the model.
3.   Objectives are refined in terms of current limitations to knowledge.
4.   Specifications of the model are finalized by removing, simplifying or combining processes that are not important to the solution being investigated.
5.   The model is built, verified, calibrated, validated and tested with sensitivity analyses (terms that are explained below).
6.   Simulation experiments follow, often in combination with the previous step. If results from the simulation experiments require a better representation of a few key processes, more research may be needed to improve the submodels of these processes.
7.   Output from the model is re-evaluated and reported with appropriate caveats for the processes that were not represented or were simplified in the model.

In regard to step 4 above, it is often convenient to describe a model of a pasture and animal production system as a group of separate but interacting submodels, or modules, such as the climate, soil, pasture (plants), animals, economic and management submodels in Fig. 3.2. The submodels of Fig. 3.2 are arranged in a progressive sequence that represents the conversion of sunlight, soil water and nutrients into animal products and, eventually, into enterprise profit. Key biological processes govern the linkage from one submodel to the next – that is, the interface between the soil, plant, animal and economic components of the system. Model building often commences by developing each module on a spreadsheet where the input data, equations and results are visible. Alternatively, the choice may be to use advanced programming software that automatically generates computer code as a flow chart is drawn and appropriate equations inserted. Whatever approach is chosen, we recommend that the submodels be progressively developed and arranged as separate modules. Another efficient way of 'getting started' is to train within an existing team of model builders who supply direction, advice and assistance to the trainee.

It is also convenient to describe the components of a system as state variables, auxiliary variables, processes and parameters. A *state variable*

Table 3.2.   A short selection of models on components of grazing systems.

Model and attributes	Supplier
WATERMOD is a mechanistic model that simulates the dynamics of soil water in agricultural and environmental systems. It has special modules for climate, crop growth and irrigation and is applicable to a range of soil types. Default parameters are available.	Greenhat Software, PO Box 1590, Armidale, NSW 2350, Australia
GRAZFEED is a static, daily model of animal production, expressed as liveweight gain, milk production or wool growth (Freer *et al.*, 1997). The user specifies: the species, breed, class and condition of animal; type of pasture; yield and digestibility of green and dead pasture; daily maximum and minimum temperature; type of supplement. It is an aid to managing sown pastures and rangelands and is a component of GRAZPLAN.	Horizon Technology, PO Box 598, Roseville, NSW 2069, Australia
DroughtPlan is a suite of decision support systems (DSS) for rangeland management in northern Australia (Cobon and Clewett, 1999). One item is a dynamic, empirical, point model of soil, plant and cattle subsystems for tussock grasslands (WINGRASP). Default inputs, including historical climate records, are supplied for locations, which can be selected from a map. A simplified version of this model is described in the next section.	Queensland Department of Primary Industries, GPO Box 46, Brisbane, Q4001, Australia
GRAZE is a complex, dynamic, mechanistic, research model for beef cattle on mixed pastures (Loewer, 1998). A Windows™ shell allows a user to specify parameters for the soil, pasture, cattle and grazing management, as well as daily weather, in a series of input files. The same shell aids in the inspection of output. It requires practice to master its attributes.	Agricultural and Biological Engineering Department, University of Florida, USA, via the internet
SPATIAL CHARACTERIZATION TOOL is an analysis system based on maps that link databases and information files to allow users to explore large-scale relationships of human activities and natural systems. It displays spatial relationships between landscapes in terms of weather, vegetation, animal populations, human populations, human infrastructures, etc.	Integrated Information Management Laboratory, TAES-Blackland Research Center, Temple, Texas, USA

Continued

describes the status of a system at a specific time, such as the amount of soil water, yield of pasture, animal liveweight, animal value and farm profit. The size of each state variable is influenced by processes that determine the flow of material to or from the state variable. For example, the processes of rainfall and transpiration influence the amount of soil water, and the processes of pasture growth and intake influence pasture yield (see Figs 3.3 and 3.4).

Table 3.2. *Continued.*

Model and attributes	Supplier
GRAZING LANDS APPLICATION is designed to allow whole-property forage inventory, herd definition, grazing scheduling, investment analysis, nutritional management and mixed animal stocking calculations. The system is the principal planning system for the United States Department of Agriculture Natural Resource Conservation Service.	Department of Rangeland Ecology and Management, Texas A&M University, College Station, TX 77843–2126, USA
NUTBAL is a static, single-case model of nutritional balance analysis of free-ranging cattle, sheep, goats and horses. Users specify the type and class of animal, physiological stage, terrain and environmental conditions, feeding regime and NIRS faecal profiling predictions of diet crude protein and digestible organic matter to predict nutrient balance, weight gain/loss and least-cost feeding recommendations.	
The Grazing Manager (TGM) is a DSS that aids operational adjustments of stocking rate throughout the year. Rainfall and use ratings for the pasture are input in the model, which estimates future shortfall in forage supply relative to projected livestock demand.	

The mathematical equations that describe processes are often called rate equations. *Auxiliary variables*, or driving variables, have a direct influence on the processes that affect the status of a system but they are not part of the flow of material through a system. For example, temperature is an auxiliary variable that may influence both pasture growth and intake. Finally, *parameters* refer to influencing factors that remain constant during a simulation, such as water-holding capacity of a soil or breed of animal. Figures 3.3 and 3.4 use special symbols to describe the soil water balance in these terms.

Model verification refers to thorough checking of the computer program to ensure that it is free of 'bugs' and performs properly within specific limits. Usually a model builder verifies a model by a series of tests, using special input data and other conditions that focus on specific components of a model and their interactions. Similarly, a simulation experiment, which is designed to determine the relative sensitivity of inputs and parameters that influence a system, is called a sensitivity analysis. Obviously, accuracy is more important with sensitive than with insensitive inputs. The relativity sensitivity of different inputs is indicated by comparing the change in output caused by a specific change in the different inputs (e.g. percentage change in output after a 5, 10 or 20% change in an input parameter). Whilst verification and sensitivity analyses are primarily the responsibility of model builders, simple exercises on these lines give model users a good appreciation of the operation and limitations of a model.

Model validation refers to how well a model mimics the system it is meant to represent. Validation is commonly demonstrated by simulating a wide range of scenarios that have been actually observed, and then by comparing predictions from a model against the observations. The validation data should be independent to the data used in developing a model. Linear regressions of observations against predictions are commonly used to make the comparisons. The closer the slope and coefficient of determination for a regression are to unity, and the intercept is to zero, the better is the validity of a model. However, there are theoretical and practical problems with validation based on regression analysis (Mitchell, 1997), and the confidence of the model builders should be recognized as a model undergoes development and modification (Harrison, 1990). Of course, serious users also develop confidence in a model through less formal validations as they compare predictions against their own observations and experiences. In practice, validation is an ongoing activity that warrants considerable effort by the model builders and independent experts, particularly when the model attempts to mimic large variation in production systems and is used as an aid to politically or financially sensitive decisions (Scanlan *et al.*, 1994). In essence a model is 'valid' when it sufficiently mimics the real world to fulfil its objectives, and when decisions based on the model are superior to those made without the model (Dent *et al.*, 1979).

Building Commercial Models

Building a commercial model goes beyond the steps in the previous section to include tasks that must meet technical and legal standards and the provision of after-sale service. High standards of program design, performance and quality control are essential since a customer will compare the convenience and operation of a DSS package with other familiar software, such as their favourite word processor or spreadsheet. Thus commercial DSS must perform in a convenient and reliable manner. A good description of the steps in DSS development is provided by Stuth *et al.* (1993), which can be condensed into the following three key steps.

1. *Feasibility analysis* – a four-way match between requirements of the market, the resulting software specifications, availability of information and human and technical resources to develop the package, and the time lines for completing the task. The time frame is usually set by the sponsor of the project or by a software publisher, and should be negotiated before the decision to proceed is made. The importance of the feasibility analysis cannot be overemphasized. There is no point in developing a product unless there is a likely market, which can be assessed by a survey of potential users. Careful planning is essential, preferably involving people who are experienced in software development, since projects for DSS development frequently experience problems because the time required for product development is underestimated. Choice of software is another early and critical decision to be made by model builders. If the model builder is free to choose, the preferred language should reflect requirements for data entry, storage and display, the availability of skilled programmers, whether or not the model will distributed as a compiled version, and the computer operating system. As previously mentioned, the computer code for each component should be arranged as separate modules, and when model development involves a team effort, one person should be responsible for version control and integrity of the code.

2. *Product development* – all measures to ensure that the product operates in a convenient and reliable manner, including interactive prototyping with potential users, and model verification and validation. Model verification and validation were explained in the previous section. Interactive prototyping refers to the process of matching the presentation and capabilities of software to the requirements of potential users. Without the acceptance of potential users a DSS will probably fail in the marketplace. Creating a 'user friendly' presentation of software that mimics pasture and animal production on a farm is a challenge because a multidimensional scenario must be described through a keyboard and monitor. The multidimensional scenario might consist of descriptions of fields in the farm, pastures in the fields, number and class of animals in herds, grazing management of herds, period type and amount of supplementary feeding, and rainfall. In addition, potential users commonly prefer the software to have keystrokes and a screen layout similar to other familiar software. Also, outputs must be clear, easily understood and suitable for further analysis or storage. One approach used by model builders to meet these requirements is to consult with a panel of potential users on a regular basis and progressively hone the software in response to suggestions from the panel. This is a time-consuming task that can lead to major changes in the program code that controls presentation, but experience has shown that model builders, who know a package intimately, are not experts in 'user friendly' presentations.

3. *Commercialization* – supply of the master copies of software, help notes and operating manuals to the publisher, legal advice on disclaimers and duty of care responsibilities, package design and presentation, the product launch, plans for promoting the package and procedures for after-sales inquiries and service. In practice, successful commercialization requires good cooperation with the publisher, since it is a blend of the professional experience and standards of the publisher with technical knowledge and experience of the model builders. Publishers tend to take the lead in presentation and distribution while the model builders are involved in promotion and after-sales service. Usually models are distributed as a compiled program, which prevents a user from seeing or altering the computer code. The code is the intellectual property of the model builder, but to share the structure of a model with the wider scientific community, model builders usually describe the mathematical equations in a conventional journal article or, in some cases, in a technical operating manual. In this way, other model builders can use or adapt equations from the compiled model to different situations, and the process of hypothesis testing continues. If a model is distributed as a commercial product it is subject to copyright law and is usually supplied with instruction manuals, and some form of version control and after-sale service. These protections may not be present when a model is distributed to users at no charge.

Example of a Soil–Plant–Animal Model

Model builders must select the most appropriate submodels and the best approach to modelling the interface between submodels (Fig. 3.2). An excellent review on these topics described many of the approaches to

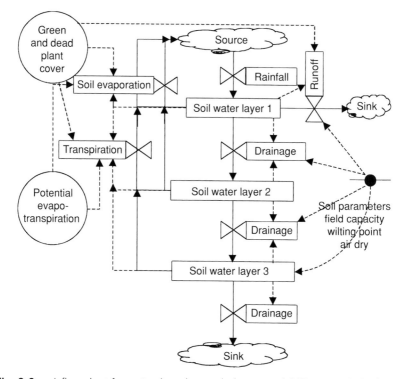

Fig. 3.3. A flow chart for a simple soil water balance model (Equation 3.1) where water is stored in three separate soil layers, each being a state variable (rectangle). Other components of the subsystem are represented as follows: processes or flows of water – a valve symbol; auxiliary or driving variables – circles; parameters – a solid dot; water or material flow – a solid arrow; information flows or influences – a dashed arrow.

modelling plant growth and diet selection and intake (Herrero *et al.*, 1998). Rather than duplicate that review, this section describes simple submodels as an introduction to modelling pasture and animal production. Each submodel can be constructed on a spreadsheet and can be parameterized by referring to field observations, local knowledge or the default values given below. The submodels also interconnect to mimic the whole system on a daily time step and simulations commence each year at the start of the local growing systems, such as 1 September in the southern hemisphere. The objective of the model is to mimic the interactions between liveweight gain, prevailing climate and choice of stocking rate for beef cattle grazing subtropical rangeland. However, it should be emphasized that this is an elementary 'getting started' model and output from the model should be considered with caution.

Soil water balance submodel

The basic soil water balance submodel, which underpins pasture production (Fig. 3.3), is given by:

$$SW_t = SW_{t-1} + Rain_t + Irrig_t - Drain_t - Runoff_t - Esoil_t - Trans_t - Ecanopy_t - Elitter_t \qquad \text{mm} \qquad (3.1)$$

where SW_t and SW_{t-1} are the soil water contents for t and $t-1$ days, respectively, and $Rain_t$, $Irrig_t$, $Drain_t$, $Runoff_t$, $Esoil_t$, $Trans_t$, $Ecanopy_t$ and $Elitter_t$ are the daily flows of rainfall, irrigation, through drainage, runoff, soil evaporation, transpiration, canopy interception and litter interception, respectively. Usually $Rain_t$ and $Irrig_t$ are supplied as input data and a soil water balance submodel calculates the remaining terms.

A water balance submodel may take a mechanistic approach based on the theory of water flow across hydraulic gradients, or use empirical relationships that operate between parameters that represent the upper and lower limits of soil water (Fig. 3.3). Further, the number of soil layers may vary from one to ten or more. Empirical models of soil water balance have been popular and reliable predictors, due in part to the conservative nature of soil water balance in dryland environments. In a drying cycle, most soil water is lost through $Esoil_t$ and $Trans_t$. Because these two processes depend on the amount of soil water present (i.e. water supply), an over- or under-prediction one day is compensated by an opposite trend the next day. However, both processes also depend on evaporative demand and on the amount and greenness of vegetation (Fig. 3.3). Locations with a high proportion of rainfall events of less than 25 mm may experience substantial evaporative losses by water adhering to tree canopies and surface litter.

A three-layer model (0–10, 10–50, and 50–100 cm) of soil water balance is described below. Since being first described (Rickert and McKeon, 1982), it has been refined and applied in modelling soil water balance for a wide range of native pasture communities (Day et al., 1997).

Runoff

When modelling runoff, model builders are faced with another interface problem: how to mimic the influence of topography, soil, vegetation and rainfall on runoff. Prediction of runoff has received a great deal of attention by hydrologists and several different runoff models have been developed, such as the modifications to the US curve number model by Littleboy et al. (1996). Do not hesitate to replace the runoff model described below (Scanlan et al., 1996) if a more appropriate model is available:

$$Runoff = Cover\_term \times (Rain - (1 - Rain\_intensity \, / \, 110) \times$$
$$sw\_deficit) \qquad (3.2)$$

where $Cover\_term$ is an index reflecting vegetation cover; $sw\_deficit$ is the soil water deficit in the top two layers (mm); $Rain$ is daily rainfall; and $Rain\_intensity$ is the maximum rainfall intensity in a 15 min period (mm h^{-1}) as described below.

Two functions are used to calculate $Cover\_term$, which is an index of the relationships between total dry matter yield of standing pasture and runoff. Firstly, the relationship between dry matter yield and proportion of ground cover, Run_cover, is given by (Fig. 3.4C):

$$Run\_cover = tsdm^{runoff\_power} \, / \, (tsdm^{runoff\_power} + yld\_tcov50^{runoff\_power}) \qquad (3.3)$$

where $tsdm$ is the total standing dry matter but not including litter; yld_tcov50 is the total standing dry matter where effective cover for runoff estimation is 50% (e.g. 1200 kg ha^{-1}); and $runoff\_power$ is a user-defined curve-shaping factor (e.g. 0.95). Secondly, the relationship between ground cover from equation 3.3 and the cover index in equation 3.2 is given by:

$$Cover\_term = (1.0 - Run\_cover)^2 \qquad (3.4)$$

which causes $Cover\_term$ to approach zero in a curvilinear manner (i.e. zero runoff) as Run_cover approaches an asymptote of 0.9 at $tsdm$ of 10,000 kg ha^{-1} (Fig. 3.4C).

Equation 3.2 also recognizes the influence of rainfall intensity on runoff, but most historical records of climate contain observations of daily rainfall without observations of rainfall intensity. An algorithm to estimate $Rain\_intensity$ in Queensland (Scanlan et al., 1996), where rainfall intensity is highest in summer and lowest in winter, is given by:

$$Rain\_intensity = MAX(100, \, Rain \times (int\_intercept +$$
$$int\_slope \times time\_of\_year)) \qquad \text{mm h}^{-1} \qquad (3.5)$$

where $int\_intercept$ (e.g. 0.9) and int_slope (e.g. 0.7) are empirical coefficients derived from the analysis of long-term records of rainfall intensity

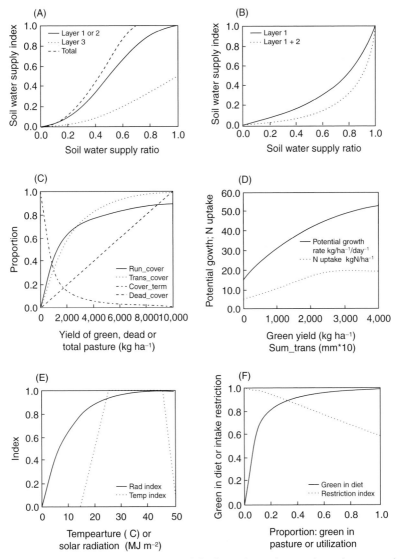

Fig. 3.4. Response surfaces for some of the key relationships in the soil water and pasture submodels. (A) Soil water supply indices for transpiration (Equations 3.16 and 3.17). (B) Soil water supply indices for soil evaporation (Equations 3.22 and 3.23). (C) Indices based on yield of standing pasture that influence runoff, potential transpiration and dead cover (Equations 3.3, 3.4, 3.11, 3.14). (D) Potential growth in relation to green yield (Equation 3.30) and nitrogen uptake in relation to accumulated transpiration (Equation 3.36). (E) Indices for radiation and temperature. (F) Green in diet in relation to green in pasture (Equation 3.55) and the intake restriction index in relation to utilization on tussock grassland (Equation 3.46).

and *time_of_year* is a factor that accounts for the seasonal pattern of rainfall. Further:

$$time\_of\_year = \text{COS}((2 \times \pi \times (day + 15)) / 365) \qquad (3.6)$$

where *day* is current day of year in the simulation. The coefficients in Equations 3.5 and 3.6 should be adjusted to reflect local conditions.

Other models with a hydrological base, such as the EPIC crop/pasture model or the PHYGROW grazing lands model, use coefficients for individual species to determine a curve number for runoff, along with a daily adjustment for moisture conditions of the soil surface (Williams *et al.*, 1984; Stuth *et al.*, 1998).

Infiltration and drainage

If there is sufficient water after runoff, each soil layer is progressively filled to field capacity. This approach assumes that water above field capacity in layers 1 or 2 drains to the layer below in a single day, and drainage from layer 3 leaves the system (Fig. 3.3). This simple process is represented for layer 1 by:

$$Infiltrate_1 = Rain - Runoff \qquad \qquad \text{mm} \qquad (3.7)$$

$$SW_{1t} = \text{MIN}(FC_1, SW_{1t-1} + Infiltrate_1) \qquad \text{mm} \qquad (3.8)$$

$$Drainage_1 = \text{MAX}(0, SW_{1t-1} + Infiltrate_1 - FC_1) \qquad \text{mm} \qquad (3.9)$$

where $Infiltrate_1$ is infiltration into layer 1, FC_1 is the field capacity (mm) of layer 1 and $Drainage_1$ is drainage from layer 1 to layer 2. Similarly, equations 3.8 and 3.9, with appropriate changes to the subscripts, can be used to partition water into layers 2 and 3, since $Drainage_1$ becomes $Infiltrate_2$ and $Drainage_2$ becomes $Infiltrate_3$. Also, the summation of $Drainage_3$ during a simulation represents water that has drained beyond the root zone of the pasture. It may enter a water table below the pasture or be used by deeper-rooted trees growing in association with the pasture (Fig. 3.3). Some models have a fourth layer below the top three soil layers to cater for deep-rooted shrubs and trees. Also, some models have an evaporative layer at the soil surface to better reflect soil evaporation and the influence of litter and organic matter at the soil surface.

Potential evapotranspiration

Both *Esoil* and *Trans* directly depend on the potential demand for evapotranspiration which is represented by daily pan evaporation. However, it is convenient to partition potential evapotranspiration into potential transpiration (*Pot_trans*), potential soil evaporation (*Pot_esoil*) and potential transpiration from trees if they are present (Day *et al.*, 1997). In this example we assume that trees are not present, and that:

$$Pot\_trans = Epan \times Trans\_cover \qquad mm \qquad (3.10)$$

where *Epan* is daily pan evaporation, *Trans_cover* is the proportion of potential evapotranspiration from green vegetation. An additional multiplier may be required in some situations, such as tussock grasslands with low dry matter yields on dry soil surfaces, to increase *Pot_trans* in response to the prevailing vapour pressure deficit (Day *et al.*, 1997). *Trans_cover* is calculated as follows:

$$Trans\_cover = 1 - EXP(Green\_sdm \times Ln(0.5) / gyld\_cov50) \qquad (3.11)$$

where *Green_sdm* is the dry matter yield of green pasture (kg ha^{-1}), and *gyld_cov50* is the yield of green pasture (e.g. 1600 kg ha^{-1}) when transpiration is 50% of *Epan* (Fig. 3.4C).

Potential soil evaporation (*Pot_esoil*) increases directly with pan evaporation (*Epan*) and decreases as plant cover increases as follows:

$$Pot\_esoil = Epan \times (1.0 - Surface\_cover) \qquad mm \qquad (3.12)$$

where

$$Surface\_cover = 1.0 - (1.0 - Trans\_cover) \times (1.0 - Dead\_cover) \qquad (3.13)$$

and

$$Dead\_cover = MIN(1.0, (Litter\_yld + Stdm\_dead) / 10,000) \qquad (3.14)$$

Equations 3.12 and 3.13 imply that potential soil evaporation is zero if either *Trans_cover* or *Dead_cover* is unity. Further, equation 3.14 implies that *Dead_cover* increases linearly with the total yield of dead pasture, up to a maximum of 10,000 kg ha^{-1} (Fig. 3.4C), which is the sum of standing dead pasture (*Stdm_dead*) and yield surface litter (*Litter_yld*).

Where interception losses by tree leaves or by litter are significant, there needs to be a mechanism that properly depicts leaf turnover and litter decomposition within the system.

Soil water supply indices for transpiration

Transpiration depends on the amount of soil water (Fig. 3.3), and a water supply index for each soil layer represents the ability of a layer to satisfy potential transpiration. All three soil layers may contribute to transpiration.

The basic variable for calculating soil water supply indices for transpiration is given by:

$$Sw\_supply\_ratio_k = MAX(0, (SW_k - WP_k) / (FC_k - WP_k)) \qquad (3.15)$$

where *Sw_supply_ratio$_k$* is the soil water supply ratio for soil layer k; and SW_k, WP_k and FC_k are, respectively, the soil water, wilting point and field capacity (mm) for layer k. In practice, FC_k refers to a field measurement of the drained upper limit and WP_k refers to a field measurement of soil water after a prolonged period of drying.

The water supply index for layers and 1 and 2 (Swi_k) is given by:

$$Swi_k = (1.0 + \text{SIN}((Sw\_supply\_ratio_k - 0.5) \times \pi)) \times 0.5 \qquad (3.16)$$

(Fig. 3.4A), and the water supply index for layer 3 is given by:

$$Swi_3 = (1.0 - \text{COS}(Sw\_supply\_ratio_3 \times \pi / 2.0)) \times roots\_layer_3 \qquad (3.17)$$

where *roots_layer₃* is a user-defined index (0.0 to 1.0) that reflects the capacity of pasture to extract water from the third soil layer (Fig. 3.4A). Typically, *roots_layer₃* ranges from 0.0 for pasture with no roots in layer 3, through 0.5 for most pasture, to 1.0 for pastures with a dense root system, such as buffel grass. Together, Equations 3.16 and 3.17 reflect the pattern of root distribution. They assume that water supply and not rooting density limits transpiration from layers 1 and 2, whereas both factors limit transpiration from layer 3, since *Swi₃* has a maximum value of 0.5 when layer 3 is at field capacity and *roots_layer₃* has a value of 0.5 (Fig. 3.4A).

The following two variables, which are used to estimate transpiration, are then calculated from Swi_k:

$$Total\_swi = Swi_1 + Swi_2 + Swi_3 \qquad (3.18)$$

and

$$Profile\_swi = \text{MIN}(1.0, Total\_swi) \qquad (3.19)$$

where *Total_swi* is the sum of the three supply indices, and *Profile_swi* is the soil water supply index for the soil profile. Since maximum value of *Total_swi* may range from 2.0 to 3.0, depending on the value of *roots_layer₃*, Equation 3.19 merely restricts the upper limit of *Profile_swi* to 1.0, a variable that reflects the ability of soil water to meet the demand for transpiration.

Characteristics of the soil surface can greatly influence these relationships. For example, if surface water ponding covers a significant proportion of the soil surface, there is not only more opportunity for infiltration but also more opportunity for evaporative losses, two opposing hydrological processes that affect soil water storage after rainfall or irrigation.

Transpiration
After the above calculations, transpiration, which was an unknown term in Equation 3.1, is given by:

$$Trans = Pot\_trans \times Profile\_swi \qquad \text{mm} \qquad (3.20)$$

Next, transpiration is removed from each soil layer as follows, provided *Total_swi* is greater than zero:

$$\Delta Sw_k = \text{IF}(Total\_swi > 0, Trans \times Sw_k / Total\_swi, 0) \qquad \text{mm} \qquad (3.21)$$

where ΔSw_k is the amount of water lost through transpiration by soil layer *k*.

Soil water supply indices for soil evaporation

Soil evaporation depends on the amount of soil water present (Fig. 3.3) and water supply indices for soil layer 1, and soil layers 1 and 2 combined, represent the ability of these layers to satisfy potential soil evaporation. Thus, only soil layers 1 and 2 contribute to soil evaporation, whereas all three layers contribute to transpiration.

Since soil evaporation might reduce the water content of layer 1 below wilting point, the lower limit for transpiration (Equation 3.15), the supply index for soil evaporation from layer 1, Es_swi_L1, is based on a user-defined air-dried moisture content:

$$Es\_swi\_L1 = 0.285 \left(\frac{Sw_1 - AD_1}{FC_1 - AD_1} \right) / \left(1.0 - 0.715 \left(\frac{Sw_1 - AD_1}{FC_1 - AD_1} \right) \right) \quad (3.22)$$

where Sw_1 is the soil water in layer 1, FC_1 is the field capacity of layer 1 (mm) and AD_1 is the moisture content of air-dried soil from layer 1 (Fig. 3.4B).

A water supply index is also calculated for layers 1 and 2 combined ($Es\_swi\_L1\&2$), but the lower limit for layer 2 is wilting point WP_2 (mm):

$$Es\_swi\_L1\&2 = 0.117 \left(\frac{Sw_1 + Sw_2 - AD_1 - WP_2}{FC_1 + FC_2 - AD_1 - WP_2} \right) /$$

$$\left(1.0 - 0.883 \left(\frac{Sw_1 + Sw_2 - AD_1 - WP_2}{FC_1 + FC_2 - AD_1 - WP_2} \right) \right) \quad (3.23)$$

where FC_k is the field capacity of layer k (mm) (Fig. 3.4B). The coefficients 0.285 and 0.117 were derived for theoretical analysis, supported by field observation of water extraction (Rickert and McKeon, 1982).

The supply index for layer 2 (10–50 cm) is the difference between the index for layers 1 and 2 combined and layer 1:

$$Es\_swi\_L2 = \text{MAX}(0, Es\_swi\_L1\&2 - Es\_swi\_L1) \quad (3.24)$$

When using these supply indices to calculate soil evaporation, as described below, soil layer 1 dries faster than layer 2.

Soil evaporation

If both Es_swi_L1 and $Es\_swi\_L1\&2$ are zero, there will be no soil evaporation and the calculations in this section should be tested to avoid a 'division-by-zero' error. Otherwise the product of the maximum supply index and potential soil evaporation (Pot_esoil, Equation 3.12) is an estimate of soil evaporation for Equation 3.1:

$$Esoil = Pot\_esoil \times \text{MAX}(Es\_swi\_L1\&2, Es\_swi\_L1, 0) \quad (3.25)$$

This water loss is partitioned across soil layers 1 and 2 according to the supply index for each layer:

$$\Delta Sw_k = \text{IF}(Esoil > 0, Esoil \times Es\_swi\_L_k \, / \\ (\text{MAX}(Es\_swi\_L1\&2, Es\_swi\_L1)),0) \tag{3.26}$$

but the lower limit of soil water is restricted to the air-dried water content for layer 1 and wilting point for layer 2.

Pasture submodel

A pasture submodel involves the interfaces between the climate, soil, plant and animal subsystems (Fig. 3.2) which are expressed through the key processes of growth, senescence, detachment and intake, although the latter process is usually a component of the animal submodel. A comprehensive pasture submodel should account for the influence of: (i) climate factors such as solar radiation, temperature, humidity, and frost; (ii) soil factors such as soil water and nutrient supply; (iii) plant factors such as plant population and development, botanical composition of pasture, and competition from trees and shrubs; and (iv) animal factors such as diet selection, intake, trampling and the impact of the grazing on plant growth.

Such a comprehensive and complex model is beyond the scope of this chapter. Rather, a simple submodel is described (Fig. 3.5), which is based on an early version (McKeon et al., 1982) of a more recent and comprehensive pasture submodel (Day et al., 1997). However, pointers for handling the omitted components are briefly mentioned.

The state variables of Fig. 3.5 are determined by the following three equations:

$$Stdm\_green_t = Stdm\_green_{t-1} + Growth_t - Death_t - \\ Intake\_green_t \qquad \text{kg ha}^{-1} \tag{3.27}$$

$$Stdm\_dead_t = Stdm\_dead_{t-1} + Death_t - Intake\_dead_t - \\ Detachment_t \qquad \text{kg ha}^{-1} \tag{3.28}$$

$$Litter\_yld_t = Litter\_yld_{t-1} + Detachment_t - \\ Decomposition_t \qquad \text{kg ha}^{-1} \tag{3.29}$$

where the subscripts refer to days $t-1$ and t, Stdm_green is yield of standing green dry matter, Stdm_dead is yield of standing dead dry matter, and Litter_yld is yield of surface litter. Further, $Growth_t$ is daily pasture growth, $Death_t$ is death of green pasture, $Intake\_green_t$ is intake of green pasture, $Intake\_dead_t$ is intake of dead pasture, $Detachment_t$ is the loss of standing dead dry matter to the soil surface and $Decomposition_t$ is the loss of surface litter through decomposition, all on day t with units of kg ha^{-1} day^{-1}.

In the previous section it was shown that Stdm_green, Stdm_dead and Litter_yld were auxiliary variables in the calculation of runoff, transpiration and soil evaporation. Simple methods for predicting growth, death, detachment and decomposition are described below as an example of a 'getting

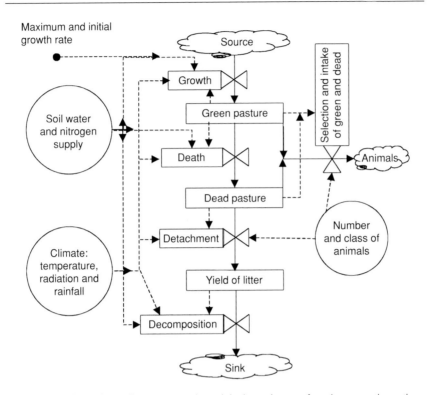

Fig. 3.5. A flow chart of a pasture submodel where the interface between the soil, climate and pasture subsystems is expressed through growth, death, detachment and decomposition, and the interface between the pasture and animal subsystems is expressed through diet selection and intake.

started' model. The default values for various parameters should be changed to reflect local conditions.

Pasture growth
In ideal conditions pastures grow at a potential rate, but in variable climates pasture growth might be constrained by supply of soil water, prevailing temperature, solar radiation or supply of soil nutrients such as nitrogen. These notions are expressed in the following model of pasture growth:

$$Pot\_growth = \mathrm{MAX}(Init\_growth, Max\_growth \times (1 - \mathrm{EXP}$$
$$(Stdm\_green \times \mathrm{Ln}(0.5) / Stdm\_green50)))\quad \mathrm{kg\ ha^{-1}\ day^{-1}}\ (3.30)$$

where potential growth, *Pot_growth*, is a function of *Stdm_green* in good growing conditions (Fig. 3.4D). It ranges between an initial growth rate, *Init_growth* (e.g. 15 kg ha^{-1} day^{-1}) and a maximum growth rate, *Max_growth* (e.g. 60 kg ha^{-1} day^{-1}), which can be measured in the field (Mott *et al.*,

1985). *Stdm_green50* is the green yield (e.g. 1500 kg ha^{-1}) that results in a growth rate that is half *Max_growth*.

Climatic limitations to growth can be expressed through a growth index (range 0 to 1):

$$Growth\_index = \text{MIN}(Profile\_swi, Temp\_index, Rad\_index) \qquad (3.31)$$

where *Profile_swi* is the soil water supply index from Equation 3.19, *Temp_index* is the temperature index for growth, and *Rad_index* is a radiation index for growth.

Temp_index is obtained from a simple step-wise function (Fig. 3.4E), which is solved for mean daily temperature and is shaped by four user-defined parameters: (i) a low temperature that is too cold for growth, *Temp1* (e.g. 14°C); (ii) a temperature at which maximum growth starts, *Temp2* (e.g. 24°C); (iii) a temperature at which maximum growth ends, *Temp3* (e.g. 45°C); and (iv) a high temperature that is too hot for growth, *Temp4* (e.g. 50°C). Values for these parameters have been given by Fitzpatrick and Nix (1970) and other reports of temperature responses for C$_3$ or C$_4$ species. The above suggestions are for C$_4$ grasses. When using a spreadsheet this function can be expressed as a nested 'IF' statement. Daily temperature (*Temp*) is given by:

$$Temp = (Temp\_max + Temp\_min) / 2 \qquad °C \qquad (3.32)$$

where *Temp_max* and *Temp_min* are daily maximum and minimum temperatures.

The radiation index, *Rad_index*, for pasture growth (Fitzpatrick and Nix, 1970) is given by:

$$Rad\_index = 1.0 - \text{EXP}(-1.0 \times Rad / 8.97) \qquad (3.33)$$

where *Rad* is daily solar radiation (Fig. 3.4D). In tropical and subtropical environments *Rad_index* is usually high and if daily measurements of solar radiation are not available, or cannot be estimated, let *Rad_index* equal 0.8 as a first approximation. Alternatively, use a radiation predictor based on longitude/latitude of the site and day of year.

When there are no climatic limitations, the upper limit to seasonal growth of unfertilized pasture is determined by the ability of the soil to supply mineralized nitrogen. This notion is expressed via the following nitrogen index:

$$N\_index = (N\_content - N\_nogrow) / (N\_maxgrow - N\_nogrow) \qquad (3.34)$$

and:

$$N\_content = 100 \times Nuptake / Sum\_growth \qquad \% \qquad (3.35)$$

where *N_maxgrow* is nitrogen content of pasture for maximum growth (e.g. 0.7%), *N_nogrow* is the nitrogen content that would limit growth (e.g. 0.4%), *Nuptake* is estimated actual yield of pasture nitrogen, and

Sum_growth is summation of growth since the start of the growing season. Further, and with reference to Fig. 3.4D:

$$Nuptake = \text{MIN}((Nuptake\_intercept + Nuptake\_slope \times$$
$$Sum\_trans), Nuptake\_max) \qquad \text{kg ha}^{-1} \qquad (3.36)$$

where *Nuptake_intercept* is the amount of nitrogen that is translocated from roots (e.g. 5 kg N ha^{-1}), *Nuptake_slope* (e.g. 0.06 kg N ha^{-1} mm^{-1}) is the nitrogen uptake in response to accumulated transpiration (*Sum_trans*), and *Nuptake_max* is maximum yield of pasture nitrogen, i.e. the product of minimum nitrogen content (*N_nogrow*) and maximum observed yield of standing dry matter. Thus, if *N_nogrow* = 0.4% and the maximum observed yield of standing dry matter is 5000 kg ha^{-1}, *Nuptake_max* is 20 kg N ha^{-1} and is indicative of the mineralization capacity of the soil.

Finally daily pasture growth (*Growth*) is calculated as follows and is added to the green standing dry matter by Equation 3.27:

$$Growth = Pot\_growth \times \text{MIN} (Growth\_index, N\_index) \qquad \text{kg ha}^{-1} \qquad (3.37)$$

where *Pot_growth* is potential growth (Equation 3.30), *Growth_index* (Equation 3.31) reflects the climatic constraints to growth and *N_factor* expresses the adequacy of soil nitrogen for growth (Equation 3.34).

Death

One approach is to consider death rate of green pasture, *Death*, as a continuous, two-stage process that is directly related to the amount of green pasture present and inversely related to the supply of soil water. Hence:

$$Death = Death\_prop \times Stdm\_green \qquad \text{kg ha}^{-1} \qquad (3.38)$$

and *Death_prop* is the proportion of green pasture that dies each day in response to water stress:

$$Death\_prop = \text{MAX}(1.0 - Death\_slope1 \times Profile\_swi,$$
$$Death\_slope2 \times (1.0 - Profile\_swi) + Death\_intercept) \qquad (3.39)$$

where *Death_slope1*, *Death_slope2* and *Death_intercept* are user-defined parameters that shape a linear increase in death rate with water stress. For rangelands in northern Australia *Death_slope1* is 9.86, *Death_slope2* is 0.013, *Death_intercept* is 0.002, and *Death_Prop* ranges from 100% day^{-1} when the soil water supply index is zero to 0.2% when the soil water supply index is unity. However, *Death_slope* and *Death_intercept* are likely to change across sites. In the more comprehensive models by Day *et al.* (1997) and Stuth *et al.* (1998), death rate is also influenced by frost and grazing.

Detachment

Loss of standing dead pasture to the soil surface involves a background rate due to wind and rain, plus trampling losses from grazing animals. A convenient and simple approach is to regard the background rate (*Detach*) as a user-defined proportion (*Detach_prop* = 0.005) of standing dead matter yield (*Dead_stdm*), but this parameter is likely to vary across locations. Then:

$$Detach = Detach\_prop \times Dead\_stdm \qquad \text{kg ha}^{-1} \qquad (3.40)$$

Trampling losses are assumed to be directly related to the amount of pasture eaten and are calculated by reference to potential utilization (*Pot_util*), a user-defined parameter that represents the proportion of total pasture growth that can be eaten. For example, if 50% of growth can be eaten (*Pot_util* = 0.5), the remainder can be lost through trampling, and:

$$Trampled = Intake \times (1.0 \ / \ Pot\_util - 1.0) \qquad \text{kg ha}^{-1} \qquad (3.41)$$

where *Trampled* is detachment of dead pasture due to trampling, and *Intake* is the amount of pasture eaten by animals, which is defined in Equation 3.50. Then, with reference to Equations 3.28 and 3.29:

$$Detachment = Detach + Trampled \qquad \text{kg ha}^{-1} \qquad (3.42)$$

Decomposition

Litter decomposition can be related to prevailing temperatures, water content of the surface soil and to stocking rate. For example:

$$Litter\_prop = Sw\_supply\_ratio_1 \times Tnorm \times Lit\_brkdwn \qquad (3.43)$$

where *Litter_prop* is the proportion of litter yield that decomposes, *Sw_supply_ratio$_1$* is the soil water supply ratio for soil layer 1 (Equation 3.15), *Tnorm* is average daily temperature normalized to 25°C, (($Temp\_max$ + $Temp\_min$) / (2×25)), *Lit_brkdwn* is a user-defined parameter (e.g. 0.04) that represents the proportion of litter decomposition at 25°C with soil layer 1 at field capacity, i.e. hot wet conditions. Thus, with reference to Equation 3.29:

$$Decomposition = Litter\_prop \times Litter\_yld \qquad \text{kg ha}^{-1} \qquad (3.44)$$

where *Litter_yld* is the yield of surface litter at day *t*− 1.

Animal submodel

This submodel deals with the interface between plants and animals (Fig. 3.2). When the submodel is confined to cattle growth, rather than reproduction, development and growth, the submodel needs to predict liveweight gain (*Lwg$_t$*, kg per head on day *t*) to satisfy the following basic equation:

$$Liveweight_t = Liveweight_{t-1} + Lwg_t \qquad \text{kg per head} \qquad (3.45)$$

where *Liveweight$_t$* and *Liveweight$_{t-1}$* are cattle liveweights at day *t* and day *t*−1, respectively.

Since liveweight gain is dependent on the intake of digestible nutrients, and cattle actively choose a diet from the pasture on offer, the challenge for the model builder is to predict the amount, botanical composition and quality of the diet (Dove, 1996). This difficult task is attempted in the GRAZFEED and GRAZE models (Table 3.2), which are suitable for relatively uniform pastures, but at this stage of development are not suited for the more complex issue of diet selection in extensive rangelands (Ash et al., 1995; Hall et al., 2000). A more comprehensive algorithm for diet selection – POPMIX, developed by Quirk and Stuth (1995) – places plant species into broad preference categories (Preferred, Desirable, Undesirable, Toxic, Emergency and Non-Consumed) and then computes the proportion of each preference class in the diet. The algorithm assumes that an animal has experience with the vegetation, has learned to avoid toxic species and is non-cognitive of non-consumed species. The 'Emergency' category accounts for species that are only eaten after the preferred, desirable and undesirable species are depleted. The PHYGROW model uses this algorithm and allows a user to categorize a species preference by an animal species according to phenological stage: fast growth, declining growth, quiescence, dormancy, dead and litter (Stuth et al., 1998).

To avoid these problems the following model sets an upper limit to liveweight gain (Pot_lwg), which is reduced by a restriction on intake imposed through to the degree of pasture utilization – the ratio of pasture eaten to pasture growth. Diet selection and intake are estimated to satisfy Equations 3.27 and 3.28. All calculations are based on a standard animal called a weaner equivalent, which is a steer of 200 kg liveweight, and performance of the standard animal needs to be related to performance in other animal classes. The following equations are in a sequence for calculating liveweight gain.

Intake and utilization

Two restrictions to intake operate; the first limits intake in response to the degree of pasture utilization, and the second limits intake when pasture yields are very low:

$$Intake\_restr1 = \text{MAX}(1.0, Intake\_util\_intercept + Intake\_util\_slope \times Utilization) \tag{3.46}$$

where Intake_restr1 is a restriction on intake due to a decline in quality of diet as utilization increases (Fig. 3.4F), Intake_util_intercept is a user-defined intercept of the utilization function, Intake_util_slope is a user-defined parameter that reduces intake in response to increasing utilization and Utilization is the proportion of growth eaten since the start of the growing season (Equation 3.53). A default value for Intake_util_intercept is 1.05 (1.2 for oats), but the value of Intake_util_slope varies across pasture types, being −0.66 for oats, −0.46 for small paddocks of tussock grassland and −0.3 for extensive tropical rangelands (Rickert and McKeon, 1984; Day et al., 1997). The second restriction is given by:

$$Intake\_restr2 = Stdm\_total / yield\_restr \tag{3.47}$$

where Stdm_total is total yield of standing pasture (Stdm_green + Stdm_tdead) and yield_restr the minimum yield of standing pasture that does not restrict intake (e.g. 230 kg ha^{-1} for cattle), a parameter that is likely to vary across pasture types and animal species.

The restriction index, which is used to calculate intake, is given by:

$$Intake\_restr = MIN(Intake\_restr1, Intake\_restr2) \tag{3.48}$$

Intake per animal (Animal_intake) is derived from the restriction index and potential liveweight gain:

$$Animal\_intake = Intake\_restr \times (Pot\_lwg /$$
$$Days\_season + 1.058) / 0.304 \qquad \text{kg per head} \tag{3.49}$$

where Pot_lwg is the user-defined liveweight gain in a good season for a standard animal grazing a specified pasture at a low stocking rate (e.g. 30, 80, 25 and 10 kg per head for spring, summer, autumn and winter, respectively) and Days_season is the number of days in a season (e.g. 91.25 days for each season). Thus, an astute manager can estimate potential liveweight gain for each season, a parameter that reflects the inherent seasonal variation in quality of a pasture for a given breed of cattle. The coefficients in Equations 3.46 and 3.49 were derived from an analysis of liveweight gain in relation to intake of native pasture in Queensland (Rickert and McKeon, 1984).

The total consumption of pasture by the herd (Intake) of cattle is give by:

$$Intake = Animal\_intake \times Stock\_equival \qquad \text{kg ha}^{-1} \tag{3.50}$$

where Stock_equival is the stocking rate in terms of standard animals per hectare. If the standard animal is a weaner steer of 200 kg liveweight, then:

$$Stock\_equival = Stocking\_rate \times$$
$$(Liveweight / 200)^{0.75} \quad \text{weaner equivalents ha}^{-1} \tag{3.51}$$

where Stocking_rate and Liveweight are the actual stocking rate (head ha^{-1}) and liveweight (kg per head) for animals on the pasture. Further, the summation of intake (Eaten) is used to calculate Utilization, the proportion of growth eaten by cattle during an annual growing cycle for pasture. Thus:

$$Eaten = \Sigma \, Intake \qquad \text{kg ha}^{-1} \tag{3.52}$$

and:

$$Utilization = Eaten / \Sigma \, Growth \tag{3.53}$$

where the annual summations commence from the start of the growing cycle (e.g. 1 September in the subtropics of the southern hemisphere).

Liveweight gain
The result from Equation 3.49 is then used to estimate liveweight gain:

$$Lwg = 0.304 \times Animal\_intake - 1.058 \qquad \text{kg per head day}^{-1} \qquad (3.54)$$

Diet selection
An estimate of diet selection is required to partition intake across the green and dead pasture. The proportion of green pasture in the diet (*Green_diet*) is given by:

$$Green\_diet = 19.0 \times Prop\_green / (Prop\_green \times (19.0-1.0) + 1.0) \qquad (3.55)$$

where *Prop_green* is the ratio of green pasture in the standing pasture (Fig. 3.4F). The coefficients in Equation 3.55 were obtained from diet selection studies by Hendricksen *et al.* (1982) but the relation is likely to change across pasture or animal types.

Having obtained the proportion of green in the diet (Equation 3.55), and with reference to Equations 3.27 and 3.28:

$$Intake\_green = Green\_diet \times Intake \qquad \text{kg ha}^{-1}\,\text{day}^{-1} \qquad (3.56)$$

and:

$$Intake\_dead = (1.0 - Green\_diet) \times Intake \qquad \text{kg ha}^{-1}\,\text{day}^{-1} \qquad (3.57)$$

where *Intake_green* and *Intake_dead* are the amounts of green and dead pasture consumed.

Economic submodel

Gross margin indicates the operating profit of a management option, and is given by:

$$Gross\_margin = Number\_sold \times$$
$$(Animal\_value - Variable\_costs) / Area \qquad \$\,\text{ha}^{-1} \qquad (3.58)$$

where *Number_sold* is the number of animals sold, *Animal_value* is the value of each animal sold, *Variable_costs* is the sum of variable or operating costs per animal associated with a management option, and *Area* is the land area for a management option. Comparison of the gross margins for different management options indicates the relative profit of the options.

Obviously, information on local costs and prices is needed for Equation 3.58, and a model should allow a user to enter, store and recall this information. Local information on variable costs is usually readily available but regular updates are needed to reflect seasonal variations in costs.

Likewise, *Animal_value* needs to be updated regularly to reflect seasonal variations as well as price premiums for markets that are characterized by specific attributes. With regard to beef cattle, *Animal_value* may vary across markets that are specified by liveweight, age, sex and breed. It is therefore convenient to maintain tables of local market specifications and for seasonal variation in prices for each market. The economic submodel can then match the herd characteristics to the tables of market specifications and prices to nominate *Animal_value*.

Future Developments

Modelling pasture and animals has come a long way in three decades. It is a widely used tool that provides direction and context to research programmes. Its future as an aid to research is assured.

In general terms farmers have been slow to adopt models of pasture and animal production as aids to farm management, because the technology seems inappropriate (Cox, 1996). Also computer ownership among farmers is often relatively low, and when one is owned mastering a DSS package tends to have a lower priority than mastering packages pertaining to financial and office management. Perhaps the underlying cause is the lack of convincing evidence that management decisions based on DSS are better and/or easier to make than decisions made in the conventional manner based on years of local experience. One approach to increasing farmer use of DSS is to have an experienced user demonstrate benefits through the analyses of management options (Buxton and Stafford Smith, 1996), thereby recognizing that DSS consists of three necessary components: hardware, software and 'liveware'. Another approach is to encourage professional advisors who service many farmer clients to use DSS, rather than individual farmers. Farm advisors need to supply good advice and are receptive to new tools that give a professional edge by providing rapid analysis of complex systems across many environments. Together these notions imply that the effectiveness of DSS should be gauged in terms of its contribution to improved management of a grazing system rather than number of sales to individual farmers.

Other limitations to use of pre-packaged DSS are the lack of spatially explicit biophysical data and understanding of relevant growth characteristics of major plant and animal species. There is a worldwide need for scientists and government agencies to organize authoring systems of critical data for the future development of DSS and integrated policy models.

The scope and range of policy models are expanding rapidly because they provide policy makers with an objective assessment of complex problems. This trend will continue, but the biophysical base to many policy models is likely to be complemented by socioeconomic outputs as governments attempt to gauge the condition and trend of ecosystems as well as the financial sustainability of rural communities (Donaldson *et al.*, 1995; Pandy and Hardaker, 1995). Indeed, future developments will better integrate hard systems technologies, such as models of pasture and animal production, with soft systems technologies to give a more holistic and realistic evaluation of management options (Stafford Smith *et al.*, 1993; Stuth *et al.*, 1993; Dent *et al.*, 1995; Park and Seaton, 1996).

Eventually, a global network of critical information and software applications via the World Wide Web will give decision makers access to a much wider range of DSS to address complex resource and policy issues. Future model developers will soon find global libraries of algorithms, interface tools and integrating computer environments which will encourage more rapid development of new models and a rich set of shared applications and experiences.

References

Ash, A.J., McIvor, J.G., Corfield, J.P. and Winter, W.H. (1995) How land condition alters plant–animal relationships in Australia's tropical rangelands. *Agriculture, Ecosystems and Environment* 56, 77–92.

Black, J.L., Davies, G.T. and Fleming, J.F. (1993) Role of computer simulation in the application of knowledge to animal industries. *Australian Journal of Agricultural Research* 44, 541–555.

Bouman, B.A.M., Keulen, H. van, Laar, H.H. van and Rabbinge, R. (1996) The 'School of de Wit' crop growth simulation models: a pedigree and historical overview. *Agricultural Systems* 52, 171–198.

Bowman, P.J., Wysel, D.A., Fowler, D.G. and White, D.H. (1989) Evaluation of a new technology when applied to sheep production systems: Part I – model description. *Agricultural Systems* 29, 35–47.

Brook, K.D. and Carter, J.O. (1994) Integrating satellite data and pasture growth models to produce feed deficit and land condition alerts. *Agricultural Systems and Information Technology* 6, 54–56.

Buxton, R. and Stafford Smith, M.S. (1996) Managing drought in Australia's rangelands: four weddings and a funeral. *Rangeland Journal* 18, 292–308.

Clarkson, N.M., Clewett, J.F., Owens, D.T. and Abrecht, D.G. (1997) Will it rain? Managing El Niño risks with the Australian Rainman computer package. *XVIII International Grassland Congress, Proceedings* 2, 24.43–24.44.

Cobon, D.H. and Clewett, J.F. (1999) *DroughtPlan CD: A compilation of software packages, workshops, case studies and reports to assist management of climate variability in pastoral areas of northern Australia.* QI99002, Queensland Department of Primary Industries, Brisbane.

Conway, G.R. (1985) Agricultural ecology and farming systems research. In: Remenyi, J.V. (ed.) *Agricultural Systems Research for Developing Countries.* ACIAR Proceedings No. 11, 43–59, Australian Centre for International Agricultural Research, Canberra.

Conway, G.R. (1994) Sustainability in agricultural development: trade-offs between productivity, stability, and equitability. *Journal for Farming Systems Research Extension* 4, 1–14.

Cox, P.G. (1996) Some issues in the design of agricultural decision support systems. *Agricultural Systems* 52, 355–381.

Day, K.A., McKeon, G.M. and Carter, J.O. (1997) *Evaluating the Risk of Pasture Degradation in Native Pastures in Queensland: Final Report for the Rural Industries Research and Development Corporation.* Department of Natural Resources, Brisbane.

Dent, J.B. and Anderson, J.R. (1971) *Systems Analysis in Agricultural Management.* John Wiley & Sons, Sydney.

Dent, J.B., Blackie, M.J. and Harrison, S.R. (1979) *Systems Simulation in Agriculture.* Applied Science Publishers, London.

Dent, J.B., Edwards Jones, G. and McGregor, M.J. (1995) Simulation of ecological, social and economic factors in agricultural systems. *Agricultural Systems* 49, 337–351.

Donaldson, A.B., Flichman, G. and Webster, J.P.G. (1995) Integrating agronomic and economic models for policy analysis at the farm level: the impact of CAP reform in two European regions. *Agricultural Systems* 48, 163–178.

Dove, H. (1996) Constraints to the modelling of diet selection and intake in the grazing ruminant. *Australian Journal of Agricultural Research* 47, 257–275.

Dyne, G.M. van (1970) A systems approach to grasslands. *Proceedings of the XI International Grassland Congress, Surfers Paradise, Australia,* A131–A143.

Ebersohn, J.P. (1976) A commentary on systems studies in agriculture. *Agricultural Systems* 1, 173–184.

Eckert, J.B., Baker, B.B. and Hanson, J.D. (1995) The impact of global warming on local incomes from range livestock systems. *Agricultural Systems* 48, 87–100.

Fisher, D.S. and Baumont, R. (1994) Modeling the rate and quantity of forage intake by ruminants during meals. *Agricultural Systems* 45, 43–53.

Fitzpatrick, E.A. and Nix, H.A. (1970) The climatic factor in Australian grassland ecology. In: Moore, R.M. (ed.) *Australian Grasslands.* ANU Press, Canberra, pp. 1–26.

France, J. and Thornley, J.H.M. (1984) *Mathematical Models in Agriculture.* Butterworths & Co., London.

Freer, M., Moore, A.D. and Donnelly, J.R. (1997) GRAZPLAN: decision support systems for Australian grazing enterprises – II. The animal biology model for feed intake, production and reproduction and the GrazFeed DSS. *Agricultural Systems* 54, 77–126.

Gillard, P. (1993) An expert system to advise Tasmanian farmers on pasture mixtures and fodder crops. *Proceedings of the XVII International Grassland Congress,* pp. 763–764.

Gustavsson, A.M., Angus, J.F. and Torssell, B.W.R. (1995) An integrated model for growth and nutritional value of timothy. *Agricultural Systems* 47, 73–92.

Hall, W.B., McKeon, G.M., Carter, J.O., Day, K.A., Howden, S.M., Scanlan, J.C., Johnston, P.W. and Burrows, W.H. (1998) Climate change in Queensland's grazing lands: II. An assessment of the impact on animal production from native pastures. *Rangeland Journal* 20, 177–205.

Hall, W.B., Rickert, K.G., McKeon, G.M. and Carter, J.O. (2000) Simulation studies of nitrogen concentration in the diet of sheep grazing mitchell and mulga grasslands. *Australian Journal of Agricultural Research* 51, 163–172.

Hall, W.H. (1997) Near-real time financial assessment of the Queensland wool industry on a regional basis. PhD Thesis, University of Queensland, Australia, 465 pp.

Harrison, S.R. (1990) Regression of a model of real-system output: an invalid test of model validity. *Agricultural Systems* 34, 183–190.

Hendricksen, R.E., Rickert, K.G., Ash, A.J. and McKeon, G.M. (1982) Beef production model. *Proceedings of the Australian Society of Animal Production* 14, 204–208.

Herrero, M., Dent, J.B. and Fawcett, R.H. (1998) The plant/animal interface in models of grazing systems. In Peart, R.M. and Curry, R.B. (eds) *Agricultural Systems: Modelling and Simulation*. Marcel Dekker Inc., New York, pp. 495–542.

Holmes, W.E. (1988) *Instructions for BREEDCOW and DYNAMA herd budgeting spreadsheets models: Versions 01–12–88*. Queensland Department of Primary Industries, Brisbane.

Howden, S.M., White, D.H., McKeon, G.M., Scanlan, J.C. and Carter, J.O. (1994) Methods for exploring management options to reduce greenhouse gas emissions from tropical grazing systems. *Climatic Change* 27, 49–70.

Hulme, D.J., Kellaway, R.C., Booth, P.J. and Bennett, L. (1986) The CAMDAIRY model for formulating and analysing dairy cow rations. *Agricultural Systems* 22, 81–108.

James, A.D., Carles, A.B., James, A.D. and Carles, A.B. (1996) Measuring the productivity of grazing and foraging livestock. *Agricultural Systems* 52, 271–291.

Jiggins, J. and Baker, M.J. (1993) From technology transfer to resource management. In: Baker, M.J. (ed.) *Grasslands for Our World*. SIR Publishing, Wellington, NZ, pp. 184–192.

Jones, R.J. and Sandland, R.L. (1974) The relation between animal gain and stocking rate. Derivation of the relation from the results of grazing trials. *Journal of Agricultural Science*, 83, 335–342.

Keulen, H. van and Wolf, J. (eds) (1986) *Modelling of Agricultural Production: Weather, Soils and Crops*. Pudoc, Wageningen, The Netherlands.

Kreuter, U.P., Rowan, R.C., Conner, J.R., Stuth, J.W. and Hamilton, W.T. (1996) Decision support software for estimating the economic efficiency of grazing land production. *Journal of Range Management* 49, 464–469.

Landsberg, R.G., Ash, A.J., Shepherd, R.K. and McKeon, G.M. (1998) Learning from history to survive in the future: management evolution on Trafalgar Station, North-East Queensland. *Rangeland Journal* 20, 104–118.

Lemberg, B., Stuth, J.W., Mjelde, J.W. and Conner, J.R. (1998) Applications of the PHYGROW model to assess hydrologic impacts of brush control in the Frio River basin. In: Potts, D.F. (ed.) *Rangeland Management and Water Resources*. American Water Resources Association, Herndon, Virginia (in press).

Littleboy, M., Cogle, A.L., Smith, G.D., Yule, D.F. and Rao, K.P.C. (1996) Soil management and production of Alfisols in the semi-arid tropics. I. Modelling the effects of soil management on runoff and erosion. *Australian Journal of Soil Research* 34, 91–102.

Loewer, O.J. (1989) Issues on modeling grazing systems. *Crop Science Society of America, Special Publication No. 16*, 127–136.

Loewer, O.J. Jr (1998) GRAZE: a beef-forage model of selective grazing. In: Peart, R.M. and Curry, R.B. (eds) *Agricultural Systems: Modelling and Simulation*. Marcel Dekker Inc., New York, pp. 301–417.

McCown, R.L., Hammer, G.L., Hargreaves, J.N.G., Holzworth, D.P. and Freebairn, D.M. (1996) APSIM: a novel software system for model development, model testing and simulation in agricultural systems research. *Agricultural Systems* 50, 255–271.

McIvor, J.G. and Moneypenny, R. (1995) Evaluation of pasture management systems for beef production in the semi-arid tropics: model development. *Agricultural Systems* 49, 45–67.

McKeon, G.M., Rickert, K.G., Ash, A.J., Cooksley, D.G. and Scattini, W.J. (1982) Pasture production model. *Proceedings of the Australian Society of Animal Production* 14, 201–204.

McKeon, G.M., Day, K.A., Howden, S.M., Mott, J.J., Orr, D.M., Scattini, W.J. and Weston, E.J. (1990) Northern Australian savannas: management for pastoral production. *Journal of Biogeography* 17, 355–372.

McKeon, G.M., Hall, W.B., Crimp, S.J., Howden, S.M., Stone, R.C. and Jones, D.A. (1998) Climate change in Queensland's grazing lands. I. Approaches and climatic trends. *Rangeland Journal* 20, 151–176.

Mitchell, P.L. (1997) Misuse of regression for empirical validation of models. *Agricultural Systems* 54, 313–326.

Morley, F.H.W. (1981) Options in pasture research. *Tropical Grasslands* 15, 71–81.

Morrison, D.A., Kingwell, R.S. and Pannell, D.J. (1986) A mathematical programming model of a crop–livestock farm system. *Agricultural Systems* 20, 243–268.

Mott, J.J., Williams, J., Andrew, M.H. and Gillison, A.N. (1985) Australian savanna ecosystems. In: Tothill, J.C. and Mott, J.J. (eds) *Ecology and Management of the World's Savannas*. The Australian Academy of Science, Canberra, pp. 56–82.

Muchow, R.C. and Bellamy, J.A. (1991) (eds) *Climate Risk in Crop Production: Models and Management for the Semiarid Tropics and Subtropics*. CAB International, Wallingford, UK.

Pandey, S. and Hardaker, J.B. (1995) The role of modelling in the quest for sustainable farming systems. *Agricultural Systems* 47, 439–450.

Park, J. and Seaton, R.A.F. (1996) Integrative research and sustainable agriculture. *Agricultural Systems* 50, 81–100.

Parton, W.J. and Ojima, D.S. (1994) Environmental change in grasslands: assessment using models. *Climatic Change* 28, 111–141.

Passioura, J.B. (1996) Simulation models: science, snake oil, education, or engineering? *Agronomy Journal* 88, 690–694.

Peart, R.M. and Curry, R.B. (1998) (eds) *Agricultural Systems Modeling and Simulation*. Marcel Dekker Inc., New York, 696 pp.

Poppi, D.P. (1996) Predictions of food intake in ruminants from analyses of food composition. *Australian Journal of Agricultural Research* 47, 489–504.

Quirk, M.F. and Stuth, J.W. (1995) Preference-based algorithms for predicting herbivore diet composition. *Acta Zootechnica* 44 (suppl.), 110.

Rickert, K.G. (1996) Stocking rate and sustainable grazing systems. In: Elgersma, A., Struik, P.C. and Maesen, L.J.G. van der (eds) *Grassland Science in Perspective*. Wageningen University Papers 96–4, Wageningen Agricultural University, The Netherlands, pp. 29–66.

Rickert, K.G. (1998) Experiences with FEEDMAN, a decision support package for beef cattle producers in south eastern Queensland. *Acta Horticulterae* 476, 227–234.

Rickert, K.G. and McKeon, G.M. (1982) Soil water balance model: WATSUP. *Proceedings of the Australian Society of Animal Production* 14, 198–200.

Rickert, K.G. and McKeon, G.M. (1984) A computer model of the integration of forage options for beef production. *Proceedings of the Australian Society of Animal Production* 15, 15–19.

Rickert, K.G. and McKeon, G.M. (1985) Models for native pasture management and development in south east Queensland. In: Tothill, J.C. and Mott, J.C. (eds) *Ecology and Management of the World's Savannas*, Australian Academy of Science, Canberra , Australia, pp. 299–302.

Rickert, K.G. and McKeon, G.M. (1988) Computer models of forage management on beef cattle farms. *Mathematics and Computers in Simulation* 30, 189–194.

Rickert, K.G. and McKeon, G.M. (1991) Modelling as an aid to systems evaluation. In: Squires, V. and Tow, P. (eds) *Dryland Farming: A Systems Approach*. Sydney University Press, Sydney, pp. 208–221.

Rickert, K.G. and Sinclair, S.E. (2000) FEEDMAN – *A feed-to-dollars beef and deer management package, Version 3.0.* Technical Manual QZ0004. Queensland Department of Primary Industries, Brisbane, 30 pp.

Scanlan, J.C., McKeon, G.M., Day, K.A., Mott, J.J. and Hinton, A.W. (1994) Estimating safe carrying capacities of extensive cattle-grazing properties within tropical, semi-arid woodlands of north-eastern Australia. *Rangeland Journal* 16, 64–76.

Scanlan, J.C., Pressland, A.J. and Myles, D.J. (1996) Run-off and soil movement on mid-slopes in north-east Queensland grazed woodlands. *Rangeland Journal* 18, 33–46.

Seligman, N.G. and Baker, M.J. (1993) Modelling as a tool for grassland science progress. In: Baker, M.J. (ed.) *Grasslands for Our World*. SIR Publishing, Wellington, New Zealand, pp. 228–233.

Sorensen, J.T. (1998) Modeling and simulation in applied livestock production science. In: Peart, R.M. and Curry, R.B. (eds) *Agricultural Systems: Modelling and Simulation*. Marcel Dekker Inc., New York, pp. 475–494.

Spedding, C.W.R. (1970) The relative complexity of grassland systems. *Proceedings of the XI International Grassland Congress, Surfers Paradise, Australia.* A126-A131.

Stafford Smith, D.M. and Foran, B.D. (1988) Strategic decisions in pastoral management. *Rangeland Journal* 10, 82–95.

Stafford Smith, D.M., Foran, B.D. and Baker, M.J. (1993) Problems and opportunities for commercial animal production in the arid and semi-arid rangelands. In: Baker, M.J. (ed.) *Grasslands for Our World*. SIR Publishing, Wellington, New Zealand, pp. 30–37.

Stuth, J.W., Hamilton, W.T., Conner, J.C., Sheehy, D.P. and Baker, M.J. (1993) Decision support systems in the transfer of grassland technology. In: Baker, M.J. (ed.) *Grasslands for Our World*. SIR Publishing, Wellington, New Zealand, pp. 234–242.

Stuth, J.W., Hamilton, W.T. and Conner, J.C. (1998) *PHYGROW Hydrologic Based Forage Production Model, Version 2. Users Guide*. Ranching Systems Group, Dept. Rangeland Ecology and Management, Texas A&M University, College Station, 120 pp.

Stuth, J.W., Freer, M., Dove, H. and Lyons, R.K. (1999) Nutritional management for free-ranging livestock. In: Jung, H.G. and Fahey, G.C. (eds) *Nutritional Ecology of Herbivores. Proceedings of the Fifth International Symposium on the Nutrition of Herbivores.* American Society of Animal Science, Savoy, Illinois.

Weston, R.H. (1996) Some aspects of constraint to forage consumption by ruminants. *Australian Journal of Agricultural Research* 47, 175–197.

White, D.H., Bowman, P.J., Morley, F.H.W., McManus, W.R. and Filan, S.J. (1983) A simulation model of a breeding ewe flock. *Agricultural Systems* 10, 149–189.

Williams, J.R., Dyke, P.T. and Jones, C.A. (1984) A modeling approach to determine the relationship between erosion and soil productivity. *Trans. ASAE* 27, 129–144.

Measuring Botanical Composition of Grasslands

R.D.B. Whalley[1] and M.B. Hardy[2]

[1]Botany Department, University of New England, Armidale, New South Wales, Australia; [2]Crop Development, Department of Agriculture, Western Cape, Elsenburg, South Africa

Introduction

The botanical composition of grassland vegetation is a reflection of many factors, including past management. Changes in these factors will be reflected in changes in composition. There are many attributes of botanical composition that can be described or measured and the objective of the description or measurement dictates the methodology. Monitoring changes over time by repeated sampling is a commonly used approach to detect environmental or management effects.

Vegetation description or measurement can be very labour intensive and time consuming. The resources invested depend on the purposes of the measurements and, essentially, the information collected is usually proportional to the resources invested but there is wide variation in the cost effectiveness of the different methods available. Scale is also important and different methods must obviously be used for vegetation measurement on a global scale compared with a small replicated experiment.

This chapter provides an overview of the methodologies available for the measurement of the botanical composition of grassland vegetation appropriate to a range of different objectives.

Scales of Measurement

Different scales of measurement of grassland vegetation require different levels of detail. Satellite technology has made it possible to distinguish grasslands from other forms of vegetation and to measure certain attributes at the global scale but there is still a gulf between the detail possible with remote sensing and that possible on the ground. There are two separate approaches when moving between scales. The first is where very detailed data are collected and then aggregated to give a big picture. The second is to collect data on a broad scale and then focus in on the detail required for a particular purpose.

Aggregation of detailed data using geographic information system (GIS) technology (Burrough, 1986) is now well developed and there are no fundamental technical problems in moving from very detailed data collected in small plots to a global scale, provided sufficient data, collected in a comparable way, are available. However, the technology to move in the other direction in order to see the fine detail in a small area, using data collected at the global scale, is still a long way away.

Global scale

Satellites can provide data over the whole of the globe within a 24 h period. Using appropriate reflectance bands (see Chapter 9) grasslands can be distinguished from other vegetation types and the rate of growth at low vegetation densities, ground cover and broad groups of species can be distinguished. Detailed botanical composition cannot at present be determined from satellite imagery but, for example, sown pastures can be distinguished from native pastures on the Northern Tablelands of New South Wales, Australia (Vickery *et al.*, 1997). Because the method of data collection is uniform over the whole world, direct comparisons can be made among different grasslands across international boundaries and over time or of the effects of different management or different seasonal conditions.

GIS technology involves digitizing a map of a region and then using computer technology to overlay detailed geographical data, which can include species composition. Detailed botanical composition data can then be aggregated to produce broader-scale maps, provided the requisite base maps and the detailed botanical composition data are available. In practice, however, there are several constraints to the use of GIS technology for this purpose. Until compatible digitized base maps are available for the whole world it is not possible to aggregate local data on a world-scale GIS database. Botanical composition of grasslands across regions must be collected in the same way for the results to be comparable across national and international boundaries. Uniform data compatible with GIS databases are simply not yet available for many of the world's grasslands and so valid aggregation to give a global picture is not yet possible.

National and regional scale

Many national and regional maps of vegetation, including grasslands, such as Beadle (1981) for Australia and Acocks (1975) for parts of southern Africa, are available. Such maps were mostly produced by ground surveys, usually by road, with periodic stops to list floristics. The surveyors used a broad vegetation classification system and simply marked the boundaries of different communities on a base map. Species lists were usually provided for the different communities with some estimates of the relative abundance of the different species. These maps have often been built up over many years, with subsequent authors correcting and improving previously published maps. One problem is that the mapping units sometimes change, and problems of nomenclature arise with taxonomic changes. This subjective classification of vegetation, with somewhat randomly collected species lists at regular or irregular intervals across the landscape, has now largely been superseded by more objective methods of site selection, quantitative data collection and data analyses. These objective methods will be dealt with in more detail later. However, there may still be some parts of the world where the subjective approach represents the only available description of national and regional grasslands.

The more detailed the data collection, the more intensively the vegetation can be sampled for species composition and classification of grasslands. In many countries black-and-white or colour aerial photographs are commercially available, either as mosaics or as overlapping individual frames that can be viewed with a stereoscope to obtain a three-dimensional perspective. The aerial photographs can then be used to select sites or transects for the ground collection of descriptive or quantitative botanical composition data, depending on the purpose of the measurements. The aerial photographs and accompanying ground-survey botanical composition data can be digitized and incorporated into a database using GIS software.

Farm scale

The simplest approach to obtaining botanical information of grasslands on a farm scale is to walk over the farm and record the species encountered with notes on their relative abundance. Depending on the size of the farm, it may be possible to record species over the whole area. For larger areas, the examination of sample sites is essential, with subsequent classification and aggregation of the data into some form of map. These maps can be valuable for planning farm operations. Searches for threatened grassland species and the identification of grassland communities with high conservation value are becoming increasingly important on farms. These species and communities are best located by either systematic or random walks, with the operator using prior knowledge of where such species and communities are most likely to occur in the landscape.

Extension services and farmers often use aerial photo mosaics as a basis for farm planning. Increasingly, with the ready availability of personal computers, a farm map can be digitized and many kinds of data, from botanical composition and pasture condition to livestock movements, included in farm GIS software. Extension services in many places provide user-friendly software so that farmers can modify and update their own GIS data for farm planning and farm record purposes.

Satellite imagery at the farm scale can be incorporated into such GIS databases. However, satellite data are expensive and special skills and equipment are necessary for their interpretation and incorporation into GIS databases.

Paddock scale

Most of the methods used to estimate botanical composition are designed for the paddock scale. This also represents the limit of the usefulness of satellite imagery, depending on the size of the paddock. Individual pixels can be located on the ground and the botanical composition related to reflectance data on specific wave bands, which can then be extrapolated to other parts of the paddock or further afield. Paddocks are often the experimental units in grassland management research where detailed botanical composition data are essential.

Many farmers are well aware of the dominant species in the different paddocks on their farms. Increasingly, there is a need for farmers to have additional information about the presence of other species, such as weeds or grassland plants of high conservation value, that may have an impact on paddock management.

Patch scale

Grasslands are almost always patchy except for newly sown pastures where the individual plants may be regularly spaced because of the method of sowing. Patches can vary in size from a few centimetres to more than 100 m across, and the smaller patches are too fine for detection by satellite imagery, though aerial photography can be very useful.

Patches can result from dung and urine voidance, in which case they may be temporary, whereas selective grazing by wild or domestic animals can produce long-term patches. The development of these patches is sometimes an early sign of weed invasion or impending land degradation and so their recognition and study become very important (Wandera et al., 1993; Lütge et al., 1998). Permanent patches can result from differences in soils or microtopography and position in the landscape. The interactions among topography, water movement, soil water availability and grazing animals affect the functioning of ecosystems and consequently the botanical composition in different parts of the landscape (Jenny, 1961; Tongway and Ludwig, 1997). Patches of high soil fertility can result from the grazing and defecation behaviour of domestic animals (e.g. Taylor *et al.*, 1984). These patches are long lived and have a different species composition than patches with lower fertility.

Measurement of botanical composition at the patch scale is becoming increasingly important in grassland management studies (e.g. Lütge *et al.*, 1998). The study of patches may include plant density or frequency measurements and patch dynamics within paddocks. It may involve the study of the population biology of individual grassland species or functional groups of species (Friedel *et al.*, 1988).

Sampling

Some form of sampling is always involved in measuring the botanical composition of grasslands. The number, size and location of sampling units and the timing of the sampling are critical. In small plot experiments, the whole population can sometimes be measured. The errors inherent in sampling vary enormously, depending not only on the spatial and temporal variation of the grassland attributes being measured but also on observer bias, and within and between the various sampling techniques. It is desirable to consult a statistician during the planning stages of any project involving grassland sampling to ensure that the sampling strategy is appropriate for the purpose and is statistically sound.

Sampling strategies

Suitable strategies depend on the characteristics of the grassland and the purposes of the measurements. The subsequent statistical analysis of the data is also governed by how samples are located in space and time.

The distribution of individuals of the species present in the grassland can affect the sampling strategy and the subsequent statistical analysis of the results. Non-random distributions are common and may confound parametric methods of statistical analysis. In contrast, the dry-weight-rank (DWR) method of botanical analysis of grasslands (Mannetje and Haydock, 1963) may not be appropriate on grasslands with random distributions (Neuteboom *et al.*, 1998). It may therefore be desirable to determine the type of distribution that occurs before deciding on sampling strategy, sample size and the statistical analysis of the results. Some species tend to be clustered while others tend to be regularly dispersed.

The distribution of species is likely to change with time, newly sown pastures having a more regular distribution of species than older pastures. It is also likely that the distribution of some species will vary over time and space with management and rainfall patterns. The nature and magnitude of non-random distributions also depends upon the scale at which the distribution is sampled.

Whether or not the distribution of an individual species in the community is random can be readily determined by observing a number of sample areas (quadrats) (see Kershaw, 1964, for details). Quadrat size should be chosen so that about three-quarters of the quadrats will contain no individuals of the species being measured. These quadrats are randomly located within the sample area and the number of quadrats containing 0, 1, 2 or 3 etc. individuals of the species are counted. The mean density is then calculated. The number of quadrats containing 0, 1, 2 or 3 etc. individuals will follow a Poisson distribution if the individuals are randomly distributed and can be tested using chi squared for the goodness of fit. If it does follow a Poisson distribution, then the mean : variance ratio should not deviate significantly from 1.

Random sample location

Random sample location is appropriate where random spatial variation occurs in the grassland vegetation and the aim is to 'average out' this variation across the whole of the sample area. Random sample location is suitable for experiments where different treatments have been applied to different parts of an area of grassland in some form of replicated experiment. Choosing sample locations seemingly at random by the operator requires caution to avoid unconscious bias in their choice. Predetermined procedures should be used: for example, the tip of the left or right boot after a predetermined number of steps or, when an obstacle is encountered, a certain number of steps sideways to the left or to the right. One disadvantage of this method is that the operator unconsciously tends to avoid areas of prickly and sharp vegetation. Grid coordinates for sampling points chosen according to a list of predetermined random numbers can be located by pacing or by the use of a tape or a knotted rope, though their use may be too time consuming. Fence posts can be used in lieu of grid references in small paddocks.

Throwing a quadrat for locating sampling sites, or some other object such as a dart with a streamer attached, is not recommended because of unconscious aiming. Furthermore, taller or stemmy patches of vegetation are likely to intercept the quadrat and result in a biased distribution.

Another sampling strategy is 'systematic random sampling'. The first sampling point is chosen at random and then subsequent locations are selected at regular intervals by pacing or at set intervals along a tape or knotted rope. For repeated sampling to detect changes in the species composition over time, a knotted rope can be stretched between two permanent markers and the quadrats located at the knots for each sampling. Strictly speaking, the sample points are not independent of one another but, provided the points are spaced widely enough so that the same plant is not sampled at two consecutive points, the sample placement is essentially random.

Fixed grid sampling

A fixed grid sample layout can be used to detect vegetation patterns within an area of grassland. This method is essentially 'systematic sampling', because the initial points of the grid are not randomly placed. The location of each sampling point needs to be precisely fixed and the different grassland communities identified and mapped (Magcale-Macandog and Whalley, 1991). Temporal changes in these patterns can be detected by repeated measurements using the same grid locations. Serious errors can occur if there is a regular spatial (e.g. topographic) pattern of variation in the grassland vegetation that could coincide with the grid. Such spatial patterns are generally obvious and appropriate sample location strategies can be used so that the results are not biased.

The sampling points in grid sampling are not independent and so standard errors of plot means cannot be calculated (Greig-Smith, 1964) if the grid sampling occurs over a number of different plots. Standard parametric statistical analyses are therefore invalid and non-parametric methods should be used. However, in practice parametric analyses are often used and this should not have very serious consequences.

Stratified random sampling

Stratified random sampling is appropriate when the grassland area is clearly patterned. More detailed studies may then be required within the different communities so detected. Sample locations can be assigned to the different communities proportional to the area (strata) occupied by each. The locations assigned to each part of the pattern are then placed randomly within the different communities. More intensive sampling of particular communities may be desirable. For instance, sheep camps may occupy only a small proportion of a paddock but a higher sample density within the sheep camp and on the sheep camp margins than in the remainder of the paddock may be necessary to sample adequately the differences in botanical composition over small distances (Robinson et al., 1983).

Size and shape of sampling units

Sampling units may differ in shape and size. In any type of grassland vegetation there may be large numbers of species present, differing in distribution, abundance and often sizes of the individuals. In addition, grasslands usually comprise both perennial and annual species and sometimes large numbers of one species of annual may appear at certain times of the year. It is obvious that if the individuals of a species are very small and there are large numbers of them, then a smaller sampling unit is necessary than for smaller numbers of larger individuals.

The distribution of individuals of the different species determines the shape of the sampling unit. If the individuals of a species are randomly distributed, then a square or circular sampling unit (quadrat) is satisfactory; but if the species of interest is highly clumped, then a rectangular quadrat will result in a lower coefficient of variation (Kershaw, 1964). If the entire species composition of the grassland is of interest, and if some species are randomly distributed while some are clumped and others are regularly dispersed, with a wide range of abundances, then a large rectangular quadrat would represent the best compromise.

A species area curve can be used to determine a quadrat size that will give adequate sampling of most of the species present in an area of grassland. The species area curve can be determined as follows:

1. Place a small quadrat (say 50 cm × 50 cm) on the ground and count the number of species enclosed.
2. Turn the quadrat over so that the sample area is doubled and count the additional species enclosed.
3. Do this repeatedly, keeping the area sampled as compact as possible, until no more species are recorded with further increases in the area.
4. Plot the number of species recorded against the total sample area (Fig. 4.1). The point of inflection of the curve (marked with an arrow) where the number of species recorded starts to decrease as the area increases is a compromise quadrat size for dealing with the majority of the species in the particular grassland sampled.

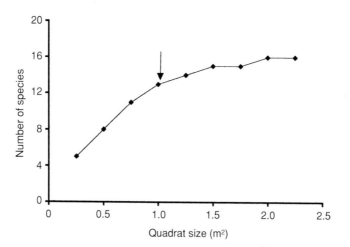

Fig. 4.1. Number of species recorded with increasing quadrat area. The arrow mark is the point of inflection that represents a compromise quadrat size for dealing with the majority of species in the grassland sampled.

This method of determining a compromise quadrat size is not appropriate in highly patterned communities, because moving from one patch of the pattern to another will result in a rapid increase in the number of species recorded as the quadrat size increases.

Types of samples

Some of the commonest types of sampling device and the ways in which they have been used will provide an introduction to the wide range of sample types available.

Quadrats

Simple quadrats of 50 cm × 50 cm or 1 m × 1 m are very commonly used for grassland studies but the size of the quadrats also depends on the vegetation type. In dense temperate grasslands, a commonly used size is 5 cm × 5 cm. These are easily constructed out of welded metal and are robust and useful in many situations. Quadrats made out of 10 × 5 mm aluminium bar are light to carry and easy to see if mislaid. It is easier to make a square or rectangular quadrat to a precise size than it is to make a circular one. Rectangular quadrats should not be too long and thin as this increases errors associated with cutting or counting plants on the quadrat edge. A suitable size for a rectangular quadrat for many grassland situations is 1.0 × 0.5 m.

Closed quadrats are often difficult to place in very tall vegetation without flattening the plants and making it difficult to determine which plants are included within the quadrat and which are not. Three-sided or open-ended quadrats are much easier to push into the grassland close to the ground with minimum disturbance of the vegetation.

A more recent variation of simple quadrats is the use of nested quadrats. This arrangement overcomes the problems associated with requiring different quadrat sizes for sampling both rare and extremely common species within the one grassland community. Clusters of nested quadrats are set out in geometrically increasing areas (e.g. 1, 2, 4, 8, 16 and 32 m^2) and species are recorded individually within these nested quadrats. In dense grassland with many species present, the size of the quadrats would be reduced. The use of nested quadrats is increasing because they are very efficient in terms of time invested relative to the large amount of information obtained, as discussed on pp. 89–91. A square shape is usually used and the corners of each sub-quadrat in the cluster are defined by marks on four diagonal cords leading outwards from a central peg.

Transects

An extension of a rectangular quadrat is a transect which may be tens of metres or even kilometres long. A transect may be either in the form of a

belt or a simple line. A belt transect usually consists of a tape or a string
stretched across the vegetation, and species or individuals occurring within
a specific distance perpendicular to the tape or string are recorded. A
simple form of belt transect in large paddocks is to drive a vehicle across
the vegetation and record species or individuals occurring between the
tyre tracks. The vehicle must be driven along a predetermined course to
avoid bias resulting from the driver avoiding difficult terrain.

With a line transect, individuals or species touching the tape or string
are recorded. If changes in the sizes of the individual plants over time are to
be followed, then the lengths of the intercepts occupied by individuals
touching the line are recorded.

Transects are very useful in detecting and quantifying vegetation
patterns within grasslands. For example, a 1000 m transect may be divided
into 50 m segments with segments overlapping by, say, 20 m. Data would be
collected from the 32 'segments' of the transect, each 50 m long, and then
used for pattern analysis.

The transects can be laid out deliberately to intersect with patches
of the grassland with different species composition and the edges of the
patches can be precisely located. If these transects with the precise location
of the edges are permanently marked, then changes in the size and/or
species composition of the patches over time can be readily quantified.

Point quadrats

The size of a quadrat can be reduced to a point so that it has a location
but no area. Points can be located randomly throughout a sample site, or
systematically to ensure even coverage (at any scale but usually within
representative parts of the area being sampled) or along a transect.
Whether each point hits leaves, a plant base, litter or bare ground can be
recorded. If 100 points are recorded and if a particular species is recorded
as a hit in ten of these points, then it can be assumed that it occupies 10% of
the area sampled. The recording of point quadrats can be rapid or slow,
depending on how they are used (as will be described later).

Many different devices have been constructed to locate points within
the area to be sampled. Some of these involve frames where the points are
a fixed distance apart and the points are slowly lowered through the
vegetation (e.g. Levy and Madden, 1933; Brown, 1954). Hits on leaves
(aerial cover) as well as plant bases (basal cover) or bare ground can be
recorded. The points in these frames are often fairly close together and if
the individual plants in the grassland are large then one hit of a species
can mean that the adjacent points hit the same plant of the same species
and the observations are not independent. In addition, because grassland
vegetation tends to occur in aggregates or clumps (Crocker and Tiver,
1948), the use of a frame will lead to correlations within the points
recorded each time the frame is located (Tidmarsh and Havenga, 1955)
and the variance will be underestimated.

An approach to eliminate this autocorrelation is to distribute the points widely across the grassland being sampled (Tidmarsh and Havenga, 1955). Methods to achieve this include the wheel point apparatus, where the spokes of a wheel are used to locate points regularly across the grassland. Usually one spoke of the wheel is marked and the data are recorded each time (or multiples of each time) the marked point hits the ground. Other methods of regularly locating points along a transect include cutting a notch in the front of the operator's boot, locating a small wire in the notch every predetermined number of paces, and recording the plant species that is hit (e.g. Mentis, 1981).

An important source of error in point quadrat data collected by different operators lies in the definition of a 'hit', particularly when estimating basal cover. The point may descend within the perimeter of a living grass tussock, but if the point is very small it may only contact dead material. In addition, the tussocks of two separate species of grass may be interwoven and it can be extremely difficult to tell just which plant base has been contacted. Tidmarsh and Havenga (1955) provided detailed diagrams of hits and misses for grassland plants with different life forms.

Theoretically points have location but no area and Goodall (1952) and Warren Wilson (1963) have investigated the relationship between area of the 'point' and the bias introduced into the results with respect to the estimation of cover. The larger the area of the 'point', the greater is the overestimation of cover. On the other hand, the smaller the area of the point, the more fragile the apparatus and the more difficult it is to use in the field. Sighting tubes with cross-hairs will reduce the effective area of the points but they are usually time consuming to use in the field. Caldwell *et al.* (1983) devised a fibre-optic point quadrat system with an effective point diameter of no more than 25 μm. The sensor is positioned at the end of a motor-driven rod that lowers the point through the canopy at a prescribed angle. When the sensor approaches a foliage element, the motor is stopped with the sensor within 1 mm of the plant part so that the operator can identify it and restart the system to proceed to the next contact. Caldwell *et al.* (1983) estimated this fibre-optic point system to be approximately twice as rapid as a conventional point quadrat system, even with motor-driven pins.

The precision of estimates of cover by species when using point quadrats is a function of the actual cover of a species and the number of points observed. For example, in a grassland with 10% cover and where one of the species present contributes only 1% of that cover, there will be a 0.1% probability of 'striking' the basal portion of that species, i.e. one chance in a thousand of striking the plant. Point quadrats are therefore not suited to sampling for rare species. In semiarid grasslands with low cover it is often recommended that 3000 points should be observed when monitoring cover by species (Tidmarsh and Havenga, 1955).

Plotless sampling methods
Several methods have been devised using the distances from randomly
distributed points to the nearest individual plant, or the nearest neighbour
to randomly chosen individuals (Mueller-Dumbois and Ellenberg, 1974;
Neuteboom *et al.*, 1992). These plotless methods can be very rapid and are
particularly useful in sparse vegetation but are very sensitive to whether the
species are randomly dispersed or not (Lamacraft *et al.*, 1983).

In the nearest-individual method, points are randomly selected and
the distance to the nearest individual of a particular species is measured.
It should also be noted that the relative abundance of species may be
estimated by identifying the nearest plant to a randomly, or systematically,
located point. The point to plant distance need not be measured.

In the point-centred quadrat method, points are randomly chosen and
axes are set up dividing the space around the point into four quadrants.
The distance to the nearest individual in each of the four quadrants is
measured, which decreases the number of points chosen and the time in
making the measurements. In sparse shrubland, range-finding devices have
been used to measure the distances to the nearest individuals.

Cores
In very dense short grasslands, cores may be collected and taken to
the laboratory for dissection and determination of the frequency or the
rank order of dry weight of the constituent species. It also allows both
above-ground and below-ground sampling of the same cores (Chapter 12).
Because of the large spatial variation in botanical composition, the location, size and number of cores is critical in terms of the statistical validity of
the results. In general terms, a large number of small cores is more efficient
than a small number of large cores. Core sampling is always destructive and
nearly always involves laboratory analyses.

Properties of Grassland Vegetation

There are several properties of species and grasslands that impinge on
the measurement of botanical composition of these communities. These
properties relate to the way in which the species present fit together to form
a community and also the species that are present in the first place. They
can affect many attributes of grassland vegetation and the ways in which
they can be measured.

Physiognomy

Physiognomy refers to the appearance of vegetation that is determined by
the life forms of the dominant and subsidiary species. Grassy vegetation can

occur as pure grasslands, with scattered trees (savanna) or with trees of various densities (woodlands) up to a grassy layer under forest trees (grassy forests) (Specht *et al.*, 1995). The physiognomy of the understorey is surprisingly uniform over a wide range of tree and shrub densities in many grassland communities. The species that comprise any vegetation, and consequently its physiognomy, are controlled by independent factors of the environment (Jenny, 1961) including management history.

Woody vegetation can be ignored or included when measuring the attributes of grasslands, depending on the purposes for which the data are being collected. However, the factors that affect the grassland structure and its species composition will often independently affect the woody vegetation. Grubb (1986) proposed a conceptual model for chalk grasslands in Europe that is relevant to many areas of grassland throughout the world. He described them as having a 'matrix' of long-lived perennial plants of various life forms with 'interstitial species' between them comprising short-lived, transient species. The matrix species are usually referred to as the dominants; if they comprise tussock grasses, then there is the potential for high species diversity with a relatively large number of interstitial species. Both the number of individuals and the number of species in the interstitium can vary from season to season, depending on management factors and rainfall, particularly in grasslands in semiarid or arid areas. Changes in the composition of the interstitial species can occur very rapidly, whereas changes in the matrix species occur more slowly. Grasslands that are dominated by annual species, of course, have a different physiognomy and can be subject to very rapid changes in response to management or to rainfall variability. The physiognomy of an area of grassland could affect the type of measurements, the timing and the methods used, depending on whether the matrix or the interstitial species are of primary interest.

Vegetation patterns

Vegetation patterns occur in grasslands at a range of scales (see p. 70) and there are essentially three approaches used to cope with them. The first is to ignore the patterns and rely on random sampling to average out the differences in species composition in various parts of the paddock. This approach is successful when the scale of the patterns is small in relation to the size of the area being sampled. However, averaging values may mask patterns that could be important. The value and methods of measuring horizontal variability are also considered in Chapter 5.

The second approach is to use some form of stratified random sampling (see p. 73) to sample adequately the different parts of the paddock that have different species composition. The sampling intensity may differ in different parts of the pattern depending on the purpose for the measurement of the species composition.

The third approach is to quantitatively measure the extent and intensity of the vegetation patterns. Fixed grid sampling (see p. 73) is an efficient means of detecting and quantifying vegetation patterns. Where the aim is to detect movement of the boundaries of patches or changes in species composition over time within the patches, a transect across and at right angles to the boundaries of the patches will provide valuable information.

Grassland Vegetation Attributes and their Measurement

There are many features of grassland vegetation that can be measured and different methodologies must be used for these attributes. Often, several methodologies are possible when measuring a particular attribute and the choice is influenced by the purposes for which the measurements are being made. Objectives of these measurements include: (i) the classification of grassland vegetation that may be important for ecological studies, for understanding agricultural potential or for predicting the responses to managerial actions; (ii) monitoring changes in grassland vegetation over time in relation to management impacts such as fertilizer applications, fire and different methods of grazing; and (iii) recording patterns associated with environmental gradients.

Diversity and species richness

'Maintaining or increasing species diversity' is a commonly stated objective for the management of natural vegetation, because of the importance of at least maintaining the species that make up the resource for the benefit and well-being of current and future generations. The terminology is often confusing and there are two components of diversity: species richness, or the number of species present; and the relative abundance or 'equitability' of the different species within the community. In addition, Scheiner (1992) defined pattern diversity, an example of which is the relative arrangement of communities within a landscape. Pielou (1975) gave a broad introduction to the general topic of diversity in plant and animal communities.

Alpha diversity
Mentis (1984) used alpha diversity to describe the two components of diversity. Three types of alpha (α) diversity are recognized: species richness (α_r), which is the number of species encountered per unit area; equitability (α_e), which is the relative abundance of each species in the community; and a combination of species richness and equitability expressed as heterogeneity (α_h). All three types of alpha diversity are conveniently measured using quadrat or point survey techniques.

The species list obtained from a sample site provides a figure for α_r. The species richness of the sample site could then, for example, be assessed depending on the number of species expected for that specific vegetation type or in comparison with other sample sites within the area being studied. Species richness is therefore a relative term.

Where all species within an area contribute more or less equally to the proportional composition of the sampled area (a rare occurrence) α_e is high. However, in most situations equitability is low as a few of the species tend to be dominants and account for the majority of the proportional composition.

Measuring α_r alone may meet some objectives but when monitoring change such a measure may be insensitive, since change may occur in the proportional contribution or frequency of some species (α_e) rather than in the number of species. For example, while the α_r of a sward may not change, the proportions of palatable and unpalatable plants could, with important implications for livestock production. Appropriate sampling techniques must therefore be employed to ensure that α_e is effectively sampled. Ultimately α_h provides the kind of information usually required for recording changes in grassland communities (i.e. a species list plus the proportional contribution or frequency of each species for each sample site).

Beta diversity

Beta (β) diversity is the amount of species turnover (or change of species composition) along an environmental gradient or between areas or communities (Gaugh, 1982). Beta diversity has sometimes been called habitat diversity. This concept is particularly useful when studying the differences in species composition resulting from different environmental impacts. These impacts may result from management strategies (e.g. variable stocking rates, frequency and intensity of fire, and fertilization rates) or abiotic factors such as moisture or elevational gradients. Appropriate sampling strategies must be employed to detect such diversity.

Species turnover is best understood by considering plant communities as groups of species whose abundances change gradually or abruptly in time and space in association with gradual or abrupt changes in environmental factors (Gaugh, 1982; Mentis, 1984). Average species turnover may be defined as the average distance along a chosen environmental gradient within which a species appears, rises to maximum abundance and then declines and disappears. In these terms, then, a change in the proportional composition of palatable and unpalatable grasses would involve less than one species turnover and would represent a lower β diversity than a change from grassland to forest, where the two communities at either end of the gradient have no species in common (Mentis, 1984). Beta diversity may be indexed using various measurements of similarity (such as percentage similarity) or distance (such as Euclidean distance) (Gaugh, 1982). Short gradients with low species turnover have low β diversity whereas longer gradients would have higher β diversity.

Gamma diversity

While the number of species encountered in a sample site is referred to as α diversity, the total number of species encountered in the entire study is called gamma (γ) diversity (Gaugh, 1982).

Other indices of diversity

The Shannon diversity index is derived from information theory; it assumes that individual species are sampled from an infinitely large population and that all species present are recorded in each sample (Kent and Coker, 1992). McIntosh's diversity index is another expression of diversity and also enables calculation of an index of dominance and of a measure of evenness. Kent and Coker (1992) give examples of how to calculate these indices.

Species richness

The 'Whittaker plot' sampling method is a nested quadrat approach that uses a $\log_{10}$ scale for determining species richness of grassland vegetation (Shmida, 1984). Species richness is initially measured in 1 m^2 (being the average number of species in 10 quadrats each of 1 m^2), then in 10 m^2, 100 m^2 and 1000 m^2 quadrats. Refer to Shmida (1984) for more detail on how the quadrats are nested. Least-squares regression is used to determine the relation between species richness and sample area. This relation can be used for comparing published species area data from other vegetation types. While the method is relatively efficient in arid and semiarid grass/shrub communities requiring 0.5 to 1.0 worker-hours per plot, it is time consuming in dense, species-rich grasslands requiring up to 6.0 worker-hours per plot (Shmida, 1984; Le Roux, 1995). Supplementary observations must also be taken if attributes such as canopy and basal cover, species dominance or equitability, and sward structure are to be measured. The method is useful in that it provides a comprehensive species list that is likely to include rare species, and is suitable for many conservation objectives.

Cover

Cover means the projection of plants or plant parts on to the soil surface. Measurements of cover can be expressed either as the percentage of the soil surface covered by the plants or plant parts or can be broken down into the species or groups of species present. It can be measured as either canopy cover or basal cover.

Canopy cover

Canopy cover is the projection of the plant canopies on to the soil surface, usually expressed as a percentage. The canopy cover of an area of grassland can change dramatically in a very short period of time, e.g. by grazing or fire, and regrowth may be slow or rapid, or may be stable, e.g. the canopy cover of the shrub component of semi-arid grass/shrub communities. Because the canopies of different individuals and different species can overlap, the total can add up to more than 100%.

Canopy cover is related to sward structure, which is considered in Chapter 5. The percentage of the area covered by bare ground, stones or litter can also be estimated at the same time.

Measurement of canopy cover in grasslands can often be difficult because the grass leaves may have a vertical or near vertical orientation. The very act of walking about in the grassland can often cause these leaves to become horizontal and therefore effectively increase the canopy cover. Care must be taken that canopy cover is not substantially affected by sampling activities.

The usual method of estimating canopy cover is to use a point quadrat frame, such as the Levy bridge (Levy and Madden, 1933; Brown, 1954), where the points can be slowly lowered through the vegetation and hits of individual leaves recorded. Where the leaves of individual species can be identified from their morphology, the contribution of the leaves of different species to the canopy cover can be estimated. The use of point quadrats to estimate canopy cover in tall grassland is impossible in windy weather and when the height is more than 0.5 m.

Canopy cover in sparse grasslands can be estimated by measuring the intercept occupied by the canopies of individual species on a line or tape stretched across the grassland. The lengths of the intercepts occupied by the canopies of individual species are then added up and expressed as a percentage of the total length to give the percentage canopy cover of each species. This method will usually lead to higher estimates of canopy cover than the careful use of pins in a point quadrat frame.

Basal cover

The basal cover represents the proportion of the ground occupied by the bases (where they are rooted to the ground) of the individual species. Because all measurements are made at ground level, there cannot be any overlap and so the total basal cover cannot be more than 100%. Again, the percentage of the area occupied by bare ground, litter or stones can be estimated simultaneously. This may be particularly important in semiarid and arid grasslands, where the percentage plant basal cover may be quite small.

Basal cover is a more stable property of vegetation than canopy cover. It is less affected by prior grazing or seasonal conditions, particularly with perennial species. Sometimes the basal cover of stoloniferous species (mat-forming grasses) is difficult to measure because basal cover actually represents the projection of the stolons on the ground, which can be difficult to measure if they have a small diameter. In addition, rosette components of grassland with radical leaves cause difficulties. Tussock grasses often have dead sections within the base and the difficult question then arises as to whether these sections should be included in the basal area or not.

Point quadrats are commonly used to measure basal cover in grassland vegetation and the limits of error, whether partitioned into individual species or expressed as total cover, depend on the amount of cover and the number of points employed. It is important that the sampling points are farther apart than the diameter of the largest units or clusters of vegetation. In addition, the points must be adequately distributed over the area surveyed. If these conditions are met, then the estimates obtained by point quadrats follow a binomial distribution. The number of points required to provide a given accuracy decreases as the percentage basal cover increases up to about 50%. Tidmarsh and Havenga (1955) provided a series of graphs which allow the limits of error to be read, given the number of sampling points and the percentage cover, so long as the basic assumptions are met.

Pantographs can be used for measuring the basal cover of individual species in a fixed quadrat and for following the changes over time. A pantograph is a mechanical device whereby a pointer is used to trace the outline of the bases of all the plants in a quadrat and a pencil follows these tracings at a reduced scale on a sheet of paper. More details are given in Chapter 6.

The line intercept method is also appropriate for measuring the basal cover of individual species or of the whole grassland. This method is impossible to use in really dense grassland.

Quadrats of, say, 0.5 m × 0.5 m divided by wires into a number of sub-quadrats can be randomly located in the grassland. Each time the quadrat is located, the percentage occupied by the individual species or individual components is estimated by adding up the squares occupied by the individual species or components. These methods can be extended to a smaller scale by using grids etched on perspex, clipping individual species to ground level, locating the grid over the top and again counting the squares occupied by the cut surfaces of the individual tillers. Similar methods include clipping individual plants and tracing the outline of the bases on transparent film, transferring the outlines to white paper using a photocopier, cutting out around the outline and measuring the area using a leaf area meter. Various attempts have been made to estimate both the precision and accuracy of these methods (Lodge *et al.*, 1981).

Density

Density is the number of individual plants per unit area of either individual species or groups of species. Measurement of the density of a single species is relatively easy for open tussock grasslands, although it can be very tedious when counting dense seedlings. However, density becomes very difficult to measure for mat grasses or other clonal species where different individuals merge together. In this case, either cover (canopy or basal) or frequency (presence–absence) is the only practicable form of measurement. Measurement of the density of a large number of species in a complex grassland community can be extremely tedious but less time-consuming techniques are available (see pp. 86–91). In general terms, species with small individuals tend to have much higher densities than species with larger individuals which gives rise to the 'minus three over two power' law (Kira *et al.*, 1953). This law is simply an expression of the maximum packing possible of individuals relative to their size in plant communities.

The opposite of density is openness, which is a measure of vigour of a pasture or related to species characteristics. Neuteboom *et al.* (1992) developed a plotless technique for measuring density and openness.

Density can be measured using quadrats (simple or nested) or plotless techniques.

Simple quadrats

Quadrats are randomly located within the grassland and the number of individuals are counted within each quadrat. An appropriate quadrat size must be chosen relative to the density and size of the individuals of the species being counted. The smaller the individuals and the higher the density, then the smaller is the quadrat; and the larger the individuals, the larger is the quadrat. A quadrat size of, say, 50×50 cm is suitable for open grasslands, whereas 20×20 cm could be suitable for denser communities. Even smaller quadrats may be necessary for very dense stands of small seedlings. It may be necessary to use several different quadrat sizes for different species in a community if there are large differences in sizes and densities. If the individuals of the species being assessed are not randomly distributed, then difficulties will be encountered in the statistical analysis of the results.

Nested quadrats

Nested quadrats, using a wide range of sizes as described in the section 'Frequency score and importance score' (see p. 89), can be used to estimate the densities of a number of species within a grassland community when there is a wide variation in the densities of the individual species.

Plotless techniques

Plotless techniques can be used for measuring the density of species in sparse grasslands but are not suitable for dense communities.

Frequency (presence/absence)

The frequency of a species is the percentage or proportion of quadrats in which it is present. Measurement of frequency is less tedious and time consuming than for density, particularly if the community is complex and information about a large number of species is required. In addition, frequency estimates are possible for clonal species where individuals cannot easily be identified. The operator searches each quadrat and records the species that are present. Arbitrary rules must be set as to whether a species is counted or not depending on whether it is rooted in the quadrat or any part of the plant is within the boundaries of the quadrat. These rules must be established when planning a survey and depend on the objectives.

Frequency data are often collected using either a number of small quadrats or a larger one (say 1 m²) divided into, say, ten smaller quadrats. This allows frequency data to be collected at intervals along a transect or at grid points located over a whole paddock. The advantage is that a frequency statistic is provided for each sampling point rather than just a presence/absence recording, giving more flexibility in the analysis of the data. There is no difference in the meaning of frequency collected using one quadrat randomly placed or a set of contiguous quadrats randomly placed, provided the conditions described below are met.

If the sub-quadrats (usually square) are arranged contiguously, then it is important that any plants that straddle the boundary between two sub-quadrats are only recorded in one. A simple way to avoid this problem is to arrange the equipment so that the distance between adjacent sub-quadrats is greater than the diameter of the largest individual plant. Each sub-quadrat is searched and the frequency is the proportion of the sub-quadrats in which a particular species occurs. In Fig. 4.2A, a dot occurs in four of the nine sub-quadrats and so the frequency is 4/9, i.e. 0.44 or 44%.

Frequency data have an upper and lower limit in that as the density of a species increases, the probability of that species occurring in a quadrat approaches one. At the other end of the scale, the probability approaches zero as the density decreases. The frequency therefore depends very little on density when the frequency is very low or very high. Selection of quadrat size is therefore critical. If several species are very common and a large quadrat is used, then each of them will have a frequency of one although there may be large differences in their relative abundance. Mueller-Dombois and Ellenberg (1974) and Bonham (1989) have suggested several rules of thumb, including having no more than ten species in each quadrat and mean frequencies should be in the range of 0.05–0.95. The quadrat size must also be appropriate to the size of individuals of the species present: 1 × 1 m is suitable for many relatively sparse grasslands, down to 20 × 20 cm for dense, short communities. It is, therefore, always necessary to indicate the quadrat size used in frequency estimates, as it affects the

(A)   (B)

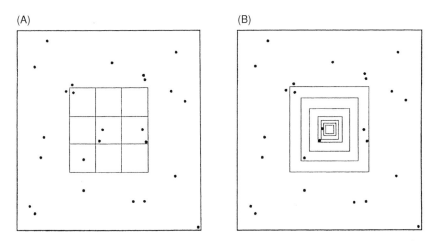

Fig. 4.2. Comparison of frequency, frequency score and importance score sampling methods in a square sampling space of 100 unit² containing 25 points. In each case, a 20 unit² quadrat is used to sample the space, which encloses six of the points, using (A) a quadrat of nine contiguous equal-area (2.2 unit²) sub-quadrats to estimate frequency, and (B) a compound quadrat of seven nested (cumulative areas of 0.2, 0.5, 1, 2, 5, 10 and 20 unit²) sub-quadrats to estimate frequency score and importance score. (From Morrison *et al.*, 1995, Fig. 1, with kind permission from Kluwer Academic Publishers.)

results. Subsequent frequency measurements in one area of grassland must always use the same quadrat size for changes over time to be measured.

Morrison *et al.* (1995) investigated the effects of different densities and a standard quadrat size divided into different numbers of sub-quadrats on the measured frequencies using computer-simulated randomly distributed points (plants). As the number of sub-quadrats increased, the size of the individual sub-quadrats decreased, clearly showing that the frequency estimates were approximately linearly related to the log of the density over the range of frequencies from 0.10 to 0.95 (Fig. 4.3A). These data also indicate that smaller quadrats are necessary for sampling species with higher densities whereas much larger quadrats must be used to sample rare species.

When a sampling quadrat is reduced to a dimensionless point, frequency becomes an absolute measure of cover. The nearest-plant method, where the plant species nearest a randomly or systematically located point is recorded, has been used as an alternative technique. The results of the nearest-plant method provide an estimate of the proportional species composition of a sample site rather than of cover. Everson and Clarke (1987) tested several methods of botanical analysis in tussock grasslands (including the quadrat, Levy bridge, step point, wheel point, metric belt transect and dry-weight-rank methods), and concluded that the wheel point method was most suitable for determining grassland species composition in terms of relative abundance in tufted grasslands.

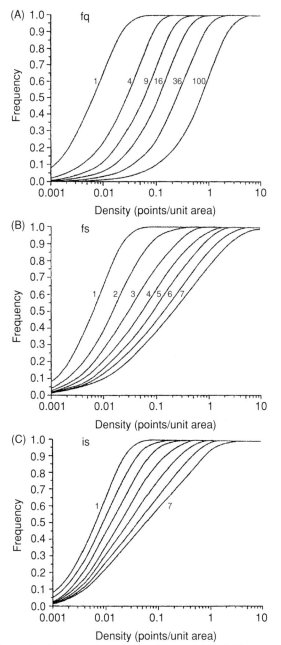

Fig. 4.3. Relationship between point density (log scale) and (A) estimated frequency (fq), (B) frequency score (fs) and (C) importance score (is) from computer simulations of randomly distributed points using a range of densities and sub-quadrat sizes. The numbers on the curves refer to the number of sub-quadrats within a 100 unit^2 quadrat used to sample the different densities. (From Morrison *et al.*, 1995, Fig. 2, with kind permission from Kluwer Academic Publishers.)

While the nearest-plant method is efficient in determining proportional species composition (or relative abundance of species) of a sample site, it has the following disadvantages: (i) rare species are not adequately sampled, so the method cannot be used to determine species richness; and (ii) since the abundance of species is calculated relative to the other species in the sample site, if one of the species were to die out completely without replacement the relative abundance of the remaining species would increase.

Frequency score and importance score

Outhred (1984) introduced two new techniques designed to overcome the problem of estimating the frequency of the species in a complex community. Both techniques are based on sampling within a nest of concentric sub-quadrats with the size increasing in a geometric or semi-geometric progression.

The first is the frequency score (Fig. 4.4), in which all the species present in the central (smallest) sub-quadrat are recorded. The area outside the smallest sub-quadrat but inside the next largest is then searched and each species present again recorded. This process is then repeated until all the species occurring in the whole nest are listed. The frequency score is the proportion of sub-quadrats in which each species occurs. In Fig. 4.2B it is 4/7, or 0.57.

The second is the importance score, which is related to the smallest sub-quadrat in which a particular species is recorded (Outhred, 1984). If a species is recorded in the smallest, central sub-quadrat, it is given an importance score of 7 (in a nest of seven sub-quadrats), 6 for the next largest and 1 if it is only recorded in the largest outside sub-quadrat. In Fig. 4.2B, the importance score is 5/7, or 0.71. Importance-score data can be collected rapidly as only newly encountered species are recorded in each sub-quadrat as they are searched progressively outwards from the centre. The location of the nest can affect the results as a rare species may be assigned a high importance score if it happens to occur where the centre of the nest is located.

Morrison *et al.* (1995) examined the efficacy of the frequency scores and the importance scores in comparison with frequency using computer simulations of randomly distributed points (plants) of different densities and a set of nested quadrats with seven sub-quadrats. Both frequency scores and importance scores were obtained using one to seven sub-quadrats across four orders of magnitude of densities (Fig. 4.3B, C).

Both the frequency scores and the importance scores were more or less linearly related to the log of density within the range of 0.1–0.95, as was the frequency (see Fig. 4.3A). However, the linear relationship extended over about two orders of magnitude for frequency score and three orders

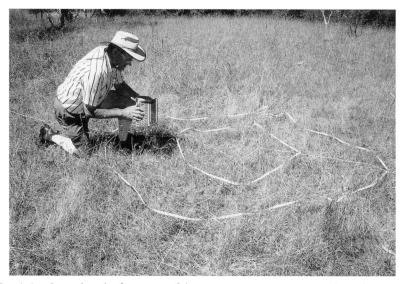

Fig. 4.4. Recording the frequency of the species present using nested quadrats in a *Themeda* grassland. Four strings are laid out at right angles and the quadrat boundaries indicated using a tape between markers on the strings. The species present in the central quadrat are recorded first and then those present in the second quadrat, that is, the space between the two tapes. The tapes are successively moved outwards and the species recorded in each annulus until all quadrats in the nest have been recorded. Nests of seven to ten quadrats are usually used in grasslands. (Photograph C. Cooper.)

for importance score, compared with only one for each sized sub-quadrat for frequency. The greater the number of sub-quadrats in the nest, the flatter the curve and the greater the range where the log of the density was linearly related to either of the scores. The importance scores were up to twice as large for any given density as the equivalent frequency scores. The importance-score data were slightly less reproducible than the frequency data because of the sensitivity to the location of the centre sub-quadrat, and at low densities the frequency data were less reproducible than the frequency-score data. Over the range of frequencies from 0.1 to 0.95, both the frequency score and the importance score were slightly less reproducible than the frequency.

Morrison *et al.* (1995) also investigated the effects of clumping and regular dispersion of the points (plants) on the frequency, frequency score and importance score. In general, clumping decreased the estimates for all three methods whereas regularity increased them. Changes in the spatial distribution of the points changed the shape of the relationship between frequency and density but it had much less effect on the relationships for the frequency score and the importance score.

Morrison *et al.* (1995) tested all three methods in the field to detect plant community patterns. Because the nested quadrat methods sample a larger area than the equivalent number of contiguous small quadrats for frequency, they are better suited to detecting the rarer species in an area of grassland and can also encompass a greater range of species sizes. By using seven sub-quadrats ranging from 1 m² to 64 m² or larger, grasses, shrubs and trees can all be included in the frequency scores or importance scores. Although considerably less time is involved in collecting importance-score than frequency-score data for the same nested quadrats, the latter method is more efficient in detecting subtleties of community patterns in the field (Morrison *et al.*, 1995).

Seedbanks

In addition to the botanical composition of the above-ground parts of a grassland ecosystem, there is also a population of viable seeds mixed in with the litter and in the surface soil. This soil seedbank may have a markedly different botanical composition compared with the above-ground plant community. Measurements of the soil seedbank, whether in terms of species composition or density, usually involves collecting soil cores and either physically separating out the seeds or germinating them (see Chapter 6).

Composition by mass

Methods of measuring the quantity of herbage mass or dry weight are described in Chapter 7. However, for many purposes it is necessary to partition the herbage mass into the individual species – that is, to measure the botanical composition by herbage mass. The most direct method is to harvest individual quadrats and physically sort into individual species or groups of species, dry and weigh them.

Clipping techniques

Clipping of quadrats followed by hand separation into individual species can be very time consuming if there are more than two or three important species in the samples or when a large number of samples are to be analysed. In addition, especially once they are cut, the recognition of single leaves of individual species (particularly grasses) becomes virtually impossible when there are many species. It may lead to a large percentage of the herbage mass being classified as unknown species. When separation into green leaf, stem and dead material as well as species is required the logistics can become virtually impossible. The accuracy of the estimates using clipping and sorting techniques is usually adequate, provided the number of samples taken is large enough, the botanical composition of the grassland is relatively simple and the material can be adequately identified. Another approach is to identify individual plants of the different species and cut them separately, putting the material of each species into a separate bag for drying and weighing. This procedure is time consuming, but does overcome the difficulty of identifying individual leaves of grasses in a mass of clipped material.

There are three major components of the herbage mass contributed by species (Lodge *et al.*, 1981). These are the number of plants per unit area (plant density), mean basal area of the individual species and the herbage mass per unit basal area. Information on all three components is desirable if the mechanism of changes in herbage mass contribution of individual species in response to management are to be properly understood. For instance, addition of fertilizers may increase the mean basal area of an individual grass species but not increase the herbage mass per unit basal area. On the other hand, another species may respond in terms of increasing the herbage mass per unit basal area without much increase in mean basal area (Lodge, 1981).

Lodge (1981), Lodge *et al.* (1981) and Lodge and Gleeson (1982) have devised a technique for estimating the three components of herbage mass for individual grass species in complex native grasslands on the Northern Tablelands and Slopes of New South Wales, Australia. Individual perennial grass plants were identified to species and clipped at ground level and the resultant herbage was later separated into green leaf, stem (including leaf bases) and dead material. The remainder of the herbage in each quadrat was also harvested. The basal area of each of the individually harvested plants was then estimated by placing a perspex sheet on the ground over each of the plants. The perimeter of each plant base was outlined and the outline transferred to a sheet of white paper, labelled, cut out with scissors and measured with an automatic leaf area meter. The relative importance of the three components contributing to herbage mass for each species was determined using the method of Henderson and Hayman (1960). In some species, the contribution of herbage mass was more sensitive to plant density; basal area was important for the herbage mass estimates of all species tested and in some the mass per unit area was significant. Lodge and Gleeson (1982) estimated that an experienced person using this technique would be able to sample four species in 23 quadrats day^{-1}. Increasing the number of species sampled individually in each quadrat would markedly decrease the number of quadrats, which could be harvested within a day.

Near-infrared reflectance spectroscopy
The use of near-infrared reflectance spectroscopy for the analysis of forages for organic and some mineral components has been available for some time (Shenk *et al.*, 1979). This technology has recently been extended to the analysis of the species composition of forage samples (Coleman *et al.*, 1985; Pitman *et al.*, 1991; Wachendorf *et al.*, 1999). Samples are

harvested from the field, dried and ground under uniform conditions and reflectance spectra are determined. The preparation of calibration equations is critical to the success of the procedure (Wachendorf *et al.*, 1999). A further limitation is that only a relatively small number of species can be distinguished within the one mixture, and that closely related species are chemically similar, and therefore are more difficult to distinguish (Coleman *et al.*, 1985). For instance, Pitman *et al.* (1991) were not able to predict adequately the proportions of several tropical legumes where a single grass dominated and the legumes were minor components of the mixture. This technique is relatively rapid compared with harvesting and hand separation, but the samples must be harvested, dried and ground and appropriate calibration equations must be available.

Estimation techniques

The use of visual estimates in the field is a very rapid procedure and allows the collection of data from a large number of quadrats. Pechanec and Pickford (1937) introduced one of the early methods using estimates, and involving a long period of training, whereby operators estimated the herbage mass of individual tussocks with repeated checks of estimates against actual weights.

Three different methods for estimating composition are commonly used:

1. *Dry-weight-rank.* The DWR method, developed by Mannetje and Haydock (1963), is the simplest procedure for estimating the proportion by dry weight of the different species in a grassland. The method involves placing quadrats in grassland and estimating which species take first, second and third (or even fourth) rank in terms of dry weight. The species occupying rank 1 is given a value of 8.04, the species with rank 2, 2.41, and rank 3, 1.0. These multipliers have been derived empirically from studies of the relation between actual and ranked dry weight composition. However, their use has been successfully validated on a large number of grasslands comprising different species and different species composition (Jones and Hargreaves, 1979; Barnes *et al.*, 1982; Scott, 1993). The above multipliers correspond to percentages of the components of 70, 21 and 9 for the first, second and third ranked species. The estimates are repeated on a number of quadrats and the values for each species are added up and expressed as a percentage of the total scores of all species.

DWR is surprisingly robust with respect to quadrat size (Mannetje and Haydock, 1963; Neuteboom *et al.*, 1998). The major requirement is that the size be large enough for most quadrats to contain at least three species. The sparser the vegetation, the larger the quadrat size in order to contain the required number of species and quadrats up to 10 m^2 have been used (Aisthorpe *et al.*, 1999). Haydock and Shaw (1975) used a 0.25 m^2 quadrat for estimating herbage mass and found that this was the largest quadrat that could be conveniently viewed as a whole in dense grassland (Figure 4.5). The choice of quadrat size rests with the observer and is a matter of compromise to obtain the most efficient use of time and the desired level of accuracy.

There are five important assumptions or requirements specific to DWR, the first four being discussed in detail by Tothill *et al.* (1992). If the first two restrictions do not apply in any situation, these authors suggest appropriate modifications:

- At least three species should be present in the majority of the sample quadrats.
- If a particular species consistently has very high percentages (> 75%) in the quadrats, then a 'cumulative ranking' (first and second rank go to the dominant species) as described by Jones and Hargreaves (1979) and Tothill *et al.* (1992) should be used.
- There should be variation among quadrats in the order in which species are ranked. If the order of ranking of the species in every quadrat is the same, then the results will indicate that the percentages of the species are 70, 21 and 9, respectively, in the area sampled if the standard multipliers are used.
- Species components, such as leaf and stem or green and dry, should not be treated as separate species as the standard multipliers are not appropriate.

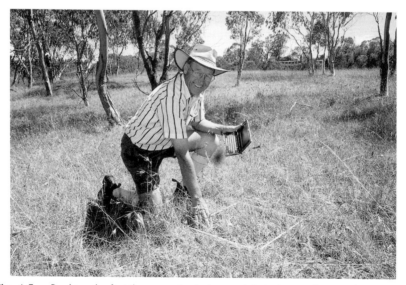

Fig. 4.5. Ranking the first three species in terms of their dry weight contribution (dry-weight-rank method) using a 0.25 m² quadrat and entering the results into a hand-held computer in a *Themeda* grassland. (Photograph C. Cooper.)

- On the basis of computer modelling, Neuteboom *et al.* (1998) suggested that DWR will not be appropriate if the species do not have some patchiness in their distribution. However, they concluded that only a small amount of patchiness is required and that in most grasslands this is probably fulfilled. This conclusion is substantiated by the successful validation of DWR on a wide range of grasslands (Jones and Hargreaves, 1979; Barnes *et al.*, 1982).

2. *Direct estimation of percentage composition.* The percentage contribution of each species to the herbage mass can be directly estimated for all of the species present in each quadrat rather than using the fixed multipliers of the DWR method. In other words, species A is recorded as being, say, 60%, species B as 25% and so on. This procedure involves a higher level of precision than simply ranking species in order and it avoids the limitations of DWR listed above (Tothill *et al.*, 1992). However, it can be difficult to use in complex grasslands because it is not easy to estimate the percentages mentally so that they add up to 100%. It is also possible to estimate components such as percentage green leaf in the quadrat.

3. *Percentage rank method.* The percentage rank method combines the simplicity of DWR with the greater accuracy of direct estimation. It is similar to DWR, in that only the first three or four species, in terms of dry weight, are 'rated', but rather than simply ranking them in order of weight, their actual percentage contribution is estimated. This also overcomes some of the limitations previously listed for DWR.

These two latter methods are of particular benefit in the following circumstances:

- One species is very dominant (> 90%).
- There are usually only two or three species in a quadrat with another minor species present in most quadrats, which would be overestimated by DWR.
- There are no dominant species, akin to the random distribution problem outlined by Neuteboom *et al.* (1998).

Estimating percentage directly, whether it be for all species or just for the three or four most important species, requires more training than simply ranking species as 1st, 2nd or 3rd (Tothill *et al.*, 1992).

Further comments on estimation techniques
The following points are pertinent to all of the above methods of estimating botanical composition.

On an individual quadrat basis, estimation techniques will never be as accurate as clipping and sorting. However, the accuracy of the latter approach is often greatly limited by the small number of quadrats, whereas estimation techniques allow for many more quadrats to be sampled. In general, 30 to 100 samples are satisfactory and with replicated small plot work acceptable results can be obtained with as few as 12 samples per plot (Waite, 1992). The larger number of quadrats opens the possibility for closer examination of variability within pastures, whether this reflects site and soil differences or reflects associations between different species (McDonald and Jones, 1997).

All techniques for estimating composition should be accompanied by estimation of standing herbage mass (presentation yield) within the same quadrats, according to the procedures discussed elsewhere (see Chapter 7). This is because if species A has an inherently lower herbage mass than species B, then those quadrats in which species A is the dominant species will have a lower herbage mass than those in which species B is dominant. If the estimation procedures assign equal weight to every quadrat, then the percentage of species A in the grassland is overestimated and that of species B is underestimated (Jones and Hargreaves, 1979).

An important source of bias in estimation techniques is associated with the different morphologies of the species comprising an area of grassland and also the different water content of different species or plants' parts. Grasses usually have ascending leaves whereas many dicots, particularly legumes, have leaves that are spread horizontally. These differences in morphology give misleading impressions of the amount of dry weight contributed by the species with different morphologies. All operators using estimation techniques should be trained in the procedures and periodically check themselves by estimating and then cutting and sorting test quadrats.

Because of the large number of field entries usually required when using visual estimation techniques, it is highly desirable that they be entered on to a hand-held computer in the field. The data can then be downloaded into a PC, where they can be processed. This saves a lot of time and also reduces the possibility of transcription errors, because data do not have to be re-entered into the computer.

In complex grassland communities, species are often present which are of little interest but make some contribution to the herbage mass. For recording purposes, these species may be bulked together into categories such as 'other dicots' while species of most interest are recorded separately. This reduces the time taken to record the quadrats but bulking should be confined to minor species. Bulking of the major species may lead to a loss of information about the behaviour of the major components of the grass-land. In certain circumstances, it may be useful to rank each quadrat in two ways simultaneously, i.e. firstly floristically and secondly on the basis of groupings that have agronomic importance. These groupings may be perennial grasses, annual grasses, legumes, other dicots and weeds.

The proportion of green leaf in the herbage mass is very important for livestock production (Mannetje, 1974). The practice of partitioning has been used whereby the herbage mass in each quadrat is visually partitioned into categories such as green leaf, dead material, stems, etc. in addition to or as an alternative to partitioning into species. This can be done when using some methods of visual estimation.

The BOTANAL package

The previous sections have outlined the advantages and limitations of three procedures for estimating composition – DWR, direct estimation of percentage and percentage ranks. It has also been pointed out that these estimates should be accompanied by estimates of herbage mass, that direct data entry is desirable and that there is potential for examining patchiness because of the large number of quadrats that can be estimated in contrast to clipping and sorting.

All these options are available in the BOTANAL package, which also allows for recording other attributes such as frequency, percentage cover or yield of green leaf (Waite and Kerr, 1996) on the same quadrats. The first BOTANAL manual (Tothill *et al.*, 1992) outlined the field procedures, the second (Hargreaves and Kerr, 1992) gave instructions on using the computer programs concerned and the third (McDonald *et al.*, 1996) outlined the procedures for the use of hand-held computers for field recording.

Classification of Grassland Vegetation

Numerical multivariate methods for classification and ordination analysis of quantitative data are commonly used for the classification of grasslands on the basis of their botanical composition and a number of suitable statistical packages are available (e.g. Belbin, 1993). A wide range of quantitative data is suitable for this type of analysis, which is not constrained by the necessity for the data to be normally distributed for the analyses to be valid. Frequency, frequency score or importance score data collected at a number of sites within grassland vegetation have commonly been used and the sites then classified into groups and the groups verified using ordination (e.g. Clarke *et al.*, 1998).

A common technique is first to list the sites with the data relating to the species within each site in a matrix, with the species in the rows and each site in the columns. The sites are then classified according to the frequencies of the species within them. The matrix is then inverted so that the sites are in the rows, with the species in the columns. The species are then grouped according to the sites in which they occur and a two-way table can be constructed giving insights into the species that are most important in the production of each group of sites. The groups can be named according to the most abundant species or dominants occurring in each site. The validity of these groupings can be verified by ordination. Further discussion about the roles of relevant classification and ordination procedures can be found in Chapter 2.

Conclusions

The reasons why the botanical composition of grasslands is measured fall into three general groups and the methodology is different for each. Some of the methodologies are well established, while others are still in the process of being developed.

The first reason is to partition the total herbage mass into the component species or groups of species. Visual estimation procedures, such as in the BOTANAL package (Hargreaves and Kerr, 1992; Tothill *et al.*, 1992; McDonald *et al.*, 1996), are usually adequate for this purpose and are now generally widely accepted.

The second is the use of specialized procedures for individual research projects involving the measurement of attributes of the species composition of grasslands. The underlying principles are well accepted and have been described in this chapter. Such objectives could involve measurements of many attributes – yield, botanical composition by weight, basal cover, canopy cover, density and frequency – sometimes over very large areas and sometimes over very small areas. The methods chosen and the intensity of measurement will vary widely, depending on the objectives and scale of operation.

There is an increasing need to measure the species composition of grasslands in terms of species abundance and species diversity for environmental purposes and this constitutes the third group of reasons. There are no generally accepted methods and either point quadrats to estimate percentage cover or frequency measures are commonly used where quantitative data are required. The use of nested quadrats to measure frequency score or importance score (Morrison *et al.*, 1995) provides extreme flexibility and the more linear relationship between frequency score and density is an advantage. This method has the capacity to produce quantitative data about the minor components of an area of grassland (of increasing importance for conservation purposes) as well as the shrub and tree components of mixed plant communities.

References

Acocks, J.P.H. (1975) *Veld Types of South Africa*, 2nd edn. Memoirs of the Botanical Survey of South Africa, No. 40, Government Printer, Pretoria, 128 pp.

Aisthorpe, R.D., Pahl, L.I., Muller, F.W. and McLennan, N.M. (1999) Adapting the comparative yield technique to monitor pasture in the mulgalands. In: *Proceedings of the VI International Rangeland Congress.* Townsville, Australia, pp. 469–471.

Barnes, D.L., Odendaal, J.J. and Beukes, B.H. (1982) Use of the dry-weight-rank method of botanical analysis in the eastern transvaal Highveld. *Proceedings of the Grassland Society of Southern Africa* 17, 79–82.

Beadle, N.C.W. (1981) *The Vegetation of Australia.* Gustav Fischer Verlag, Stuttgart, 690 pp.

Belbin, L. (1993) *PATN Reference Manual and Users Guide.* CSIRO, Division of Wildlife and Ecology, Canberra, 287 pp.

Bonham, C.D. (1989) *Measurements for Terrestrial Vegetation.* Wiley, New York, 338 pp.

Brown, D. (1954) *Methods of Surveying and Measuring Vegetation.* Bulletin Number 42, Commonwealth Agricultural Bureau of Pastures and Field Crops, Hurley, UK, 223 pp.

Burrough, P.A. (1986) *Principles of Geographic Information Systems for Land Resource Assessments.* Oxford University Press, Oxford, 193 pp.

Caldwell, M.M., Harris, G.W. and Dzurec, R.S. (1983) A fiber optic point quadrat system for improved accuracy in vegetation sampling. *Oecologia* 59, 417–418.

Clarke, P.J., Gardener, M.R., Nano, C.E. and Whalley, R.D.B. (1998) *The Vegetation and Plant Species of Kirramingly.* Division of Botany, University of New England, Armidale, New South Wales, 44 pp.

Coleman, S.W., Barton II, F.E. and Meyer, R.D. (1985) The use of near infrared reflectance spectroscopy to predict species composition of forage mixtures. *Crop Science* 25, 834–837.

Crocker, R.L. and Tiver, N.S. (1948) Survey methods in grassland ecology. *Journal of the British Grassland Society* 3, 1–26.

Everson, C.S. and Clarke, G.P.Y. (1987) A comparison of six methods of botanical analysis in the montane grasslands of Natal. *Vegetatio* 73, 47–51.

Friedel, M.H., Bastin, G.N. and Griffin, G.F. (1988) Range assessment and monitoring in arid lands: the derivation of functional groups to simplify vegetation data. *Journal of Environmental Management* 27, 85–97.

Gaugh, H.G. (1982) *Multivariate Analysis in Community Ecology.* Cambridge University Press, Cambridge, 298 pp.

Goodall, D.W. (1952) Some considerations in the use of point quadrats for the analysis of vegetation. *Australian Journal of Science* 5, 1–41.

Greig-Smith, P. (1964) *Quantitative Plant Ecology*, 2nd edn. Butterworths Scientific Publications, London, 256 pp.

Grubb, P.J. (1986) Problems posed by sparse and patchily distributed species in species-rich plant communities. In: Diamond, J.M. and Case, T.J. (eds) *Community Ecology.* Harper and Row, New York, pp. 207–225.

Hargreaves, J.N.G. and Kerr, J. (1992) *BOTANAL – A Comprehensive Sampling and Computing Procedure for Estimating Pasture Yield and Composition. 2. Computational Package.* Tropical Agronomy Technical Memorandum No. 79, CSIRO Division of Tropical Crops and Pastures, St Lucia, Queensland, 83 pp.

Haydock, K.P. and Shaw, N.H. (1975) The comparative yield method for estimating dry matter yield of pasture. *Australian Journal of Experimental Agriculture and Animal Husbandry* 15, 663–670.

Henderson, A.E. and Hayman, B.I. (1960) Methods of analysis and the influence of fleece characters on unit area of wool production of Romney lambs. *Australian Journal of Agricultural Research* 11, 851–870.

Jenny, H. (1961) Derivation of state factor equations of soils and ecosystems. *Proceedings of the Soil Science Society of America* 25, 385–388.

Jones, R.M. and Hargreaves, J.N.G. (1979) Improvements to the dry-weight-rank method for measuring botanical composition. *Grass and Forage Science* 34, 181–189.

Kent, M. and Coker, P. (1992) *Vegetation Description and Analysis: a Practical Approach.* Belhaven, London, 363 pp.

Kershaw, K.A. (1964) *Quantitive and Dynamic Ecology.* Edward Arnold, London, 183 pp.

Kira, T., Ogawa, H. and Shinozaki, K. (1953) Intraspecific competition among higher plants. I. Competition–density–yield inter-relationships in regularly dispersed populations. *Journal of the Institute of Polytechnology, Osaka City University Series D* 4, 1–16.

Lamacraft, R.R., Friedel, M.H. and Chewings, V.H. (1983) Comparison of distance based density estimates for some arid rangeland vegetation. *Australian Journal of Ecology* 8, 181–187.

Le Roux, N.P. (1995) Grasslands of Umtamvuna Nature Reserve, KwaZulu-Natal: description and recommendations for monitoring. MSc Agric. thesis, University of Natal, Pietermaritzburg, South Africa.

Levy, E.B. and Madden, E.A. (1933) The point method of pasture analysis. *New Zealand Journal of Agriculture* 46, 267–279.

Lodge, G.M. (1981) The role of plant mass, basal area and density in assessing the herbage mass response to fertility of some perennial grasses. *Australian Rangeland Journal* 3, 92–98.

Lodge, G.M. and Gleeson, A.C. (1982) The importance of plant density, plant basal area and plant mass per unit basal area as factors influencing the herbage mass of some native perennial grasses. *Australian Rangeland Journal* 4, 61–66.

Lodge, G.M., Taylor, J.A. and Whalley, R.D.B. (1981) Techniques for estimating plant basal area and assessing the herbage mass of some native perennial grasses. *Australian Rangeland Journal* 3, 83–91.

Lütge, B.U., Hardy, M.B. and Hatch, G.P. (1998) Soil and sward characteristics of patches and non-patches in the Highland Sourveld of South Africa. *Tropical Grasslands* 32, 64–71.

Magcale-Macandog, D.B. and Whalley, R.D.B. (1991) Distribution of *Microlaena stipoides* and its association with introduced perennial grasses in a permanent pasture on the Northern Tablelands of N.S.W. *Australian Journal of Botany* 39, 295–303.

Mannetje, L. 't (1974) Relations between pasture attributes and liveweight gains on a subtropical pasture. In: *Proceedings of the XII International Grassland Congress.* Moscow, Vol. 3, pp. 299–304.

Mannetje, L. 't and Haydock, K.P. (1963) The dry-weight-rank method for the botanical analysis of pasture. *Journal of the British Grassland Society* 18, 268–275.

McDonald, C.K. and Jones, R.M. (1997) Measuring spatial variation within pastures. In: *Proceedings of the XVIII International Grassland Congress.* Winnipeg and Saskatoon, Canada, Paper 26–1.

McDonald, C.K., Corfield, J.P., Hargreaves, J.N.G. and Toole, J.G. (1996) *BOTANAL – A Comprehensive Sampling and Computing Procedure for Estimating Pasture Yield and Composition. 3. Field Recording Direct to Computer* 2nd edn. Tropical Agronomy Technical Memorandum No. 88, CSIRO Division of Tropical Crops and Pastures, St Lucia, Queensland, 37 pp.

Mentis, M.T. (1981) Evaluation of the wheel-point and step-point methods of veld condition assessment. *Proceedings of the Grassland Society of Southern Africa* 16, 89–94.

Mentis, M.T. (1984) *Monitoring in South African Grasslands*. South African National Scientific Programmes Report No. 91, Council for Scientific and Industrial Research – Foundation for Research Development, Pretoria, 55 pp.

Morrison, D.A., Le Brocque, A.F. and Clarke, P.J. (1995) An assessment of improved techniques for estimating the abundance (frequency) of sedentary organisms. *Vegetatio* 120, 131–145.

Mueller-Dumbois, D. and Ellenberg, H. (1974) *Aims and Methods of Vegetation Ecology*. John Wiley and Sons, New York, 547 pp.

Neuteboom, J.H., Lantinga, E.A. and Loo, E.N. van (1992) The use of frequency estimates in studying sward structure. *Grass and Forage Science* 47, 358–365.

Neuteboom, J.H., Lantinga, E.A. and Struik, P.C. (1998) Evaluation of the dry weight rank method for botanical composition analysis of grassland by means of simulation. *Netherlands Journal of Agricultural Science* 46, 285–304.

Outhred, R.K. (1984) Semi-quantitative sampling in vegetation survey. In: Myers, K., Margules, C.R. and Musto, I. (eds) *Survey Methods for Nature Conservation*. CSIRO, Canberra, pp. 87–100.

Pechanec, J.P. and Pickford, G.D. (1937) A weight estimate method for the determination of range or pasture production. *Journal of the American Society of Agronomy* 29, 894–904.

Pielou, E.C. (1975) *Ecological Diversity*. John Wiley & Sons, New York, 165 pp.

Pitman, W.D., Piacitelli, C.K., Aiken, G.E. and Barton II, F.E. (1991) Botanical composition of tropical grass–legume pastures estimated with near-infrared reflectance spectroscopy. *Agronomy Journal* 83, 103–107.

Robinson, G.G., Whalley, R.D.B. and Taylor, J.A. (1983) The effect of prior history of superphosphate application and stocking rate on faecal and nutrient distribution on grazed natural pastures. *Australian Rangeland Journal* 5, 79–82.

Scheiner, S.M. (1992) Measuring pattern diversity. *Ecology* 73, 1860–1867.

Scott, D. (1993) Constancy in pasture composition? In: *Proceedings of the XVII International Grassland Congress*. New Zealand Grassland Association, Palmerston North, New Zealand, pp. 1604–1606.

Shenk, J.S., Westerhaus, M.O. and Hoover, M.R. (1979) Analysis of forage by infrared reflectance. *Journal of Dairy Science* 62, 807–812.

Shmida, A. (1984) Whittaker's plant diversity sampling method. *Israel Journal of Botany* 33, 41–46.

Specht, R.L., Specht, A., Whelan, M.B. and Hegarty, E.E. (1995) *Conservation Atlas of Plant Communities in Australia*. Centre for Coastal Management, Lismore, New South Wales, 1061 pp.

Taylor, J.A., Hedges, D.A. and Whalley, R.D.B. (1984) The occurrence, distribution and characteristics of sheep camps on the Northern Tablelands of NSW. *Australian Rangeland Journal* 6, 10–16.

Tidmarsh, C.E.M. and Havenga, C.M. (1955) *The Wheel-Point Method of Survey and Measurement of Semi-Open Grasslands and Karoo Vegetation in South Africa*. (Memoir No. 29). Botanical Survey of South Africa, The Government Printer, Pretoria, 49 pp.

Tongway, D.J. and Ludwig, J.A. (1997) The conservation of water and nutrients within landscapes. In: Ludwig, J.A., Tongway, D.J., Freudenberger, D.O., Noble, J.C. and Hodgkinson, K.C. (eds) *Lanscape Ecology: Function and Management*. CSIRO Publishing, Collingwood, New Zealand, pp. 13–22.

Tothill, J.C., Hargreaves, J.N.G., Jones, R.M. and McDonald, C.K. (1992) *BOTANAL – A Comprehensive Sampling and Computing Procedure for Estimating Pasture Yield and Composition. 1. Field Sampling.* Tropical Agronomy Technical Memorandum No. 78, CSIRO Division of Tropical Crops and Pastures, St Lucia, Queensland, 24 pp.

Vickery, P.J., Hill, M.J. and Donald, G.E. (1997) Satellite derived maps of pasture status: association of classification with botanical composition. *Australian Journal of Experimental Agriculture* 37, 547–562.

Wachendorf, M., Ingwersen, B. and Taube, F. (1999) Prediction of the clover content of red clover- and white clover-grass mixtures by near-infrared reflectance spectroscopy. *Grass and Forage Science* 54, 87–90.

Waite, R.B. (1992) The application of visual estimation procedures for monitoring pasture yield and composition in exclosures and small plots. *Tropical Grasslands* 30, 314–318.

Waite, R.B. and Kerr, J.D. (1996) Measuring yields of green leaf blade in pastures by visual estimation techniques. *Tropical Grasslands* 30, 314–318.

Wandera, F.P., Kerridge, P.C., Taylor, J.A. and Shelton, H.M. (1993) Changes in productivity associated with replacement of *Heteropogon contortus* by *Aristida* species and *Chrysopogon fallax* in the savannas of south east Queensland. *Proceedings of the XVII International Grassland Congress.* New Zealand Grassland Association, Palmerston North, New Zealand, pp. 352–353.

Warren Wilson, J. (1963) Errors resulting from thickness of point quadrats. *Australian Journal of Botany* 11, 178–188.

Measuring Sward Structure

E.A. Laca[1] and G. Lemaire[2]

[1]Department of Agronomy and Range Science, University of California, Davis, California, USA; [2]INRA, Station d'Écophysiologie des Plantes Fourragères, Lusignan, France

Introduction

Successful and efficient sward measurements can only be achieved with prior definition of object and purpose, and with proper methods. Thus, three basic questions can be posed. What is sward structure? Why does one measure it? How does one measure it? This chapter approaches sward structure measurements from two broad perspectives: plant growth and grazing.

Sward structure has usually been defined and measured as the distribution and arrangement of above-ground plant parts within a community. Norman and Campbell (1989) defined canopy structure as the 'amount and organization of aboveground plant material'. Traditionally, in studies of both sward growth and grazing, emphasis was put on the characterization of vertical structure within the canopy, with horizontal replications used just to obtain reliable estimates of average community variables such as leaf density per horizontal stratum, or leaf area index.

Usually, sward structure is measured to provide mechanistic explanations for higher-order phenomena such as growth rate, light interception by canopies, susceptibility to pathogens, diet quality and intake rate by herbivores. As intermediary factors that determine ecological and agronomic characteristics of species, which are subject to genetic control, sward structure variables are also measured as objectives for selection. Sward structure is a crucial determinant of primary and secondary productivity of grazed ecosystems; thus, its measurement is necessary for full understanding of these processes. Sward measurements are time consuming and expensive and may be destructive. Therefore, more practical guidelines are necessary to determine when sward structure measurements are required. We identify three experimental situations where measurements of sward structure are imperative: (i) when sward structures are treatments, to corroborate that desired sward structure treatments have been obtained; (ii) when sward structure is the response variable of interest, to test specific hypotheses about differences between treatments; and (iii) when sward structure is hypothesized to be an explanatory factor, to explore cause-and-effect relationships.

Initially, sward structure measurements focused on plant growth and competition. In the 1960s and subsequently, sward measurements were linked to intake rate by grazing animals. Black and Kenney (1984) provided a clear demonstration of the role of sward structure on intake rate of sheep. Using similar approaches, Gross *et al.* (1993) extended the demonstration to multiple species of mammalian herbivores.

This chapter discusses methods to study sward structure with two foci: (i) sward structure is the result of a series of plant morphogenesis parameters, and determines basic tissue and nutrient flow rates in grazed ecosystems; and (ii) both vertical and horizontal patterns of sward structure are relevant because of the limited spatial range of plant–plant interactions, and because large mammalian grazers select forages vertically and horizontally from bite to landscape scales. Given that sward structure can be defined and measured in a potentially infinite number of ways, we take a functional approach and explain the most important aspects of growth and defoliation that shape some definitions and measurements for the study of grassland ecosystems.

Sward Structure and Herbage Growth

Herbage growth can be considered as the result of: (i) acquisition of resources as C and N by individual plants; (ii) use of these resources for growth; and (iii) senescence which leads to accumulation of dead tissues as litter, followed by the recycling of C and N. Sward structure and herbage growth are highly interdependent because structure results from the growth pattern of individual plants within the sward and it affects the rate at which resources are acquired by individual plants and the sward as a whole.

Light interception and herbage growth

Gross herbage production is firstly determined by the amount of light intercepted by the sward. The proportion of incident photosynthetically active radiation (PAR_0) that is absorbed by a sward, i.e. the absorption efficiency (E_a), is determined by sward variables, such as LAI (leaf area index), mean inclination angle of laminae, and optical properties of leaf tissues such as transmittance and reflectance of visible wavelengths. Using the Monsi and Saeki (1953) approach, the relationship between mean daily absorption efficiency (E_a) and the sward LAI is:

$$E_a = K_1(1 - e^{-K_2 LAI})$$ (5.1)

The value of K_1 is determined by the optical properties of leaves. A K_1 value of 0.95 can be used for many species (Varlet-Grancher *et al.*, 1989). Coefficient K_2 is a light extinction coefficient that depends on the geometrical structure of the canopy. A K_2 value of 0.5–0.6 can be used for erect species such as *Festuca arundinacea* (Belanger *et al.*, 1992) and 0.8–0.9 for more horizontal leaves such as *Medicago sativa* (Gosse *et al.*, 1982) or *Digitaria decumbens* (Sinoquet and Cruz, 1993).

Absorption efficiency E_a can be measured directly using sunfleck ceptometers (Decagon Devices Inc., Pullman, Washington, USA) placed at the top of the canopy (incident PAR, or PAR_0) and at soil level (transmitted PAR, or PAR_t). The difference between PAR_0 and PAR_t represents the intercepted PAR, or PAR_i. For the determination of the absorbed PAR (PAR_a), it is necessary to measure the quantity of PAR reflected by the sward (PAR_r) by using the same ceptometer above the canopy but facing the soil. E_a can be calculated as follows:

$$E_a = PAR_a / PAR_0 = (PAR_0 - PAR_t - PAR_r) / PAR_0$$ (5.2)

E_a can be estimated instantaneously and therefore its value depends on sun elevation and the proportion of diffuse and direct radiation. Canopy structure can have an important impact on instantaneous light absorption efficiency. Usually E_a is averaged during the day and then canopy structure has less impact. If only instantaneous measurement of E_a can be made, it is best done at midday during the period of maximum incident PAR in order to better represent average daily absorption efficiency.

Using the approach of Monteith (1972), it is possible to relate directly the sum of above-ground biomass produced daily (dW/dt) in a sward during a given period to the sum of PAR absorbed daily (PAR_a) by the crop during the same period:

$$\Sigma(dW / dt) = a\Sigma(PAR_a) = a\Sigma(E_a PAR_0)$$ (5.3)

The coefficient a represents the radiation use efficiency (RUE) of the sward, which is relatively constant throughout a regrowth period (Gosse *et al.*, 1986; Belanger *et al.*, 1992). For most temperate grass species, RUE with non-limiting N nutrition in the absence of water stress is about 2.0 g dry matter (DM) MJ^{-1} PAR (Belanger *et al.*, 1992). For tropical grasses, values of RUE of 2.2–2.5 g DM MJ^{-1} are common (Sinoquet and Cruz, 1993). However, use of Equation 5.3 for herbage growth analysis requires an estimation of how light absorption and light use efficiency of the sward vary according to environmental constraints (N nutrition level, water stress and temperature).

In the absence of direct measurements of E_a, it is possible to use Equation 5.1 to estimate the daily efficiency of light absorption. This requires determination of LAI of the sward and estimation of the light extinction coefficient K_2, which reflects sward geometrical structure (mean leaf angle). Methods for estimating LAI have to be appropriate for the research objectives. For growth analysis of monospecific swards, use of Equations 5.1, 5.2 and 5.3 does not require sophisticated analysis of the sward structure; a simple destructive determination of total LAI should be sufficient.

The estimation of the extinction coefficient of Equation 5.3 requires more attention. For the majority of temperate grasses published values of K_2 (e.g. Belanger *et al.*, 1992) provide relative convergent estimates which can be confidently used for evaluating the daily efficiency of light absorption, because integration of E_a throughout the day makes the influence of canopy structure less important.

When the objective is to describe competition for light between different species in a complex sward, the use of a multilayer representation of the sward becomes necessary. The geometrical structure of a mixed canopy can be described by vertical distribution of leaves and leaf angle for each species involved (Nassiri *et al.*, 1996). Density of leaf area (LAD) in each canopy layer is then used to calculate light profiles and absorption of light by each species (Kropff, 1993). However, in grass–clover mixtures it is necessary to obtain the relationship between plant height and LAD in order to allow for differences in leaf area distribution between the two species (Faurie *et al.*, 1996). The inclined point quadrat method (Warren-Wilson, 1960, 1963) remains the best available method to obtain values for leaf area density, leaf dispersion, leaf angle distribution and extinction coefficient for each species present in each of the 5 cm layers of a mixed canopy. Using these values in a light extinction model, it is therefore possible to estimate the proportion of incident PAR absorbed by each species of a grass–clover mixture (Nassiri, 1998).

Plant morphogenesis and herbage growth

Plant morphogenesis can be defined as the dynamics of appearance and expansion of plant form in space (Chapman and Lemaire, 1993). It can be expressed in terms of rate of appearance and expansion in size of new plant organs and their rate of senescence. For grasses, as shown by Lemaire and Chapman (1996), relationships can be found between the three main morphogenetic characteristics of leaf appearance rate (LAR), leaf elongation rate (LER) and leaf life span (LLS), and the main sward structural characteristics of mature leaf size, maximum number of leaves per tiller and tiller density. Thus, two swards can have the same LAI and the same growth potential but very different canopy structures, possibly leading to different rates of herbage intake by herbivores. LAR plays a central role because of its direct influence on sward structure. Plant species with high LAR tend to produce swards with higher tiller density and larger tillers than species with low LAR.

Measurement of LAR is done by labelling tillers (Davies, 1993). A very satisfactory field method consists of randomly marking tillers with plastic-coated wire and recording the number of leaves that emerge on each tiller during a given period of time. The emergence of leaves can be recorded as emerging leaves or as fully developed leaves. The rate of leaf appearance is more often expressed by its reciprocal, the phyllochrone, which represents the time elapsed between the appearance of two successive leaves on the same tiller. Because of the strong influence of temperature on leaf appearance rate, the phyllochrone is usually expressed in degree-days. As discussed by Davies (1993), the precision in the determination of LAR depends on length of time between observations and on the number of tillers marked. For clover or lucerne plants, LAR is recorded on the main shoot axis as the number of leaves reaching a given leaf development stage during a given period of time.

Measurement of LER can be obtained by recording the length of every leaf on marked tillers on two successive dates. Length is measured between the tip of a leaf and the ligule of the preceding leaf. LER can be calculated at individual leaf level as the difference in leaf length divided by the time elapsed between two successive measurements. Another expression of LER at individual tiller level can be obtained as the sum of the length increments of all leaves (Gastal *et al.*, 1992). In general, the measurement of LER is associated with the measurement of LAR and can be performed on the same tiller. The use of a Linear Variable Differential Transducer allows the recording of ontogenic variation of elongation of individual leaves (Gallagher *et al.*, 1976). This allows the determination of duration of the elongation of an individual leaf (leaf elongation duration, LED). Thus the variation in mature leaf length, which is an important sward structural characteristic, can be analysed in terms of variation in LER and/or in LED.

Leaf senescence flux is one of the major components of leaf tissue turnover and determines herbage use efficiency in grazed swards (Lemaire and Chapman, 1996). The proportion of leaf tissues lost by senescence in continuously grazed swards is greatly determined by the average leaf life span (Mazzanti and Lemaire, 1994). Therefore, determination of the effects of environmental and management variables on LLS for the main species within a sward can be an important objective for grazing studies. Chapman and Lemaire (1993) described a method for *in situ* determination of the leaf life span on labelled tillers as the time elapsed between the accumulation of new leaf tissues and the accumulation of the dead leaf tissues after a defoliation. Duru *et al.* (1997) developed this method for comparing leaf life span of different monocotyledonous and dicotyledonous species. Such a determination of leaf life span can be made on the same marked tiller sample used for LAR and LER determination, so the dynamics of accumulation of dead leaf material in a sward, which constitutes an important parameter of sward structure, can be directly determined by tissue turnover techniques.

Sward Structure and Grazing

Vertical sward structure and grazing

In homogeneous swards, where no vertical or horizontal selection by the grazing animal takes place, bite dimensions result from the interaction of sward height, stiffness of plant units, and harvesting behaviour of the animal. Bite weight and sward susceptibility to defoliation cannot be predicted only on the basis of herbage mass; both sward height and density must be taken into account. These structural sward characteristics are related to LAI, which in turn determines light absorption and herbage growth. Thus, the vertical distribution of LAI influences both growth and rate of tissue removal by grazing animals.

Correlations between variables such as amount or proportion of green leaf in the grazed horizon and diet quality and quantity of grazers improve with increasing sward heterogeneity (O'Reagain and Oven-Smith, 1996). The presence of stems and pseudostems can hinder the bite formation process; thus, spatial distribution and height of these organs are important determinants of defoliation. Tropical swards and bunchgrasses can generally exhibit a high degree of heterogeneity in terms of vertical and horizontal distribution of quality and quantity of forage. Thus, it is likely that bite formation processes in these swards are more complex than in temperate swards. Nevertheless, empirical studies confirm the positive relationships between distribution of green leaf laminae in the canopy, bite weight and intake rate.

Horizontal sward structure and grazing

Competition among plants and forage selection by herbivores are strongly influenced by horizontal patterns in the sward. Bergelson (1990) showed that *Senecio vulgaris* has a greater population growth rate when planted among clumped *Poa annua* than when planted among randomly distributed *P. annua*, because the clumped distribution promotes intra vs. interspecific competition. However, *S. vulgaris* planted among *P. annua* clumps was more susceptible to herbivore damage. Sheep are able to more than double the selectivity for clover over grass when grass and clover are planted in strips instead of mixed together (Clark and Harris, 1985; Ridout and Robson, 1991). The evidence indicates that both plant community dynamics and herbivore strategy depend on horizontal structure.

Typically, grasslands are spatially heterogeneous because resources are patchy and plant characteristics differ among patches. Grasslands with the same total herbage mass and botanical composition can vary widely in horizontal spatial structure. Ramet size and density are important sward structure characteristics that vary over space (for definition of ramet see Chapter 6). Under conditions of limiting light, short dense ramets may be competitively inferior to tall sparse ones. However, tall tillers are more easily consumed by livestock, and tend to be more susceptible to lack of water (Coughenour, 1985). Although some tropical species may escape grazing damage after they exceed a certain height, they must go through the susceptible intermediate stages. This view does not negate the fact that susceptibility of tillers to herbivore damage depends not only on absolute and relative tiller dimensions but also on absolute and relative nutritional quality and palatability.

Experimental results and models illustrate the need to take into account horizontal heterogeneity to explain observed variation in aggregated measures of bite weight and intake rate (Ungar and Noy-Meir, 1988). Therefore, intake rate and feeding behaviour should be influenced more by the selected areas than by the sward as a whole. Penning *et al.* (1991) found that animals grazing clover were not completely restricted by average sward height as it declined, because they always had distinct ungrazed areas available. Bite weight in clover swards reflected height of the selected patches, and was not related to average sward height.

The importance of vegetation heterogeneity in determining grazing behaviour and intake poses new practical and theoretical questions. The definition of heterogeneity and ways of measuring it must be relevant to the herbivore–plant interaction. Degree of heterogeneity is strictly dependent on the scale at which it is measured. From the animal's point of view, heterogeneity depends on the scale at which the forager perceives its environment, and on the scale at which it can perform its behaviours (Laca and Ortega, 1996). From the point of view of the plant, heterogeneity is important at scales ranging from the area of direct influence of individual plants to distances involved in dispersal of propagules.

Measuring Sward Structure in Three Dimensions

We classify methods depending on whether they focus on vertical or horizontal structure. Under vertical structure, we consider both vertical distribution of characteristics and overall sward structure at a point on the horizontal plane. Under horizontal structure we consider methods to detect spatial patterns of characteristics determined by vertical structure methods. Usually, vertical patterns are assumed to be predictable gradients, whereas horizontal patterns can range from uniform to random to patchy at multiple scales. These assumptions are reflected in the organization of the following sections of this chapter.

Vertical structure

Clipping methods

LAI can be estimated from *in situ*, non-destructive methods, or from destructive harvests. Destructive measurements require harvesting of above-ground biomass on a given area and subsampling on a fresh or dry weight basis, for determination of the leaf area:plant mass ratio (LAR) using an appropriate leaf area meter[1]. This is very time consuming and subject to large sampling variation that necessitates many measurements. LAI is calculated as the product of sward mass (W), determined on harvested quadrats, and sward leaf area ratio determined on subsamples. Because of the generally negative allometric relationship between LAR and the standing sward biomass (Duru *et al.*, 1997; Lemaire and Gastal, 1997) these two variables are not independent. Therefore, variations in sward mass could be compensated partly by inverse variations in LAR leading to a reduced variation in LAI. It is important to reduce errors in measuring LAR. Reduction of subsampling error requires careful mixing of harvested material and adequate definition of subsample size in order to optimize time requirements vs. precision. The shortest possible delay between harvesting and leaf area determination reduces errors by avoiding leaf rolling due to water loss.

Vertical distribution of plant parts, species, etc. can be determined by stratified clipping. This is a comprehensive and time-consuming method. The main problem with this method is to maintain all elements of the canopy in place during and after clipping. If plant parts are not secured in place before clipping, pieces of laminae that normally hang into lower horizons will either fall to the bottom or be collected with the material in higher horizons. Barthram (1992) devised a pliers-like instrument to clamp a thin and long section of canopy in place for later separation of horizons by clipping. This method seems to be quite successful. A similar technique consists of clamping the canopy on a small circular or square area (e.g. 10×10 cm) by hand and wrapping it with paper into a tight cylinder (E.A. Laca, California, 1990, unpublished). This cylinder can later be sliced with a sharp knife into the desired horizons. A good description and references for earlier stratified clipping methods can be found in Rhodes (1981).

Point quadrat

The point quadrat technique (Warren-Wilson, 1960, 1963) is widely used. Although clever and extremely useful, improvements over the original

---

[1] Delta-T Devices, or LI-COR Inc.

method are based on the same principles, whereby amount of foliage, LAI, mean leaf angle and other canopy characteristics can be calculated as a function of number of contacts between canopy elements and a straight line (point quadrat) that penetrates the canopy. As a non-destructive method, the point quadrat technique has the advantage that successive determinations can be made on the same site. This enables more precise analyses of sward dynamics and spatial variation of light penetration.

The point quadrat technique has many potential pitfalls, but when used properly it can be accurate and precise. Use of a single angle of point quadrat pins of 32.5° leads to an estimate of sward LAI to within ± 10%, while the use of two measurement angles of 13° and 52° allows a precision of ± 2% (Grant, 1993). Rhodes (1981) offered a good review of the advantages and limitations of this method. Some of the limitations of this technique stem from the following:

- Needles are not true points but have a certain thickness.
- Ground may be sloping or uneven, thus presenting the question of whether to orient the quadrats with respect to the horizontal or to the ground.
- Foliage orientation is not random, particularly in species that exhibit clear solar tracking such as some legumes.
- Detection and identification of contacts without disturbing the canopy may be impossible.
- The method is extremely time consuming.

Caldwell *et al.* (1983) designed an automated fibre-optic point quadrat system that increases accuracy, eliminates subjectivity in recognition of contacts, and reduces time costs of the sampling process. The system uses a very precise infrared beam mounted on a steel rod that is driven into the canopy by an automatic motor. When the tip of the rod gets within 1 mm of a plant part the beam is reflected and sensed by the rod, and the motor stops. The operator records plant part, species and height of the contact, then restarts the motor that drives the rod. This system is approximately twice as rapid as the conventional point quadrat with motor-driven pins.

Foliage orientation methods

Foliage orientation is defined by two angles: leaf inclination (angle between perpendicular to the leaf and the vertical) and azimuth (angle between horizontal projection of main leaf axis and north). Overall orientation is described by the proportion of the total leaf area (or leaf area within a stratum) that has a certain inclination and azimuth. For simplicity, inclination and azimuth can be partitioned into classes (Norman and Campbell, 1989). Measurements of orientation can be extremely time consuming and subject to errors. The most commonly used instrument is a hand-held compass-protractor that measures both angles simultaneously. At least 1000 randomly selected measurements are considered necessary.

However, Moran *et al.* (1989) were able to detect differences in lucerne foliage orientation due to water stress by measuring 12–16 leaflets in each of two plots in a treatment.

Light transmission methods

A more recent non-destructive method to estimate LAI has been developed from analysis of light transmission through the canopy. Canopy gap fraction analysis (Welles and Norman, 1991) is conceptually similar to point quadrat analysis in the sense that light replaces pins. The proportion of sky visible through the canopy at various angles can be measured by either a fisheye (Bonhomme and Chartier, 1972) or a linear light sensor (Walker *et al.*, 1988) and is mathematically converted to LAI (Campbell and Norman, 1989). This indirect estimation of LAI implies that leaves are randomly distributed in the canopy and have a random azimuth orientation, which is usual for grasslands. The LAI-2000 Plant Canopy Analyser[2] allows the measurement of the canopy gap fraction by using a filtered sensor with limited view angles. This commercial system provides an estimation of the LAI and mean leaf angle. These two parameters can be measured rapidly on several sites to take their spatial variation into account, and the measures can be repeated at exactly the same places to study the dynamics of leaf area development. Nevertheless, the size of the probe may cause disturbance to the sward, limiting its use to tall canopies and making it unsuitable for very short and dense swards.

Near-infrared reflectance (NIR) methods

An alternative method of LAI estimation uses near-infrared reflectance. This method is based on the difference between absorption and reflectance of light of green leaves in the visible (400–700 nm) and NIR (700–2000 nm) ranges and is used in remote sensing studies for calculation of ground cover. Allirand *et al.* (1997) found that a simple portable sensor which directly measures the red/far-red ratio[3] of the reflected radiation allowed rapid estimation of LAI. But the signal has to be calibrated to allow for variation in the reflectance of bare soil and dead leaf litter due to change in humidity. Moreover, the signal saturates as the LAI becomes higher than 2 or 3 and such a method has to be restricted to periods of leaf area expansion, just after sowing or severe defoliation.

Laser methods

Denison and Russotti (1997) combined the inclined-point quadrat with laser-induced chlorophyll fluorescence to develop an instrument that automatically measures LAI of green leaves and other tissues. The instrument

---

[2] LI-COR Inc., Lincoln, Nebraska, USA
[3] Skye Instruments SKR 110

can read both laser angle and first hit on green leaves under most light and weather conditions. Unlike the point quadrat, the laser only detects whether a leaf has been hit or not, but does not indicate the vertical location of the leaf in the canopy. Tests with sudan grass, wheat and maize showed good correlations ($r^2 = 0.76$ to 0.98, slope $= 0.93$ to 1.02) between laser and harvest estimates of LAI. This instrument has a great potential to facilitate measurements of green LAI and its relationship with pasture growth and consumption by herbivores. The fact that it is fast and that it can be fully automated will increase workers' ability to consider spatial and temporal patterns of sward condition in grazing studies. Denison (1997) presented a theoretical analysis of the sources and magnitude of error by using this technique. Non-random leaf arrangements and crops in rows tend to increase error, but under such conditions errors can be maintained below 15% by using an appropriate range of azimuth angles for the laser beam.

Horizontal structure

The structure or pattern along the horizontal dimensions can be a key determinant of animal strategies and plant community dynamics. Spatial heterogeneity is a multidimensional and complex concept. We focus, for example, on spatial patterns of botanical composition, quantity of herbage removed and proportion of plants killed by disturbances on a horizontal plane.

Because of its complexity and relatively new emphasis, spatial heterogeneity and the associated terminology are not fully defined, though some definitions can be found in Kolasa and Rollo (1991) and Turner and Gardner (1991). In this chapter the following terms and concepts are used:

- Spatial heterogeneity is the presence of different values of a given vegetation descriptor measured in different locations at (practically) the same time.
- Grain size is the resolution or finest level of measurement in a study.
- Extent is the area encompassed by the study.

Spatial heterogeneity is scale dependent (i.e. it varies with grain size). For example, the botanical composition of a grassland can be highly heterogeneous when measured with a small quadrat, but homogeneous when measured with a larger one, because the larger quadrat may always include very similar proportions of small patches (Palmer, 1988). Natural spatial variability is characterized by different degrees of heterogeneity at different scales (Palmer, 1988). Typically, spatial variance increases with increasing resolution and extent of the measurements (O'Neill *et al.*, 1991).

Identification of the scales at which ecosystems show heterogeneity is essential for understanding and identifying underlying ecological processes. Patch size, for example, reflects scale of heterogeneity. Many quantitative techniques are available for description of spatial pattern and test of hypotheses (Legendre and Fortin, 1989; Turner and Gardner, 1991). This chapter concentrates on intermediate scales relative to plant size (10^{-1} m to 10 m). Competition and defoliation are most important at these scales, which are defined by the size of the plants, their dispersal radius and the foraging mechanisms that determine ungulate selectivity from bites to feeding sites.

Pattern, scale and sampling

Whereas the study of vertical structure focuses on techniques used to measure sward attributes at different heights on a given location, the study of horizontal structure focuses on sampling, recording locations (geo-referencing) and analysis techniques to detect and quantify horizontal arrangements of the different vertical structures. This quantification goes beyond the documentation of spatial variance. Measurements for eco-logical and nutritional assessment of pasture and rangelands should be performed with at least a minimum consideration of spatial sampling requirements, and should be geo-referenced. Thus, data obtained will allow the traditional mean-based assessment, as well as determination of patchiness of quantity and quality of forages.

Spatial variance is not equivalent to pattern. The same amount of spa-tial variance in sward vertical structure can theoretically be arranged in an infinite number of patterns. Thus, a variety of horizontal patterns can be identified and quantified. Palmer (1988, 1992) presented enlightening summaries of some of the dimensions of spatial variability. In the context of sward structure, pattern and scale are important because the effects of aver-age values and variance of variables such as LAI or sward height are strictly dependent on spatial distribution. Light penetration, photosynthesis response to light, plant competition, functional response of herbivores and other ecological processes that depend on LAI and herbage mass are non-linear. Therefore, one should not expect the same overall responses from a sward where patches of high and low LAI are finely interspersed as from swards where leaf area-saturated patches are separated by large gaps. The same rationale applies for almost all sward characteristics.

Results of measurements of sward structure depend on scale. Scale is given by the extent and resolution (grain) of the method used. Methods that have low resolution, such as stratified clipping with lawn mowers (using different size wheels), have smaller variance than hand clipping or point quadrats, but may average over the spatial scale within which animals select forages, thus masking the options perceived by the forager. Explicit consid-eration of resolution and extent of the study in relation to potential sward structure methods is crucial. Usually, high-resolution methods are time consuming and expensive, and thus limit the extent of measurements. Some methods, such as point quadrat, clipping, leaf protractors and sward stick (Barthram, 1986), yield values that represent very small areas of the canopy (high resolution) in the order of $10^{-2} - 1\ m^2$. Other methods give readings that already integrate sward characteristics over areas in the order of $1–10^2\ m^2$, such as small mowers, laser-based LAI methods and light transmission methods. Common remote sensing methods have resolutions coarser than $10^2\ m^2$.

Whereas the resolution of the selected method sets the maximum resolution feasible, the actual resolution of spatial patterns that can be measured depends on the spatial sampling scheme. As a rule of thumb, sampling resolution is at least three times the distance between adjacent sampling locations. Thus, if sampling locations are 1 m apart, the smallest patches and patterns detectable are larger than 3 m. Samples can be placed on transects or grids, with a random component to avoid potential pitfalls of systematic arrangements. Spatial sampling is a complex field beyond the scope of this chapter.

Geo-referencing

Assessment of spatial patterns requires that locations of all measurements be recorded. These locations can be identified in relation to an arbitrary origin, such as a permanent stake or landmark, or in real-world coordinates. Global positioning systems (GPS) allow efficient recording of coordinates, but for most studies where the necessary resolution is less than 5 m, the cost of the equipment can be high, particularly if it is necessary to navigate to positions predetermined by a sampling scheme with a random component. In this case, the GPS approach would require real-time differential correction. Even so, navigation would be extremely time consuming. The best solution would involve a uniform grid to which random components are added as deviations from known nodes.

Geo-referencing can be greatly facilitated by using less expensive GPS in conjunction with traditional and new surveying equipment. New range meters[4] do not require special reflectors or need to occupy the location whose position is being determined. E.A. Laca and Jeffrey S. Fehmi (California, 1998, unpublished data) have used these range meters to record locations grazed by livestock within 1 m without any disturbance to the animals. The same instrument was used to navigate to the recorded locations to measure characteristics of the sward in the selected areas. The ability to download the information from the laser instrument to a laptop computer permitted simultaneous recording of position, time and grazing behaviour.

---

[4] For example, Criterium 300, Laser Technoplogy Inc., Engelwood, Colarado. http://www.lasertech.com/

Measurement and analysis of horizontal structure

Goals for analyses of horizontal vegetation structure in one or two dimensions can be classified into four categories (Legendre and Fortin, 1989): (i) detection of presence of spatial auto-correlation or structure in the sward; (ii) description of spatial structure; (iii) test of causal models that include space as a predictor; and (iv) estimation of values in unmeasured sites and mapping.

Legendre and Fortin (1989) and Turner and Gardner (1991) gave excellent overviews of the many techniques available to accomplish these goals. Rossi *et al.* (1992) presented an in-depth, accessible explanation of geostatistical tools for studying spatial structure, and Palmer (1988) offered clear explanation of the use of fractal geometry to describe spatial patterns of plant communities. In this section some of the methods are briefly described. The choice of method depends on the goals of the analysis, nature of the spatial pattern detected, nature and spatial distribution of sampling units, and whether the data are uni- or multivariate (Turner and Gardner, 1991). Auto-correlation, spectral analysis and blocking techniques are best suited for patterns that repeat in space, whereas semi-variance and moving-window analyses are suitable for non-uniform patterns. Depending on the scope of the analysis, some of these methods require that the data be stationary, with constant mean and variance over space. Stationarity can be achieved by statistically removing polynomial or other trends. All methods of spatial analysis require numerous samples. As a rule of thumb, auto-correlation and semi-variance should not be used when there are fewer than 30 pairs of points available for a given distance between points.

Auto-correlation can be calculated as Moran's I (Legendre and Fortin, 1989), a statistic that is conceptually similar to Pearson's correlation coefficient. Moran's I can be calculated for each of a series of distances classes, and indicates whether sward structure at a point or quadrat is statistically dependent on values at points located at a given distance. The best way to describe patterns with Moran's I is to construct a correlogram, a graph of I vs. distance. Characteristic shapes of the correlogram are associated with specific types of spatial structure, but the relationship is not one-to-one (Legendre and Fortin, 1989). Thus, it is theoretically possible for more than one type of spatial structure to yield the same correlogram. Yet, comparison of empirical correlograms with correlograms generated from simulated spatial patterns can be used to test for presence of a specific pattern. A complete discussion of the use of correlograms to study spatial patterns is given by Legendre and Fortin (1989).

Semi-variance is the average of squared differences between all possible points separated by a given distance. When points at a given distance are independent, semi-variance equals the overall variance in the data set, which indicates a random pattern at the given spatial scale. As with auto-correlation coefficients, semi-variance is best inspected as a semi-variogram showing the log of semi-variance as a function of log of distance. The pattern of change of semi-variance vs. distance can suggest intensity and scale of patchiness of the vegetation (Palmer, 1988). Slope of the semi-variogram is related to the fractal dimension of the spatial pattern at each scale. A slope near zero evinces a fractal dimension of 2.0 (for transect data), and indicates that spatial pattern at that scale is random or homogeneous. An intermediate slope that yields a fractal dimension between 1.0 and 2.0 indicates patchiness, whereas a steeper slope and a fractal dimension of 1.0 indicates a predictable trend. Fractograms that convey similar information can be constructed on the basis of semi-variograms or by direct calculation of fractal dimensions.

Neuteboom *et al.* (1992) used the relationship between frequency of plant absence and quadrat radius to describe the structure of swards. As quadrat size declines, the proportion of quadrats without plants (absence frequency) approaches the proportion of bare ground in the sward. In a manner conceptually similar to the variogram, the pattern of decrease in absence frequency with increasing quadrat radius reflects the spatial pattern of gaps and plants. As with correlograms, different spatial patterns can yield the same absence frequency curve, thus derivation of definite numbers of gaps of a given size can be misleading. This absence frequency method has the advantage of being faster than the point quadrat method and it yields more complete information about the openness of the sward.

Spectral analysis is particularly suitable for detection of multiple scale patterns that repeat over space. The total spatial variance is partitioned into sinusoidal components. This method requires large data sets with equally spaced points and does not allow for missing values. Spectral analysis is not suitable for aperiodic patterns. Non-uniform aperiodic data can be inspected by wavelet analysis, a method related to spectral analysis.

Studying horizontal spatial patterns of swards is extremely time consuming because of the large number of samples necessary to compute spatial statistics, particularly when direct measurements of vertical sward structure are desired at each sampling point. This difficulty can be partially surmounted by double-sampling (Bonham, 1989) and similar methods that combine precise, time-consuming techniques (e.g. clipping, point quadrat) with faster correlated measurements (e.g. visual estimation, remote sensing) in a subset of points. A larger number of points is surveyed with the faster techniques and those attributes that are difficult to measure are derived on the basis of relationships established from the subset of points measured by both methods.

Conclusion

Sward structure is a determinant of plant growth, community dynamics, grazing and production processes. Measurement of sward structure is not an essential component of all experimentation on grasslands but may be desirable or even essential when seeking to understand underlying processes. Methods to measure it should be designed and chosen on the basis of specific hypotheses or research questions. A variety of techniques is available to determine vertical canopy structure at a point or sample area. Usually, the accuracy and precision of the data obtained are in direct relation to effort and cost of the method used. However, novel modifications of traditional methods have significantly increased sampling efficiency and reduced costs. We emphasize the importance of considering both vertical and horizontal structure of swards, because both are essential determinants of plant growth, competition and herbivory processes. Non-linear relationships between resource availability and trophic processes are pervasive. Thus, one should expect differences in productivity, stability and dynamics of plant and animal communities when vertical and horizontal patterns are different, even if all average sward characteristics are similar.

Acknowledgement

This work is partially based on research supported by grant IS-2331-93C from US–Israel Binational Fund for Agricultural Research and Development, and award 9701033 from NRI Competitive Grants Program/USDA to EAL.

References

Allirand, J.M., Chartier, M., Andrieu, B., Gosse, G., Varlet-Grancher, C. and Coulmier, D. (1997) Estimation de faibles indices foliaires d'une culture de luzerne par mesure de reflectance hemisphérique dans le rouge clair (660 nm) et le rouge sombre (730 nm). *Agronomie* 17, 83–95.

Barthram, G.T. (1986) Experimental techniques: the HFRO sward stick. In: *Biennial Report 1984–85*. Hill Farming Research Organisation, Penicuik, UK, pp. 29–30.

Barthram, G.T. (1992) New equipment for determining the vertical distribution of herbage mass in pastures. In: *Proceedings, Third BGS Research Conference, British Grassland Society, September 1992*. British Grassland Society, Reading, UK, pp. 17–18.

Belanger, G., Gastal, F. and Lemaire, G. (1992) Growth analysis of a tall fescue sward fertilized with different rates of nitrogen. *Crop Science* 32, 1371–1376.

Bergelson, J. (1990) Spatial patterning in plants: opposing effects of herbivory and competition. *Journal of Ecology* 78, 937–948.

Black, J.L. and Kenney, P.A. (1984) Factors affecting diet selection by sheep: II. Height and density of pasture. *Australian Journal of Agricultural Research* 35, 565–578.

Bonham, C.D. (1989) *Measurements for Terrestrial Vegetation*. Wiley, New York, 338 pp.

Bonhomme, R. and Chartier, P. (1972) The interpretation and automatic measurement of hemispherical photographs to obtain sunlit foliage area and gap frequency. *Israel Journal of Agricultural Research* 22, 53–61.

Caldwell, M.M., Harris, G.W. and Dzurec, R.S. (1983) A fiber optic point quadrat system for improved accuracy in vegetation sampling. *Oecologia* 59, 417–418.

Campbell, G.S. and Norman, J.M. (1989) The description and measurement of plant canopy structure. In: Russell, G., Mashall, B. and Jarvis, P.G. (eds) *Plant Canopies: Their Growth, Form and Function.* Society of Experimental Biology, Cambridge, UK, pp. 1–19.

Chapman, D.F. and Lemaire, G. (1993) Morphogenetic and structural determinants of plant regrowth after defoliation. In: Baker, M.J. (ed.) *Grasslands for Our World.* SIR Publishing, Wellington, New Zealand, pp. 55–64.

Clark, D.A. and Harris, P.S. (1985) Composition of the diet of sheep grazing swards of differing white clover content and spatial distribution. *New Zealand Journal of Agricultural Research* 28, 233–240.

Coughenour, M.B. (1985) Graminoid responses to grazing by large herbivores: adaptations, exaptations, and interacting processes. *Annals of the Missouri Botanical Garden* 72, 852–863.

Davies, A. (1993) Tissue turn-over in swards. In: Davies, A., Baker, R.D., Grant, S.A. and Laidlaw, A.S. (eds) *Sward Measurement Handbook.* British Grassland Society, Reading, UK, pp. 183–215.

Denison, R. (1997) Minimizing errors in LAI estimates from laser-probe inclined-point quadrats. *Field Crops Research* 51, 231–240.

Denison, R. and Russotti, R. (1997) Field estimates of green leaf area index using laser-induced chlorophyll fluorescence. *Field Crops Research* 52, 143–149.

Duru, M., Lemaire, G. and Cruz, P. (1997) The nitrogen requirement of major agricultural crops: grasslands. In: Lemaire, G. (ed.) *Diagnosis of Nitrogen Status in Crops.* Springer-Verlag, Heidelberg, pp. 59–72.

Faurie, O., Soussana, J.F. and Sinoquet, H. (1996) Radiation interception, partitioning and use in grass–clover mixtures. *Annals of Botany* 77, 35–45.

Gallagher, J.N., Biscoe, P.V. and Safell, R.A. (1976) A sensitive auxanometer for field use. *Journal of Experimental Botany* 27, 704–716.

Gastal, F., Belanger, G. and Lemaire, G. (1992) A model of leaf extension rate of tall fescue in response to nitrogen and temperature. *Annals of Botany* 70, 437–442.

Gosse, G., Chartier, M., Varlet-Grancher, C. and Bonhomme, R. (1982) Interception du rayonnement utile à la photosynthèse chez la luzerne: variations et modelisation. *Agronomie* 2, 583–588.

Gosse, G., Varlet-Grancher, C., Bonhomme, R., Chartier, M., Allirand, J.M. and Lemaire, G. (1986) Production maximale de matière sèche et rayonnement solaire intercepté par un couvert végétal. *Agronomie* 6, 47–56.

Grant, S.A. (1993) Resource description: vegetation and sward components. In: Davies, A., Baker, R.D., Grant, S.A. and Laidlaw, A.S. (eds) *Sward Measurement Handbook.* British Grassland Society, Reading, UK, pp. 69–97.

Gross, J.E., Shipley, L.A., Hobbs, N.T., Spalinger, D.E. and Wunder, B.A. (1993) Functional response of herbivores in food-concentrated patches: tests of a mechanistic model. *Ecology* 74, 778–791.

Kolasa, J. and Rollo, C.D. (1991) Introduction: the heterogeneity of heterogeneity: a glossary. In: Kolasa, J. and Pickett, S.T.A. (eds) *Ecological Heterogeneity.* Ecological Studies 86, Springer-Verlag, New York, pp. 1–23.

Kropff, M.J. (1993) Mechanisms of competition for light. In: Kropff, M.J. and Laar, H.H. van (eds) *Modelling Crop–Weed Interactions*. CAB International, Wallingford, UK, pp. 33–61.

Laca, E.A. and Ortega, I.M. (1996) Integrating foraging mechanisms across spatial and temporal scales. In: West, N.E. (ed.) *Fifth International Rangeland Congress*. Society for Range Management, Salt Lake City, Utah, pp. 129–132.

Legendre, P. and Fortin, M.J. (1989) Spatial pattern and ecological analysis. *Vegetatio* 80, 107–138.

Lemaire, G. and Chapman, D. (1996) Tissue flows in grazed plant communities. In: Hodgson, J. and Illius, A.W. (eds) *The Ecology and Management of Grazing Systems*. CAB International, Wallingford, UK, pp. 3–36.

Lemaire, G. and Gastal, F. (1997) On the critical N concentration in agricultural crops. 1. N uptake and distribution in plant canopies. In: Lemaire, G. (ed.) *Diagnosis of the Nitrogen Status in Crops*. Springer-Verlag, Heidelberg, pp. 3–34.

Mazzanti, A. and Lemaire, G. (1994) The effect of nitrogen fertilisation on herbage production of tall fescue swards continuously grazed by sheep. 2. Consumption and efficiency of herbage utilisation. *Grass and Forage Science* 49, 352–359.

Monsi, M. and Saeki, T. (1953) Uber den Lichtfaktor in den Planaegesellshaften und seiner Bedeutung für die Stoff Produktion. *Japanese Journal of Botany* 14, 22–52.

Monteith, J.L. (1972) Solar radiation and productivity in tropical ecosystems. *Journal of Applied Ecology* 9, 747–766.

Moran, M.S., Pinter, P.J., Clothier, B.E. and Allen, S.G. (1989) Effect of water stress on the canopy architecture and spectral indices of irrigated alfalfa. *Remote Sensing of Environment* 29, 251–261.

Nassiri, M. (1998) Modelling interactions in grass–clover mixtures. PhD thesis, University of Wageningen, The Netherlands.

Nassiri, M., Elgersma, A. and Lantinga, E.A. (1996) Vertical distribution of leaf area, dry matter and radiation in grass–clover mixtures. In: Parente, G., Frame, J. and Orsi, S. (eds) *Grassland and Land Use System. Proceedings of the 16th General Meeting of the European Grassland Federation*, Grado, pp. 269–274.

Neuteboom, J.H., Lantinga, E.A. and Van Loo, E.N. (1992) The use of frequency estimates in studying sward structure. *Grass and Forage Science* 47, 358–365.

Norman, J.M. and Campbell, G.S. (1989) Canopy structure. In: Pearcy, R.W., Ehleringer, J., Mooney, H.A. and Rundel, P.W. (eds) *Plant Physiological Ecology. Field Methods and Instrumentation*. Chapman & Hall, New York, pp. 301–325.

O'Neill, R.V., Gardner, R.H., Milne, B.T., Turner, M.G. and Jackson, B. (1991) Heterogeneity and spatial hierarchies. In: Kolasa, J. and Pickett, S.T.A. (eds) *Ecological Heterogeneity*. Springer-Verlag, New York, pp. 85–96.

O'Reagain, P.J. and Oven-Smith, R.N. (1996) Effect of species composition and sward structure on dietary quality in cattle and sheep grazing South African sourveld. *Journal of Agricultural Science, Cambridge* 127, 261–270.

Palmer, M.W. (1988) Fractal geometry: a tool for describing spatial patterns of plant communities. *Vegetatio* 75, 91–102.

Palmer, M.W. (1992) The coexistence of species in fractal landscapes. *The American Naturalist* 139, 375–397.

Penning, P.D., Rook, A.J. and Orr, R.J. (1991) Patterns of ingestive behaviour of sheep continuously stocked on monocultures of ryegrass or white clover. *Applied Animal Behaviour Science* 31, 237–250.

Rhodes, I. (1981) Canopy structure. In: Hodgson, J., Baker, R.D., Davies, A., Laidlaw, A. and Leaver, J. (eds) *Sward Measurement Handbook*. British Grassland Society, Hurley, UK, pp. 141–158.

Ridout, M.S. and Robson, M.J. (1991) Diet composition of sheep grazing grass/ white clover swards: a re-evaluation. *New Zealand Journal of Agricultural Research* 34, 89–93.

Rossi, R.E., Mulla, D.J., Journel, A.G. and Franz, E.H. (1992) Geostatistical tools for modeling and interpreting ecological spatial dependence. *Ecological Monographs* 62, 277–314.

Sinoquet, H. and Cruz, P. (1993) Analysis of light interception and use in a pure and mixed stands of *Digitaria decumbens* and *Arachis pintoi*. *Acta Oecologia* 14, 327–339.

Turner, M.G. and Gardner, R.H. (1991) Quantitative methods in landscape ecology: an introduction. In: Turner, M.G. and Gardner, R.H. (eds) *Quantitative Methods in Landscape Ecology*. Springer-Verlag, New York, pp. 3–14.

Ungar, E.D. and Noy-Meir, I. (1988) Herbage intake in relation to availability and sward structure: grazing processes and optimal foraging. *Journal of Applied Ecology* 25, 1045–1062.

Varlet-Grancher, C., Gosse, C., Chartier, M., Sinoquet, H., Bonhomme, R. and Allirand, J.M. (1989) Mise au point: rayonnement solaire absorbé ou intercepté par un couvert végétal. *Agronomie* 9, 419–439.

Walker, G.K., Blackshaw, R.E. and Dekker, J. (1988) Leaf area and competition for light between plant species using direct sunlight transmission. *Weed Technology* 2, 159–165.

Warren-Wilson, J. (1960) Inclined quadrats. *New Phytologist* 59, 1–8.

Warren-Wilson, J. (1963) Estimation of foliage denseness and foliage angle by inclined point quadrats. *Australian Journal of Botany* 11, 95–105.

Welles, J.M. and Norman, J.M. (1991) Instrument for indirect measurement of canopy architecture. *Agronomy Journal* 83, 818–825.

Plant Population Dynamics in Grasslands

6

M.J.M. Hay[1], R.M. Jones[2] and D.M. Orr[3]

[1]AgResearch, Palmerston North, New Zealand; [2]CSIRO Tropical Agriculture, St Lucia, Australia; [3]Queensland Department of Primary Industries, Tropical Beef Centre, Rockhampton, Australia

Introduction

Instability of the botanical composition of grasslands is one of the primary concerns of grassland managers. Although it is relatively simple to measure botanical change, such information documents only the occurrence of change and provides no reasons as to why or how change occurred. Thus progress in development of management strategies favouring maintenance of particular species and limitation of invasion of weed species, especially in the face of environmental variability, requires knowledge of the factors determining population fluctuations. One approach towards such understanding is to obtain quantitative information on demography.

Population dynamics or demography of plants (or animals) is concerned with the numbers of individuals within the population and the way in which these numbers change with time (Harper, 1977). The key processes are birth, death and migration. Demographic studies therefore involve collection of quantitative data on individuals sampled within populations.

Some knowledge of the life history of the species of interest is a prerequisite for demographic studies. Demographic studies then quantify the changes in numbers in various life history stages over time and allow for calculation of the fecundity/recruitment rates necessary for population stability. Figure 6.1 provides a generalized flow diagram of the life history of grassland species, indicating the options that species may deploy, in various 'degrees' of combination, in order to maintain themselves. Basically populations can recruit from sexual reproduction or vegetative (clonal) growth.

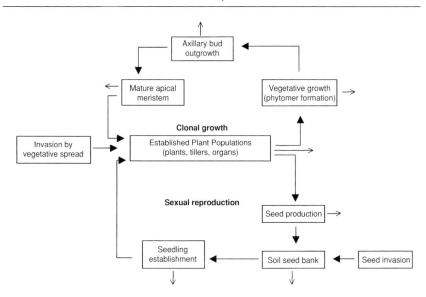

Fig. 6.1. A generalized life cycle of a plant species showing population recruitment via sexual reproduction and clonal growth pathways. Mortality losses (→) occur at all stages of the life cycle.

The relative degree of recruitment from either pathway can vary with environment; for example, in temperate pastures *Trifolium repens* perennation is through development of new stolons – seedlings are rarely seen and are of negligible consequence (Chapman, 1983, 1987), whereas in subtropical environments seedling and stolon recruitment are both important (Jones, 1982).

For annual species, demography is simplified as only the sexual pathway has to be considered and individuals rarely, if ever, survive into a second year. Also many important perennial species of grasslands are non-clonal and their demography can also be monitored considering only the sexual reproductive pathway, e.g. *Medicago sativa*, *Trifolium pratense*. However, as most clonal species utilize both pathways, as mentioned previously for *T. repens* and later for the grasses *Heteropogon contortus* and *Astrebla* spp., the relative importance of each pathway has to be determined for specific environments.

Where a species primarily utilizes clonal growth for perennation it can confer potential for extreme longevity to a genotype, lateral mobility and development of many individuals (clonal fragments) of the same genotype. This in turn means that the choice of unit (or individual) for study becomes an important methodological issue when studying demography of clonal grassland species. For example, plants (e.g. interconnected aggregations of tillers in grasses) are not usually a suitable unit because their size can fluctuate markedly over short intervals and identification within the sward can be difficult. These factors complicate the demographic study of clonal plants and so clonal and non-clonal pathways are discussed separately.

The various steps within Fig. 6.1 can be further broken down into more detailed components; for example, between seed set and seedling recruitment, there may be seed dispersal, survival, dormancy and predation. The transitions between each of the stages are influenced by a range of environmental and management factors with sensitivities peculiar to each transition. It is the understanding of the factors influencing the transitions from stage to stage in the life history that provides opportunities for designing management practices to bring about demographic changes, favouring desired species at the expense of undesirable species.

For the purposes of this chapter, density is defined as the number of units of study (plants, seeds, etc.) per unit area. Persistence of a species is defined as maintenance over time of a population density within managerially acceptable limits for the species.

This chapter firstly comments on methods of measurement of demography of the sexual pathway, then covers the demography of clonal growth and finally presents guidelines as to when demographic studies are useful.

Demography of the Sexual Reproductive Pathway

Survival of mature plants

This section details methods particularly suited to non-clonal species with readily identifiable individual plants but also to some clonal species which form discrete individuals, e.g. perennial tussock grasses. Measuring plant persistence of perennials is usually done only once or twice a year. In environments where the growing and dormant seasons are identifiable, convenient times are near the beginning and end of the growing season. At the start of the growing season it is usually easy to identify plants that have persisted through the dormant season. Measuring twice a year enables identification of whether plant death occurs during the growing season or the dormant season.

To measure persistence of plants it is necessary to identify and record the fate of individual plants. This is achieved by marking individual plants within fixed quadrats located within the pastures. These quadrats are preferably marked by pegs at each corner – for example, 5 cm × 5 cm wooden pegs driven firmly into the ground so that they can be located but do not interfere with or get dislodged by grazing or slashing. Alternatively, weldmesh sheets, pegged on to the soil after sowing or after heavy grazing, enable the quadrat to be easily divided into sub-quadrats to assist in identifying plants (Gardener, 1981). Each of these quadrats can be identified by a numbered tag. Metal pegs, such as lengths of galvanized pipe, can also be used as markers and, if necessary, relocated by a metal detector. In tall pastures it is desirable to have a tall marker near the quadrats as it can be very difficult to find short pegs in a tall pasture. The tall markers should be not closer than 2 m to the fixed quadrat as they can attract cattle, which rub against them and atypically trample adjacent vegetation. Quadrats of 1.0×0.5 m, with extensions that fit around the fixed pegs, can be used. Coloured strips of adhesive insulation tape 1 cm wide can be wrapped around the four sides of the quadrat at 10 cm intervals. This assists in visual identification of the x and y coordinates of observed plants.

Individual plants are then marked and their coordinates recorded. Marking can be done by using plastic rings, such as used on legs of pigeons, or plastic-covered copper insulation wire. Alternatively, small 10 cm lengths of wire may be used as follows. One end is pushed into the soil, while the other end, covered with coloured plastic, has previously been formed into a 'V' about 1 cm across. The marker is sited so that the plant is in the middle of the 'V'. Different-coloured plastic can be used for different cohorts (a cohort being defined as a discrete group of similarly aged individuals). It is unwise to rely on markers alone and not to measure coordinates, as rings can be removed by birds or grazing animals, or covered by soil or litter. It is also possible to use a plastic overlay for each quadrat. The plastic is clipped over the metal quadrat frame and positions of plants are marked with a waterproof pen, using a different colour for the records for different years on the one sheet (Jones and Bunch, 1988a).

The position of each plant is recorded on a new row on a data sheet specific to that quadrat, along with the dated initial recording, x and y coordinates and the colour of the marker ring. At each subsequent observation, entries are made in a new column; the plant is recorded as live and coded observations can be entered to show the vigour of the plant, whether it has seeded, etc. The same sheet should be taken out into the field when the next recordings are taken. Alternatively, data can be entered into a spreadsheet in the field using a laptop computer. If taproot size of a selection of plants is measured at the same time, it is possible to derive a relationship between taproot size and plant age, as done for *Chamaecrista rotundifolia* by Jones *et al.* (1998). Such relationships will vary with site but they offer the potential of going into another pasture and estimating the proportion of the total density that can be attributed to plants of different ages.

Although perennial tussock grasses grow clonally, each tussock can be regarded as a single entity and so slight adaptation of the above techniques permits assessment of their demography. However, individual tussocks often fragment into separate segments with increasing age (Samuel and Hart, 1995). Where this occurs, it is advisable to record each segment and identify segments as part of one individual plant at the initial recording. At subsequent recordings, that plant is considered to be alive if one or more segments of that tussock remain alive. This segmentation of tussocks caused by the birth and death of individual segments also means that individual tussocks 'move' within the quadrat. Consequently, when locating tussocks through coordinates care must be taken not to lose the identity of individual tussocks with time. This movement of tussocks is particularly important on clay soils, which swell and then dry out with seasonal rainfall and which can cause the position of tussocks to change between recordings. Another consequence of fragmentation of tussocks is that the basal diameter of tussocks is not always a useful basis for estimation of plant age.

In pasture communities that are open (i.e. plants are spatially separated and distinct), it is possible to use photographs to record individual quadrats, taking sequential photographs in the same way, with the camera pointing vertically towards the ground on each occasion. However, top-growth often obscures the base of grass tussocks, making this method imprecise for long-term, detailed studies of plant dynamics. A more precise method is to map the outline of the base of individual tussocks contained within permanently located quadrats. Where plant densities are low, as in *Astrebla* (Mitchell grass) grasslands where plant densities are usually fewer than five tussocks m^{-2}, permanent quadrats are commonly 1×1 m in size and the position of individual plants, within 16 grid cells each 25×25 cm, can be hand drawn at a smaller scale, on a sheet of paper (Orr and Phelps, 1994). Where plant density is higher, pantographs should be used to measure survival of individual tussocks (Orr *et al.*, 1997). When using a pantograph, the permanent quadrats are commonly 50×50 cm in size. The pantograph operates by simultaneously moving the flexible arm of the pantograph around the base of individual tussocks while the second arm records the tussock, on a smaller scale, on a sheet of paper (Fig. 6.2). By measuring the diameters of tussocks, it is possible to calculate the basal area

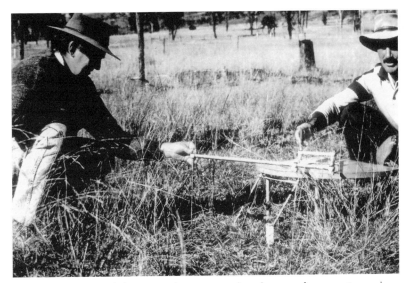

Fig. 6.2. A pantograph being used to measure basal cover of grasses in a subtropical native grassland.

of these species by converting each tussock diameter to an area and summing the areas of all tussocks in each quadrat (Orr *et al.*, 1997).

With either method, the previous chart is used with a piece of tracing paper over the top to record the current data. In this way, a recording can be made on each tussock present at the previous recording. The current data chart then becomes the previous chart for the next recording. Once field sampling is complete, it is possible to identify seedling plants that have been recruited and whether tussocks survive the period between recordings by comparing successive pairs of charts. Pantographs can also be used to mark point plants with a single taproot, though the pantograph may be less useful where the species being studied can develop high densities. For example, *Stylosanthes scabra* (shrubby stylo) can reach densities in excess of 250 small plants m^{-2}, making the identification of individual plants very difficult when using this system.

Once field recordings have been completed, records of individual plants are then entered on a spreadsheet. Each plant in each quadrat is assigned an identifying number and a new number is assigned to each new plant in each quadrat. The record for each plant in each quadrat in each treatment occupies one line so that data from each recording continues that line in the spreadsheet until that plant dies. Any seedling plant recruited is added to the record of the quadrat in which it occurs by inserting a new line into the spreadsheet. For tussock grasses, a new line can be added for each individual segment as the tussock fragments.

More recently, a mobile system for recording plant population data has been developed based on digital image processing equipment suitable for personal computers (Roshier *et al.*, 1997). In this system, a video camera is carried on a gantry attached to a vehicle which carries the computer. This system can offer savings in field and data handling time. While this system is well suited to open arid and semiarid pastures, it is unsuited to mesic pastures.

Data on plant survival and seedling recruitment are used to produce a life table, as illustrated in Table 6.1, where the two life tables illustrate how persistence of siratro (*Macroptilium atropurpureum*) was affected by stocking rates. Over a 10-year period, individual siratro plants persisted for much longer at the lighter grazing pressure and after 6 years there was a marked drop in annual recruitment of new plants at the higher stocking rate.

For non-clonal species Deevey survivorship curves (Fig. 6.3) can be a useful tool to identify the stage of plant growth at which the greatest rate of mortality occurs. A Deevey Type I curve indicates that the rate of mortality is greatest in older individuals of the population, whereas a Type II curve indicates a constant rate of mortality within the population age structure and a Type III curve shows that mortality is greatest in young individuals. However, a single survivorship curve does not characterize a species (Watkinson, 1997) as grazing management and environmental conditions can strongly modify curves (Mack and Pyke, 1983). For example, all three

Table 6.1. Life tables of *Macroptilium atropurpureum* growing under a high (3.0) or low (1.7) stocking rate (heifers ha^{-1}) giving numbers and longevity of crowns m^{-2} from ten cohorts as measured early each growing season from 1971 to 1981 (from Jones and Bunch, 1988a).

Season of crown appearance	Year of measurement										Half-life (months)
	1971/2	1972/3	1973/4	1974/5	1975/6	1976/7	1977/8	1978/9	1979/80	1980/1	
(a) 3.0 heifers ha^{-1}											
Pre 1971/72	8.3	2.8	0.2	—	—	—	—	—	—	—	5
1972/73		3.1	0.3	—	—	—	—	—	—	—	4
1973/74			1.2	0.4	0.1	0.1	—	—	—	—	9
1974/75				2.1	1.2	0.6	0.3	—	—	—	14
1975/76					1.9	0.5	0.1	—	—	—	6
1976/77						1.4	0.4	0.1	—	—	6
1977/78							0.3	—	—	—	—[a]
1978/79								0.8	0.4	0.1	9
1979/80									1.1	0.1	3
1980/81										0.2	—
Total all crowns	8.3	5.9	1.7	2.5	3.2	2.6	1.1	0.9	1.5	0.4	
(b) 1.7 heifers ha^{-1}											
Pre 1971/72	5.5	4.0	1.9	1.4	1.3	0.9	0.5	0.3	0.3	0.2	21
1972/73		2.3	0.7	0.5	0.5	0.3	0.3	0.2	0.2	—	27
1973/74			1.6	0.4	0.3	0.3	0.3	0.1	0.1	—	18
1974/75				2.6	1.3	1.2	1.0	0.8	0.8	0.5	23
1975/76					2.1	1.6	1.1	0.7	0.5	0.4	21
1976/77						2.7	1.8	1.1	0.9	0.8	24
1977/78							1.4	0.9	0.8	0.6	19
1978/79								2.4	1.7	1.4	13
1979/80									5.0	3.0	12
1980/81										4.0	10
Total all crowns	5.5	6.3	4.2	4.9	5.5	7.0	6.4	6.5	10.3	10.9	

[a]Half-life not given where all plants died within 12 months or where the initial count was below 0.5 plants m^{-2}.

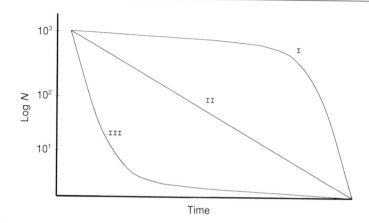

Fig. 6.3.   Examples of types I, II and III Deevey survivorship curves, which are the plot of the logarithm of number of surviving individuals (log N) against time.

curves have been documented for the legume *M. atropurpureum* (Jones and Bunch, 1988b; Jones *et al.*, 1993a).

Measuring seed set and seed fall

Because of the difficulty of measuring true seed set and seed predation, most studies on pasture species have measured effective seed input by directly measuring soil seed reserves.

Seed production

Seed production is difficult to measure in grazed pastures, especially at higher grazing pressure, where animals are continually removing seed heads and where many species flower and seed over an extended period of time. In lightly grazed pastures with a short growing season, it is possible to measure seed production of grasses, assuming that there is minimum removal of seed by animals. This can be done by counting the number of seed heads m^{-2} of each species and measuring numbers of sound seeds per seed head (McIvor *et al.*, 1996). In open pastures Gardener (1981) measured direct seed drop of *Stylosanthes hamata* by sweeping pods from the soil surface at the end of seeding, though this did not account for seed ingested by grazing animals. Seed traps and sticky tape have been used to measure seed set in ecological studies, but these techniques could be difficult to use in grazed pastures.

In ungrazed pastures, it is possible to measure seed production by collecting seed that falls into funnels located above the soil surface (Campbell, 1995). By collecting seed at intervals (say, fortnightly) during the period of seed production, it is possible to measure seasonal production as well as total seed production.

Seed predation
Seed predation can be an important source of seed loss in pastures, with small mammals, birds and ants all being able to remove large quantities of seed. By placing out known numbers of seed on small seed-free areas it is relatively simple to document that seed predation occurs and to show that seed of some species is removed in preference to others. Mott and McKeon (1977), for example, showed that ants preferred grass seed to legume seed in northern Australia. It is more difficult to quantify the role of predation in the loss of seed that occurs between seed set and seedling emergence.

Seed in faeces
After ingestion, seed of many species passes through the digestive tract of animals and is voided in faeces. Some seed is lost during passage, though losses are generally least with small seed and hard-seeded legumes and are less with cattle than with sheep or goats (Simao Neto et al., 1987). Seed levels in faeces change markedly with season as most species have defined reproductive periods. Additionally the timing and quantity of seed production may vary with grazing management. Therefore a comparison of faecal seed levels from different grazing treatments at only one point in time may not adequately represent the relative importance of transfer via the faeces among treatments (Jones et al., 1991). Seed voided in faeces is recovered as part of the soil seed reserve but measurements of viable seed in faeces may assist in understanding how different species spread. Seed reserves of up to 100 seeds g^{-1} dry dung have been measured for T. repens (Jones, 1982) and up to 30 seeds g^{-1} for S. scabra (McIvor et al., 1993). Both these legumes have been observed to establish well in the field from seed in faecal patches.

Furthermore, faecal seed may be an important pathway for the spread of weeds with edible fruits. For example, Grice (1996) suggested that spread of the shrub Ziziphus mauritiana in northern Australia can take place through dung of cattle or wallabies.

If dung beetles are active, faecal samples should be collected early in the morning from fresh dung dropped that night. Each sample is divided into two. One section is used to measure the moisture content. After drying, this section can also be used for other analyses, such as the proportion of C_3 and C_4 plants in the diet (see Chapter 15). The second sample is weighed while wet, and the recovered seed can then be expressed as seeds g^{-1} of dry dung.

There are two approaches to measuring seed levels in faeces. Seed can be washed out from faeces or viable seed can be germinated and seedlings identified. The procedures are described below in the section on seed or seedling recovery.

Seed produced in grazed pastures can also be dispersed through wind and adhesion to the coat of animals.

Measuring seed banks

Effective soil seed reserves are a key factor in those species that persist through seedling recruitment. There is considerable information on seed reserves in both temperate (e.g. Rice, 1989) and tropical pastures (e.g. McIvor and Gardener, 1994). Seed banks are crucial for annual species, and this is reflected in the many studies carried out on the seed reserves of annual legumes such as *Trifolium subterraneum* (Taylor *et al.*, 1984). However, in the long term, seed banks are also essential for most perennial species, even the long-lived *Astrebla* spp. (Orr, 1998). Sometimes the species composition of the seed banks reflects above-ground botanical composition (e.g. Jones *et al.*, 1991) but in many cases it does not (e.g. McIvor and Gardener, 1994).

Seeds of some species remain viable for only a few months, and so regular sampling may be required to understand the seasonal trends in increase and decrease of seed reserves, as shown for annual *Sorghum* spp. in tropical Australia (Andrew and Mott, 1983). Seed banks of other species, such as hard-seeded legumes, can persist for many years. In long-term studies samples may be collected only once a year, at the end of the seeding period. However, where there is a distinct period of seeding, there may be a case for sampling twice a year, immediately before and after seed fall. This gives the minimum and maximum soil seed reserves.

For species that rely on seed banks for persistence, there is likely to be some seed set within established pastures in most years. Thus the seed reserve will be composed of seed of different ages, similar to the plant life table discussed earlier, but it is impossible to identify seed of different ages in samples collected from the field. Applying different radioactive isotopes to seed in different years, prior to detachment from plants, could enable the subsequent identification of the age of individual seeds recovered from the soil. However, such procedures require special analytical equipment and may not be permitted in grazed pastures unless special safety protocols are followed. If there are years without any new seed set, changes in the soil seed bank can be used to estimate the rate of rundown. Alternatively, a known quantity of seed of a designated species can be sown into an area where it does not occur. The fate of seed and longevity of seed reserves can then be followed by annually recording and removing seedlings and measuring soil seed levels (Taylor *et al.*, 1984; Jones *et al.*, 1998).

Sampling for soil seed reserves
Sampling of soil seed reserves can be done using soil cores or collecting sods of a known size. Soil coring is quicker than sod sampling and has the

advantage of reducing sampling bias due to spatial variability through increasing the number of samples taken. A preliminary sampling study could enable some assessment of the number of cores required, but spatial variability from species to species and site to site would make such preliminary studies a daunting prospect. We have usually taken 30–50 cores of 7 cm diameter per paddock, depending on paddock size. This has been adequate to describe long-term changes with time (Jones and Bunch, 1988b), even though the total area sampled (1846 cm^2 with 48 cores) was still very low. In small plot studies, which are usually more even and with more replicates, fewer cores can be taken per plot but ten cores of this size would be a minimum.

Many forms of corer can be used and we have found that a corer with a foot-operated lever to help to expel cores is particularly useful. If soil conditions are suitable, it is possible to remove the core carefully and then slice it into sections so that seed reserves can be measured in different layers. Many studies have taken samples to 5 cm although most seed is usually in the top 2 cm. A higher proportion of seed at depths below 2 cm may indicate that the seed has been set many years ago (Jones, 1982).

Depending on the soil type, it can be easier to take core samples from moist soil but this means there is a risk of germination occurring if seed is not recovered soon after sampling. One way of eliminating this problem is to store the soil samples in a cool room until they are processed. As it takes much longer to process soil samples than to collect them, this type of storage is recommended. If soils are sampled when dry, storage at ambient temperature can help to break seed dormancy.

Seed or seedling recovery

There are two approaches to measuring seed reserves: separating out seed, or germinating seed and identifying the seedlings. The separation procedure is best suited to cases where the interest is limited to one or very few species with easily recognizable seeds and to species (such as most legumes) with markedly hard seed which may prevent germination. There are many variations on the procedure, but the steps usually involve washing over a sieve known to be fine enough to retain the seed being measured, separating seed from soil by use of a solvent, aspirating to remove large pieces of organic matter, and a final stage of sorting seed from pieces of organic matter of the same size and density (e.g. Jones and Bunch, 1988c). Considerable care is needed. The procedure will always give a result, but if operators are careless there is no way of knowing how much seed has been lost. When commencing studies of this type for the first time, recovery of test samples, with known numbers of viable seed, should be undertaken as a check.

Recovered seed can be separated into that which visually appears 'normal' or 'abnormal'. Samples can be checked for germination, although it must be recognized that the recovery procedure is likely to break dormancy of some seed and possibly even cause some death of soft seeds. Thus testing after recovery may underestimate the percentage of hard or dormant seed. The viability of 'abnormal' seed is invariably low.

The second approach to measuring seed reserves involves germination and seedling identification. Advantages of using a germination method over a separation method include ease of handling small seeds (which can be difficult to recover and count) and greater confidence when dealing with species whose seeds are difficult to distinguish. However, considerable preliminary work is involved in identifying seedlings. Unknown seedlings can be grouped and given identification numbers, and representative seedlings can be grown on and identified. The soil from each core or a group of cores can be spread out on a tray and regularly watered. After the first wave of germination, which may last for some 8 weeks, has ended, samples should be left to dry out for a similar time period. The dry periods help to control growth of algae and may stimulate germination. The samples should then be thoroughly mixed before watering again for the second and subsequent cycles, as the first cycle usually only germinates part of the viable seed (Jones *et al.*, 1991). As a general rule, plan for several cycles. For example, Orr (1999) showed that most grasses germinated in either the first or second cycle while substantial germination of broad-leaved species continued until the fourth cycle.

While the pots or trays can be watered by hand, it is hard to do this evenly and keep the soil moist but not saturated, especially under hot conditions. The best option is to apply water through a misting system (Orr *et al.*, 1996). Alternatively, soil can be spread as a thin layer on top of a sterile salt-free sand base which is kept moist by placing the pots in standing water (e.g. McIvor and Gardener, 1994). This procedure has worked well with lighter soils and with a sand base of the appropriate texture.

Care is needed in interpreting data on seed banks. For example, seed banks may be historical and have minimal influence on current botanical changes. Alternatively, it is possible to have large seed banks that have little consequence for persistence. For example, Jones (1989) showed that the tropical legume *Desmodium intortum* could accumulate some thousands of seeds m^{-2}, yet there was very little recruitment of plants from seedlings and *D. intortum* persisted primarily through stolon rooting.

Seedling establishment and survival

Measurements of seedling survival, as for plant survival, necessitate the use of fixed quadrats. If the objective is to document the total number of seedlings that emerged, this will usually involve several counts over the growing season. In regions with a distinct and reliable seasonal rainfall, as in Mediterranean environments and the seasonally dry tropics, most of the seedlings may emerge during the first major rainfall event of the wet season (e.g. McIvor and Gardener, 1994). If there is adequate rainfall for these to survive they will usually dominate any seedlings that emerge later. In areas with more unreliable rainfall, there are often major germination events that fail to survive dry periods following the isolated rainfall event that stimulated germination.

If there are few germination events and they are widely spaced, it is possible to get a reasonable measure of survival from each event without tagging seedlings. This is done by counting seedlings after each emergence event and then by a final count of the different-sized seedlings at the end of the year. However, in most situations it is impossible to identify seedlings from the different cohorts at the end of the growing season.

If seedlings are sparse, they can be tagged and recorded as described under plant survival. If seedlings are dense, with some hundreds m^{-2} and with possibly several separate emergence events, use of fixed quadrats can become very time consuming. We have used two ways of dealing with this situation. Firstly, in dense strikes, tagging of individual seedlings can be restricted to a small area of the fixed quadrat. Secondly, a small number of representative seedlings can be tagged, their coordinates measured and their survival followed. In each case all the remaining seedlings in the quadrat can be counted and their survival estimated from the smaller sample.

Survival of seedlings that emerge from sowing into a seedbed is often far higher than survival of seedlings that emerge in an established pasture, as competition from established plants is removed and in many cases stored soil water and mineral nitrogen is available for growth. Because of this, it is often convenient to follow plant survival in seedbeds right from seedling emergence, but to consider recruitment in established pastures in two phases – as seedling emergence and survival in the first growing season and as plants after the start of the second season.

Supporting measurements

Supporting studies and measurements can aid interpretation of the measurements described in the previous sections. Some studies, such as the breakdown of seed dormancy, can be carried out in the glasshouse or under controlled conditions. Other studies, such as on seed predation by ants and breakdown of hard seed in different environments, are best done in the field. Small enclosures can be used to follow the effect of seasonal exclusion of stock on seed set. Plants grown within steel tubes driven into the soil can be a useful tool to aid understanding of the role of shoot and root competition in limiting seedling growth and survival in established pastures (Cook and Ratcliff, 1984). The extent of defoliation of each plant at the time of recording can be estimated by developing a set of photographic standards (Orr, 1980).

Demography of Clonal Species

Clonal growth

As mentioned in the introduction, demography of clonal species is more complicated than that of non-clonal species as usually both sexual and vegetative growth recruitment pathways have to be assessed (e.g. Dammon and Cain, 1998). This section deals solely with the vegetative or clonal growth pathway of recruitment. Bell (1984) defined clonal species as 'those perennials that spread and multiply by vegetative means'. A prerequisite for clonal growth is the iterative modular construction of plants (Harper and White, 1974). We define the iterative unit as a phytomer, each comprising internode, node, leaf, axillary meristem and root primordium, and thereby possessing the potential to form an independent plant. Clonal fragments (plants) comprise a system of branching stems, with each stem consisting of a string of phytomers, all derived from the apical meristem of the stem. Clonal growth involves production of new phytomers at stem apical meristems, death of phytomers at the basal end of the primary stem and birth and death of apices (branches) which form from the axillary meristems of phytomers. Death of a primary stem phytomer releases (if present) the lateral branch originating at that phytomer as an independent plant of the same genotype (see Figure 1 in Chapman, 1983). Therefore a single genotype may be represented by several physiologically and physically independent plants.

The processes of clonal growth have consequences that complicate demographic studies. Firstly, the fragmentation processes mean that the population is structured at a genetic level and at a plant phenotype (clonal fragment) level. Secondly, the fragmentation processes also provide the possibility for sudden change in both the size of individual plants and also the mean plant size of a population. Thirdly, large temporal variability in the size of individual clonal fragments raises the question of what meaningfully constitutes the individual for demographic study, i.e. tussocks, genotypes, clonal fragments, apical meristems, stolons, rhizomes, phytomers, leaves or other specific organs. Fourthly, movement in space over time, especially for species with laterally spreading stems or rhizomes, makes it possible for genotypes to have a patchy distribution, either separate from or closely intermingled with other genotypes. Collectively these factors can make it difficult to distinguish and follow the development of either genotypic or phenotypic individuals within populations.

Understanding the dynamics of clonal populations may require information of more than one level of organization. For instance, relatively infrequent sampling of populations, for characterization of genetic composition, might have to be combined with seasonal measurements of the clonal fragments such as continual monitoring of births and deaths of meristems and phytomers.

This section will focus primarily on clonal demography in mesic (temperate, moist) grasslands where clonal growth is the dominant pathway of recruitment. Methods of measuring changes in the genetic composition of clonal populations will be considered before dealing with phenotypic changes.

Changes in the genetic composition of populations

A common question is: does the genetic composition of the current population differ from that of the sown seed line?

McLellan *et al.* (1997) gave an excellent account of the problems that clonal populations pose when estimates of genotypic variation (number and frequency of genotypes) or genetic variation (number and frequency of alleles, expected heterozygosity) are required.

The genetic composition of clonal populations can be assessed by various methods.

Common garden

This approach involves taking a random sample of plants from the field at a point in time and transplanting them into a common garden along with a similar number of randomly selected genotypes from the original seed line. The field must be stratified so that the distance between plant samples is sufficient to avoid multiple sampling of genotypes. After a period sufficient for the phenotype to reflect the common garden rather than its previous environment, plant traits are assessed and the field and seed lines compared (e.g. Brock and Caradus, 1996). This method has been a fundamental tool of genecology but has drawbacks. Firstly, persistence of phenotypic variation carried over from the field is common (Seliskar, 1985) and uncertain in duration, but can be up to 2 years (Evans and Turkington, 1988). Secondly, the common garden is a single environment that may favour plastic convergence, thus masking genetic diversity (Sultan, 1987). Hence, while the common garden approach has a major advantage of requiring low technological resources, care is required in interpreting results.

Allele frequency methods

This approach can be particularly useful to establish whether or not the genetic structure of a population changes in response to treatment or environmental perturbations. Marker properties of the population, associated with one or more alleles, are measured in the test population before and after treatment, e.g. frequency of cyanogenic presence in leaves of *T. repens* (Williams, 1987).

Isozyme or allozyme electrophoresis can also be used to identify the frequency of alleles within populations. Where alleles at several different loci are determined the method can also have value for identification of genotypes, but care is required as different genotypes may possess the same subset of multilocus alleles, leading to an underestimation of genotypic variation (Ellstrand and Roose, 1987). However, Parks and Werth (1983) provided a method to infer the number of genotypes from isozyme data.

Molecular biology techniques

McLellan *et al.* (1997) provided a very good introduction to the usefulness of DNA analysis methods. In general, such techniques, although expensive, provide an accurate picture of the number of genotypes in a population but do not measure allelic variation. Berry *et al.* (1991) gave technical details and discussed this methodology.

Clonal demography at the phenotype level

These studies concern the numerical changes in the population of the vegetative units rather than the fate of individual genotypes. Generally the processes involved in clonal growth result in high temporal variability in the size and structure of any particular clonal fragment or 'plant'. Consequently, as identification of individual clonal fragments in the field is difficult, clonal fragments are rarely used in these studies (although some useful exceptions are described below). Most studies concentrate on a unit of growth referred to in the ecological literature as the ramet. A ramet usually comprises an apical meristem and the phytomers directly differentiated from it – the structure that grassland agronomists refer to as the tiller of grasses or the stem or stolon of laterally spreading species. Unfortunately, the term ramet is also sometimes used to represent individual phytomers and so care should be exercised whenever the terminology is encountered.

Interest in use of tillers or stems/stolons for demographic studies arises because the apical meristems are the sites of initiation of new leaves and axillary buds and tillers/stems are readily identified *in situ* in the field. Where there is consistency in growth of all apices of a population, the productive consequences of management or environmental change may be adequately understood by assessing demography of tillers/stems. However, where recruitment of tillers/stems is limited by the availability of viable axillary buds or root primordia, rather than favourable conditions for outgrowth, or where there is large variation in the characteristics of growth within the population of tillers/stems, the phytomer may be the required unit of study.

In mesic grasslands it is population density (number of individuals per unit area) that is of interest. Thus all demographic studies of clonal growth involve measurements of population density over the assessment period, and this topic will be considered initially. This will be followed by a discussion of the value of repeated measurements/observations of identified individuals.

Population density

Jewiss (1993) provides detailed information on both non-destructive and destructive techniques of measuring population density. Measurements are periodic (non-continuous) and assess the state of the population at a point in time. Inherent in all such measurements are sampling procedures that cope with the heterogeneity of pastures. Heterogeneity may be transient (e.g. that resulting from dung deposition or previous variability in grazing intensity; McIvor *et al.*, 1993), permanent (e.g. that associated with variation in soil type, or not visually apparent, such as the association of particular genotypes of *T. repens* with different perennial grass species; Turkington and Harper, 1979). Variability will not be a problem in all pastures, but careful thought is required to ensure that a 'mean value' does not hide variation that assists the understanding of demographic processes.

Non-destructive assessments are limited to vegetation units, such as tillers or leaves that are easily identified, and may be done in randomly chosen areas or in fixed sites repeatedly counted. Non-destructive techniques are commonly used where the plot size is small, thereby precluding use of destructive sampling, but suffer the disadvantages that they are demanding as they require kneeling at ground level for long periods, adjacent areas may be damaged, and handling of the forage may induce atypical growth.

Destructive assessments involve either cutting to ground level or removal of turves or cores for subsequent monitoring in the laboratory. Dissection of herbage material cut to ground level yields information on density and size of tillers/stems or leaves. Similarly areas within removed turves can be sampled by cutting to ground level and measuring tiller/stem density as above. Alternatively, turves may be washed to remove soil so that intact connected tillers/stems (clonal fragments or plants) can be separated out, thereby enabling assessment of the density and characteristics of the clonal population and/or the tiller/stem population (e.g. Brock *et al.*, 1988, 1996; Brock and Fletcher, 1993). In addition such samplings can be used to characterize physiological attributes of populations. For example, Newton *et al.* (1992) used a bioassay (Newton and Hay, 1992) to assess the potential of the bank of axillary buds to contribute to future growth of *T. repens* and subsequently captured this information in a clonal population model (Louie *et al.*, 1998). However, the destructive nature and the size (up to $300 \times 300 \times 50$ mm) of turf sampling necessary for adequate sampling of laterally spreading species such as *T. repens* means that there is often a requirement to minimize the number of turves sampled. In this situation Hay *et al.* (1989, 1991) lifted two to six turves for sampling of clonal fragments (plants) for characterization and undertook a separate sampling that better accounted for spatial heterogeneity within pastures, using 5 cm diameter cores (Mitchell and Glenday, 1958) to assess density.

Morphological details of the extent of fragments, size of organs and connective tissues provide insights into the potential within the population for storage, physiological integration and future resource capture. Successive measurements may also provide insights into changes in rate processes that give rise to seasonal cycles of clonal growth. This in turn allows identification of seasonal phenomena that impact on populations, with implications for management policies. For example, in *T. repens* in New Zealand pastures, accelerated rates of senescence of basal stolon tissues in spring increases the rate of fragmentation of clonal fragments, approximately halving mean fragment size. This decreases the carbohydrate reserves of fragments and tolerance to applied nitrogen in spring, especially under lax defoliation regimes (Brock *et al.*, 1988).

The processing of turf samples for clonal fragment characterization is very labour intensive. For instance, each of the monthly samplings of *T. repens* reported in Brock *et al.* (1988) involved five staff working for a week. However, such work does not need expensive instrumentation.

Density of rhizomes

Demography of rhizomatous species is complicated by the difficulties inherent in the monitoring of underground organs and is therefore limited to obtaining measures of the net effects of birth/death/migration processes at sequential samplings on rhizome density and on the rhizome characteristics of plants in the population. Sheath (1980) sequentially sampled turves ($300 \times 300 \times 200$ mm), washed out and sampled intact plants and made separate, parallel harvests of shoots to ground level in 0.1 m^2 quadrats. The aim was to assess the effects of season and defoliation on the density of rhizomes, roots and shoots of *Lotus pedunculatus* and on the characteristics of plants. Information obtained was used to typify the growth habit of the species in specific environments and provide insights as to the processes likely to influence persistence.

Population fluxes

Sequential estimates (as described above) of density of plants, tillers or leaves provide information on the net effect of changes in birth and death over time. As such they give no information on the gross rates of birth and death of these organs (Watkinson *et al.*, 1979). Such information is obtained by monitoring identified individuals within the population. Net changes in population density result when birth and death rates change relative to each other. The measurement of these changes provides a focus for developing appropriate strategies to manipulate the population. For instance, in *Lolium perenne* populations, management during spring to optimize the birth of tillers from axillary buds at the base of reproductive tillers is important because these tillers then form the basis for summer/autumn production (Matthew, 1992).

Knowledge of the gross rates of birth and death of organs and how these rates vary with environmental change is particularly important in grazed grasslands, as standing biomass often remains almost constant and so it is the flux of organs that underpins both productivity and population stability.

The review of Davies (1993) should be read before commencing studies on population flux in mesic grasslands. We will not repeat that information but rather comment on the principles of measuring population flux. In general, sequential observations of a number of individually identified tillers/stems are made such that rates of leaf and tiller appearance (birth) and death can be calculated on a per unit area basis. Earlier studies (Langer *et al.*, 1964; Garwood, 1969) achieved this by marking and following all grass tillers within a defined sample area, including young tillers upon birth. The major advantage of this approach is that the sample is representative of the age distribution of tillers in the population. However, Davies (1993) indicates that the usefulness of this method is severely limited by the considerable time required to get accurate information.

The method usually employed now involves repeated monitoring of randomly located individual tillers, coupled with complementary but separate samplings of tiller density. This method assumes that the sampled tillers are representative of the whole population and so care must be taken not to oversample the more easily accessible tillers – for example, those on the edges of clumps. As sampled tillers age there is a requirement to re-sample at intervals no greater than two leaf appearances to ensure the age distribution of the sample remains representative of the population, particularly during the reproductive phase (Davies, 1993). Davies (1993) makes specific mention of the difficulties encountered when working with white clover. Care is required to categorize stems according to maturity (e.g. Brock *et al.*, 1988) in both density and flux measurements, or to ensure that all categories of stem are included in the samples. Technically this is very difficult to do in the field. Wilman and Simpson (1988) and Hay *et al.* (1993), respectively, identify differing growth and defoliation rates of young branch as opposed to parent stems.

A common criticism of any technique that repeatedly handles plants is that it may lead to atypical growth, which means that the sample becomes unrepresentative of the population. However, in grazed pastures, where there is frequent defoliation and treading, such effects are usually not significant (Hodgson and Ollerenshaw, 1969).

Use of Demographic Studies

Modelling of persistence

Conceptual or qualitative modelling of demography is fundamental to understanding the persistence of pasture plant species. Although we have outlined procedures for measuring many different demographic attributes, such as plant survival, the importance of each attribute can only be assessed by relating back to the pathways of recruitment indicated in Fig. 6.1.

A major purpose of demographic studies is to gather sufficient data to enable development of a comprehensive model of the population dynamics of a species. Such a model, usually qualitative rather than fully quantitative, assists prediction of the effects of differing environments or management on persistence of the species (e.g. Orr, 1998). This use of demography is considered in more detail by Jones and Mott (1980). Once there is a good understanding of demography of a species, it is possible to make a better interpretation of some simple measurements in other experiments with the same species. For example, once the demography of *Siratro* was reasonably well understood, it was possible to take measurements of soil seed reserves and seed input at the end of an experiment and use these to predict the long-term effect of continuation of the treatments (Jones and Mott, 1980).

Although this chapter is primarily about taking measurements of plant demography, there is an important role for careful observations. These will usually provide insight of how environments or different experimental treatments affect factors such as seed set, seedling regeneration and even plant survival. A watch should also be kept for other factors, such as insect attack, presence of diseases and selective grazing, which may affect persistence. Such observations help to pinpoint the attributes of the recruitment pathways important for persistence and hence can identify the important parameters for measurement.

Quantitative modelling

As many factors influence persistence it is difficult to construct mathematical models that can quantitatively predict the effect on persistence of a specified sequence of events. Quantitative models will be most successful where there is a relatively reliable period of growth and seed set followed by a long dry season – such as occurs with annual species in Mediterranean environments (Galbraith *et al.*, 1980) and the seasonally dry tropics (Torsell and Nicholls, 1978). However, quantitative models have also been developed for *T. repens* persistence in complex subtropical environments (Hill *et al.*, 1989) and in temperate climates where clonal processes dominate (Louie *et al.*, 1998). Similarly, a model is being developed for the short-lived perennial *C. rotundifolia* (Jones *et al.*, 1993b) which has to cope with the problems of describing plant death, seed set, seed loss, seedling recruitment and seedling survival in subtropical environments with very variable rainfall. Some of the problems that have been encountered in deriving appropriate functions are discussed by Jones *et al.* (1998). Quantitative modelling is difficult and a decision to move from qualitative to quantitative modelling will be unusual.

There are at least three benefits arising from building quantitative models. Firstly, development of the model is a very effective way of finding out where current data is inadequate. Secondly, the models may play a useful role in development of new cultivars. For example, an objective may be to develop a new cultivar that has greater persistence through dry periods. This might be achieved via several mechanisms: better plant survival, more seed set, slower breakdown of hard seed, more vigorous seedlings, etc. Once a reasonably accurate mathematical model is developed it is possible to compare the effects of changing different attributes – for instance, the effect of improving plant survival by 20% can be compared with that of decreasing the breakdown rate of hard seed by assessing persistence using a 50-year rainfall data set. Although the output of such a model should never be pursued as the sole selection criterion, it has obvious potential for use in development of more persistent cultivars. Thirdly, the model can be used to predict the effects of likely changes in management or environment. For example, models that predict climate change due to global warming could be used in conjunction with a persistence model to predict likely changes in the area to which a species is adapted.

Associated studies

Many pasture demographic studies are undertaken as a means of obtaining information to elucidate how a treatment or management impacts upon pasture production or persistence. For instance, Vertes *et al.* (1988) used both tagged stolon observations and morphological measures of plants extracted from destructive turf samplings to assess how treading by cattle influenced *T. repens* growth. Alternatively, studies using demographic methodology can provide valuable independent estimates of grazing preference and animal intake (Davies, 1993; Grant and Marriott, 1994). Additionally, studies using demographic techniques are used to track how interspecific interactions and disease epidemiology impact on the populations of pasture species (Grant and Marriott, 1994).

Plant demographic measurements can supplement pasture information collected at a coarser scale. For example, at the plant community scale, pasture composition measured in native *Heteropogon contortus* pasture has indicated that burning once each spring for 3 years progressively reduced the contribution of the undesirable perennial grass *Aristida ramosa*. Concurrent demographic measurements indicated that burning initially reduced the size of individual tussocks and eventually resulted in the death of *A. ramosa* plants (Orr *et al.*, 1997).

Interpretative uses

Most demographic studies on natural communities are only concerned with understanding demography in relation to variation in uncontrollable factors such as climate and soils. However, in most grassland situations there is perhaps even more interest in studying demography in relation to controllable factors such as grazing intensity, fertilizer, irrigation and burning. This is because there is the possibility of manipulating management once the demographic pathways are understood. For example, demographic studies can identify the seasonal period when recruitment or death processes are particularly significant for the population. This in turn can lead to suggested management strategies, such as management to favour tiller recruitment from flowering tillers in *L. perenne* under moist conditions in spring (Matthew, 1992). Additionally, detailed studies may identify phenomena occurring in one season that explain population behaviour in a later season; for example, burial of stolons of *T. repens* in winter forms the base for recovery after drought in the following autumn (Hay *et al.*, 1987).

Aspects to Consider before Starting Demographic Study

Considerable prior thought in clarifying objectives is required before commencing plant demographic studies in order to ensure that meaningful information is obtained. Once the objectives are clarified it is easier to decide on the type and intensity of measurements to make. It is also essential to recognize the time scales required to obtain meaningful information. For example, development of a meaningful life table for some tropical perennial grasses requires data over a time scale of at least 10 years. Furthermore, for some arid species, such as *Astrebla* spp., seedling recruitment occurs episodically so that measurement should be taken over a sufficient time scale to encounter such events. It should also be stressed that many demographic measurements are very time consuming. Thus the long time scale often required and the detailed and time-consuming nature of the work mean that demographic measurements should not be undertaken without considerable prior thought and planned commitment of resources.

The decision as to when to commence population studies of germplasm within plant improvement programmes is more complex. Studies that commence when germplasm is undergoing preliminary evaluation are very likely to be premature. However, population studies undertaken during later stages of cultivar development can elucidate mechanisms for persistence and assist in developing recommendations for management, as in the case of *Desmanthus virgatus* (Burrows and Porter, 1993).

As demographic studies are site specific, a very detailed demographic study under one stocking rate and method of grazing in one environment may be of limited use in predicting what would happen under different management systems or environments. Hence it is suggested that it could often be more desirable to undertake fewer measurements but repeat them under contrasting management situations or environments (Jones and Mott, 1980). Alternatively, if there are resources to carry out detailed studies at only one or two sites or environments, then some less time-consuming measurements (such as soil seed banks) at other sites will assist in the extrapolation of the detailed studies.

References

Andrew, M.H. and Mott, J.J. (1983) Annuals with a transient seed bank: the population biology of indigenous sorghum species of tropical north-west Australia. *Australian Journal of Ecology* 8, 265–276.

Bell, A.D. (1984) Dynamic morphology: a contribution to plant population ecology. In: Dirzo, R. and Sarubhan, J. (eds) *Perspectives on Plant Population Ecology.* Sinauer, Sunderland, Massachusetts, pp. 48–65.

Berry, R.J., Crawford, T.J. and Hewitt, G.M. (1991) *Genes in Ecology.* Blackwell, Oxford, 534 pp.

Brock, J.L. and Caradus, J.R. (1996) Influence of grazing management and drought on white clover population performance and genotypic frequency. In: Woodfield, D.R. (ed.) *White Clover: New Zealand's Competitive Edge.* Agronomy Society of New Zealand Special Publication No. 11, Palmerston North, New Zealand, pp. 79–82.

Brock, J.L. and Fletcher, R.H. (1993) Morphology of perennial ryegrass (*Lolium perenne*) plants in pastures under intensive sheep grazing. *Journal of Agriculture Science, Cambridge* 120, 301–310.

Brock, J.L., Hay, M.J.M., Thomas, V.J. and Sedcole, J.R. (1988) Morphology of white clover (*Trifolium repens* L.) plants in pastures under intensive sheep grazing. *Journal of Agricultural Science, Cambridge* 111, 273–283.

Brock, J.L., Hume, D.E. and Fletcher, R.H. (1996) Seasonal variation in the morphology of perennial ryegrass (*Lolium perenne*) and cocksfoot (*Dactylis glomerata*) plants and populations in pastures under intensive sheep grazing. *Journal of Agricultural Science, Cambridge* 126, 37–51.

Burrows, D.M. and Porter, F.J. (1993) Regeneration and survival of *Desmanthus virgatus* 78382 in grazed and ungrazed pastures. *Tropical Grasslands* 27, 100–107.

Campbell, S.D. (1995) Plant mechanisms that increase *H. contortus* and decrease *A. ramosa* in burnt pastures in south-east Queensland. PhD thesis, University of Queensland, Brisbane, Australia.

Chapman, D.F. (1983) Growth and demography of *Trifolium repens* stolons in grazed hill pastures. *Journal of Applied Ecology* 20, 597–608.

Chapman, D.F. (1987) Natural reseeding and *Trifolium repens* demography in grazed hill pastures. *Journal of Applied Ecology* 24, 1037–1043.

Cook, S.J. and Ratcliff, D. (1984) A study of the effects of root and shoot competition on the growth of green panic (*Panicum maximum* var. *Triochoglume*) seedlings in an existing grassland using root exclusion tubes. *Journal of Applied Ecology* 21, 971–982.

Dammon, H. and Cain, M.L. (1998) Population growth and viability analyses of the clonal woodland herb, *Asarum canadense*. *Journal of Ecology* 86, 13–26.

Davies, A. (1993) Tissue turnover in the sward. In: Davies, A., Baker, R.D., Grant, S.A. and Laidlaw, A.S. (eds) *Sward Measurement Handbook*. British Grassland Society, Reading, UK, pp. 183–215.

Ellstrand, N.C. and Roose, M.L. (1987) Patterns of genotypic diversity in clonal plant species. *American Journal of Botany* 74, 123–131.

Evans, R.C. and Turkington, R. (1988) Maintenance of morphological variation in a biotically patchy environment. *New Phytologist* 109, 369–376.

Galbraith, K.A., Arnold, G.W. and Carbon, B.A. (1980) Dynamics of plant and animal production of a subterranean clover pasture grazed by sheep. 2. Structure and validation of the pasture growth model. *Agricultural Systems* 6, 23–44.

Gardener, C.J. (1981) Population dynamics and stability of *Stylosanthes hamata* in grazed pastures. *Australian Journal of Agricultural Research* 32, 63–74.

Garwood, E.A. (1969) Seasonal tiller populations of grass and grass/clover swards with and without irrigation. *Journal of the British Grassland Society* 24, 333–344.

Grant, S.A. and Marriott, C.A. (1994) Detailed studies of grazed swards – techniques and conclusions. *Journal of Agricultural Science, Cambridge* 122, 1–6.

Grice, A.C. (1996) Seed production, dispersal and germination in *Cryptostegia grandiflora* and *Ziziphus mauritiana*, two invasive shrubs in tropical woodlands of northern Australia. *Australian Journal of Ecology* 21, 324–331.

Harper, J.L. (1977) *Population Biology of Plants*. Academic Press, London, 892 pp.

Harper, J.L. and White, J. (1974) The demography of plants. *Annual Review of Ecology and Systematics* 5, 419–463.

Hay, M.J.M., Chapman, D.F., Hay, R.J.M., Pennell, C.G.L., Woods, P.W. and Fletcher, R.H. (1987) Seasonal variation in the vertical distribution of white clover stolons in grazed swards. *New Zealand Journal of Agricultural Research* 30, 1–8.

Hay, M.J.M., Brock, J.L. and Thomas, V.J. (1989) Density of *Trifolium repens* plants in mixed swards under intensive grazing by sheep. *Journal of Agricultural Science, Cambridge* 113, 81–86.

Hay, M.J.M., Newton, P.C.D. and Thomas, V.J. (1991) Nodal structure and branching of *Trifolium repens* in pastures under intensive grazing by sheep. *Journal of Agriculture Science, Cambridge* 116, 221–228.

Hay, M.J.M., Kim, M.C., McLean, R.W. and Gonzalez-Rodriguez, A. (1993) Defoliation of young branch and parent stolons of white clover in rotationally grazed pastures. In: *Proceedings of the XVII International Grassland Congress*, 1. Palmerston North, New Zealand, pp. 120–121.

Hill, M., Archer, K.A. and Hutchison, K.J. (1989) Towards developing a model of persistence and production of white clover. In: *Proceedings of the XVI International Grasslands Congress*. Nice, France, pp. 1043–1044.

Hodgson, J. and Ollerenshaw, J.H. (1969) The frequency and severity of defoliation of individual tillers in set-stocked swards. *Journal of the British Grassland Society* 24, 226–234.

Jewiss, O.R. (1993) Shoot development and number. In: Davies, A., Baker, R.D., Grant, S.A. and Laidlaw, A.S. (eds) *Sward Measurement Handbook*. British Grassland Society, Reading, UK, pp. 99–120.

Jones, R.M. (1982) White clover (*T. repens*) in subtropical south-east Queensland. I. Some effects of site, season and managements practices on the population dynamics of white clover. *Tropical Grasslands* 16, 118–127.

Jones, R.M. (1989) Productivity and population dynamics of silverleaf desmodium (*Desmodium uncinatum*) and greenleaf desmodium (*D. inortum*) and two *D. inortum* × *D. sandwicense* hybrids at two stocking rates in coastal south-east Queensland. *Tropical Grasslands* 23, 43–55.

Jones, R.M. and Bunch, G.A. (1988a) The effect of stocking rate on the population dynamics of siratro in siratro (*Macroptilium atropurpureum*)–setaria (*Setaria sphacelata*) pastures in south-east Queensland. I Survival of plants and stolons. *Australian Journal of Agricultural Research* 39, 209–219.

Jones, R.M. and Bunch, G.A. (1988b) The effect of stocking rate on the population dynamics of siratro in siratro (*Macroptilium atropurpureum*)–setaria (*Setaria sphacelata*) pastures in south-east Queensland. II Seed set, soil seed reserves, seedling recruitment and seedling survival. *Australian Journal of Agricultural Research* 39, 221–234.

Jones, R.M. and Bunch, G.A. (1988c) *A Guide to Sampling and Measuring the Seed Content of Pastures Soils and Animal Faeces.* Technical Memorandum No. 88, Division of Tropical Crops and Pastures, CSIRO, Brisbane, Australia.

Jones, R.M. and Mott, J.J. (1980) Population dynamics in grazed pastures. *Tropical Grasslands* 14, 218–224.

Jones, R.M., Noguchi, M. and Bunch, G.A. (1991) Levels of germinable seed in topsoil and cattle faeces in legume–grass and nitrogen fertilized pastures in south-east Queensland. *Australian Journal of Agricultural Research* 42, 953–968.

Jones, R.M., Kerridge, P.C. and McLean, R.W. (1993a) Population dynamics of siratro and shrubby stylo in south-east Queensland as affected by phosphorus, soil type, stocking rate and rainfall. *Tropical Grasslands* 27, 63–74.

Jones, R.M., McDonald, C.K. and Bunch, G.A. (1993b) Persistence of roundleaf cassia in grazed pastures. In: *Proceedings of the XVII International Grasslands Congress,* III. Rockhampton, Australia, pp. 1902–1903.

Jones, R.M., McDonald, C.K. and Bunch, G.A. (1998) Ecological and agronomic studies on *Chamaecrista rotundifolia* cv. Wynn as related to modelling of persistence. *Tropical Grasslands* 32, 153–165.

Krauss, E., Lambers, H. and Kollöffel, C. (1993) The effect of handling on the yield of two populations of *Lolium perenne* selected for differences in mature leaf respiration rate. *Physiologia Plantarum* 89, 341–346.

Langer, R.H.M., Ryle, S.M. and Jewiss, O.R. (1964) The changing plant and tiller populations of timothy and meadow fescue swards. *Journal of Applied Ecology* 1, 197–208.

Louie, K., Clark, H. and Newton, P.C.D. (1998) Analysis of differential equation models in biology: a case study for clover meristem populations. *New Zealand Journal of Agricultural Research* 41, 567–576.

Mack, R.N. and Pyke, D.A. (1983) The demography of *Bromus tectorum*: variation in time and space. *Journal of Ecology* 71, 69–73.

Matthew, C. (1992) A study of seasonal root and tiller dynamics in swards of perennial ryegrass (*Lolium perenne* L.). PhD thesis, Massey University, New Zealand.

McIvor, J.G. and Gardener, C.J. (1994) Germinable soil seed banks in native pastures in north-eastern Australia. *Australian Journal of Agricultural Research* 34, 1113–1119.

McIvor, J.G., Jones, R.M. and Taylor, J.A. (1993) Tropical pasture establishment. 4. Population dynamics of sown species in developing pastures. *Tropical Grasslands* 27, 302–313.

McIvor, J.G., Singh, J.P., Corfield, J.P. and Jones, R.J. (1996) Seed production by native and naturalised grasses in north-east Queensland: effects of stocking rate and season. *Tropical Grasslands* 30, 262–269.

McLellan, A.J., Prati, D., Kaltz, O. and Schmid, B. (1997) Structure and analysis of phenotypic and genetic variation in clonal plants. In: de Kroon, H. and Groenendael, J. van (eds) *The Ecology and Evolution of Clonal Plants.* Backhuys Publishers, Leiden, The Netherlands, pp. 185–210.

Mitchell, K.J. and Glenday, A.C. (1958) The tiller population of pastures. *New Zealand Journal of Agricultural Research* 1, 305–313.

Mott, J.J. and McKeon, G.M. (1977) A note on the selection of seed types by harvester ants in northern Australia. *Australian Journal of Ecology* 2, 231–235.

Newton, P.C.D. and Hay, M.J.M. (1992) A technique for evaluating the potential for growth of shoot and root buds of white clover (*Trifolium repens*). *Journal of Agricultural Science, Cambridge* 119, 179–183.

Newton, P.C.D., Hay, M.J.M., Thomas, V.J. and Dick, H.B. (1992) Viability of axillary buds of white clover (*Trifolium repens*) in grazed pasture. *Journal of Agricultural Science, Cambridge* 119, 345–354.

Orr, D.M. (1980) Effects of sheep grazing *Astrebla* spp. grassland in central western Queensland. II. Effects of seasonal rainfall. *Australian Journal of Agricultural Research* 31, 807–20.

Orr, D.M. (1998) A life cycle approach to the population ecology of two tropical grasses in Queensland, Australia. In: Cheplick, G.P. (ed.) *Population Biology of Grasses.* Cambridge University Press, Cambridge, pp. 366–388.

Orr, D.M. (1999) Effects of residual dormancy on the germinable soil seed banks of tropical pastures. *Tropical Pastures* 33, 18–21.

Orr, D.M. and Phelps, D.G. (1994) *Basal Area Change in* Astrebla *Grassland – in Harmony with Trends in Seasonal Rainfall.* Working Paper, 8th Biennial Conference, Australian Rangeland Society, Katherine, pp. 215–216.

Orr, D.M., Paton, C.J. and Blight, G.W. (1996) An improved method for measuring the germinable soil seed banks of tropical pastures. *Tropical Grasslands* 30, 201–205.

Orr, D.M., Paton, C.J. and Lisle, A.T. (1997) Using fire to manage species composition in *Heteropogon contortus* (black speargrass) pastures. 1. Burning regimes. *Australian Journal of Agricultural Research* 48, 795–802.

Parks, J.C. and Werth, C.R. (1983) A study of spatial features of clones in a population of bracken fern, *Pteridium aquilinum* (Dennstaedtiaceae). *American Journal of Botany* 80, 537–544.

Rice, K.J. (1989) Impacts of seed banks on grassland community structure and population dynamics. In: Leck, M.A., Parker, V.T. and Simpson, R.L. (eds) *Ecology of Soil Seed Banks.* Academic Press, San Diego, California, pp. 221–231.

Roshier, D., Lee, S. and Borreland, F. (1997) A digital technique for recording of plant population data in permanent plots. *Journal of Range Management* 50, 106–109.

Samuel, M.J. and Hart, R.H. (1995) Observations on the spread and fragmentation of blue grama clones in disturbed rangelands. *Journal of Range Management* 48, 508–510.

Seliskar, D.M. (1985) Effect of reciprocal transplanting between extremes of plant zones on morphometric plasticity of five plant species in an Oregon salt marsh. *Canadian Journal of Botany* 63, 2254–2262.

Sheath, G.W. (1980) Effects of season and defoliation on the growth habit of *Lotus pedunculatus* Cav. cv. 'Grasslands Maku'. *New Zealand Journal of Agricultural Research* 23, 191–200.

Simao Neto, M., Jones, R.M. and Ratcliff, D. (1987) Recovery of pasture seed ingested by ruminants. 1. Recovery of six tropical pasture species fed to cattle, sheep and goats. *Australian Journal of Experimental Agriculture* 27, 239–246.

Sultan, S.E. (1987) Evolutionary implications of phenotypic plasticity in plants. *Evolutionary Biology* 21, 127–178.

Taylor, G.B., Rossiter, R.C. and Palmer, M.J. (1984) Long term patterns of seed softening and seedling emergence from single seed crops of subterranean clover. *Australian Journal of Experimental Agriculture and Animal Husbandry* 24, 200–212.

Torsell, B.W.R. and Nicholls, A.O. (1978) Population dynamics in species mixtures. In: Wilson, J.R. (ed.) *Plant Relations in Pastures.* CSIRO, East Melbourne, pp. 217–232.

Turkington, R. and Harper, J.L. (1979) The growth distribution and neighbour relationships of *Trifolium repens* in a permanent pasture. II. Inter- and intra-specific contact. *Journal of Ecology* 67, 219–230.

Vertes, F., Le Corre, L., Simon, J.C. and Rivere, J.M. (1988) Effets du piétinement de printemps sur un peuplement de trèfle blanc pur ou en association. *Fourrages* 116, 347–366.

Watkinson, A.R. (1997) Plant population dynamics. In: Crawley, M.J. (ed.) *Plant Ecology.* Blackwell Scientific Publications, Oxford, pp. 359–400.

Watkinson, A.R., Huiskes, A.H.L. and Noble, J.C. (1979) The demography of sand dune species with contrasting life cycles. In: Jefferies, R.L. and Davy, A.J. (eds) *Ecological Processes in Coastal Environments.* Blackwell Scientific Publications, Oxford, pp. 95–112.

Williams, W.M. (1987) Genetics and breeding. In: Baker, M.J. and Williams, W.M. (eds) *White Clover.* CAB International, Wallingford, UK, pp. 343–419.

Wilman, D. and Simpson, D. (1988) The growth of white clover (*Trifolium repens*) in five sown hill swards grazed by sheep. *Journal of Applied Ecology* 25, 631–642.

Measuring Biomass of Grassland Vegetation

7

L. 't Mannetje

Department of Plant Sciences, Wageningen University, Wageningen, The Netherlands

Introduction

Biomass of grassland vegetation refers to above-ground herbaceous material, commonly referred to as 'dry matter (DM) yield'. Research workers and managers of grassland vegetation are interested in this to determine the amount of available forage for animals or to measure the effects of management (e.g. fertilization, grazing, cutting) on the vegetation, whether the vegetation is for agricultural or amenity purposes. Vegetation biomass is important also for assessment of grassland or rangeland condition and for evaluation of new germplasm and cultivars.

The economic value of grassland vegetation is for animal production, although grassy sports fields also have commercial value. Grassland vegetation for the feeding of animals is commonly referred to as 'forage' or 'herbage' and a distinction can be made between these two terms. 'Herbage' can be regarded as herbaceous biomass in general, e.g. as used in ecological studies of grassland vegetation, whereas 'forage' refers to animal feed in keeping with the term 'foraging': the animal's actions of selecting and ingesting herbaceous feed. The term 'pasture' is sometimes used for feed, but this is confusing, as 'pasture' also stands for a grazed grassland field.

The agronomic value of standing forage is most directly related to its DM yield in (near) monospecific swards. In mixed swards the value of standing forage depends also on the botanical composition. In both monospecific and heterogeneous swards the value of measuring standing forage may be enhanced by measurements of nutritive value. Herbage or forage can be divided into botanical species (Chapter 4), into groups of species (grasses, legumes, weeds or other species), or into standing green and dead material and litter. The quantity of grassland vegetation present at any one time can be used to calculate changes, such as herbage growth, utilization by grazing animals, or deterioration. Although the basic techniques of measuring the amount of vegetation present can be used for each of these purposes, the procedures and intensity of sampling will differ, depending on the objectives of the measurements.

Most grassland used for agricultural purposes is stocked by animals for at least part of the time and in many cases year-long. Grazing affects grassland production because of defoliation, treading and fouling. Much of the grazing takes place in the growing season and that makes forage exceptional as an agricultural commodity: it is harvested whilst it grows and the harvestable product is at the same time the photosynthetic material that produces it. Harvesting takes place frequently or at least several times in a year. For these reasons measuring yield of forage is more difficult than that of other agricultural commodities.

Many grassland areas, particularly in the tropics, contain shrubs and trees. Some of these are edible, but all of them interact with the ground layer of the vegetation. They create shade, affect pasture DM yields, or, in some cases, alter the nitrogen economy of the habitat (Wilson *et al.*, 1986) and the feeding value of the understorey herbage (Samarakoon *et al.*, 1990; Belsky, 1994).

Instead of DM yield, vegetation mass can also be expressed as organic matter (OM). OM yield has the advantage that it is true herbage yield without soil contamination, which often occurs in herbage samples as a result of mechanical cutting, raking up of grass or rain splash. Contamination increases weight and distorts chemical analyses. Where samples have to be used for mineral analysis, care needs to be taken to avoid contamination of the samples, or to clean the material beforehand with minimum losses of minerals. If contamination is unavoidable, the cut material should not be used for chemical analyses, but separate pluck samples should be taken for that purpose. However, plucked samples can still be contaminated by soil from rain splash.

In intensive animal production systems, grassland yield, although initially sampled as DM or OM, is often expressed in terms of feeding units based on net energy value. Several systems are in use (Van der Honing and Alderman, 1988), e.g. VEM ('fodder units milk') or VEVI ('fodder units intensive beef production') in The Netherlands, ME ('metabolizable energy') in the UK, and UF ('unité fourragère') in France. In the USA and many Latin American countries the TDN ('total digestible nutrient') system is used, which is based on digestible energy. In some countries the original SE ('starch equivalent') is still in use.

Sampling

An understanding of the type and magnitude of errors and bias is essential to make the best choice of sampling method within the limitations of available resources. Agronomic and ecological aspects of sampling procedure and the shape, size and number of sampling units to be discussed in this section are related to density, height, botanical composition and spatial variability of the sward. The sampling unit and the frame used to delineate the area are both called *quadrat*, irrespective of the shape.

Sampling procedures

Factors affecting the choice of method are the accuracy desired, which itself depends on the purpose for which the data are needed, and the scale of operations. Greater accuracy will usually be required for the comparison of treatments, such as fertilizer levels, or for advanced germplasm evaluation than for the description of an area of grassland. For small plots, measured in square metres, a different method may be used than for paddocks, or for areas encompassing a region. The sampling procedure must also be adapted to the homogeneity of the sward, its physiognomy, density, height and species composition and to the resources available. DM yield is not a fixed parameter; it changes on a daily basis. For measurements to be meaningful, sampling must be carried out in as short a time span as possible. A careful assessment should be made of the cost–benefit balance before sampling is undertaken on the basis of labour, time and finance going into sampling and the expected outputs in terms of results and their accuracy. There is no point in doing a very rough estimate of DM yield if the data must show small differences in the effects of rates of fertilizer, or differences between cultivars of the same species. On the other hand, for an estimate of the DM yield of an area in terms of tonnes per hectare, accuracy to the level of 100 kg ha^{-1} is not important.

The sampling procedure selected also depends on whether data are required for one or more purposes. For example, it is possible to estimate DM yield and botanical composition in one operation (Chapter 4 and p. 160 this chapter) and it may be necessary to obtain information on the chemical composition or nutritive value of the forage (Chapter 11). In small plot work it can then be more efficient to cut samples by hand, sorting the material into different species, drying, weighing and grinding each component separately, than it is to use an indirect non-destructive procedure for DM yield followed by separate samplings for botanical composition and/or nutritive value. On the other hand, in a large grazing experiment the most efficient methodology is likely to be a combined indirect method for DM yield and botanical composition (Chapter 4 and

p. 160 this chapter) and taking pluck samples for chemical and nutritive value assessments (Chapter 11).

If the data are to be used to measure changes in DM yield, such as growth, utilization, decomposition or damage by wildlife, accuracy becomes an important issue. In these cases, where the interest is in the difference between two yield measurements, a larger number of sampling units is needed than for a single estimate that simply describes the state of the vegetation (Boyd, 1949). The difficulties of measuring changes in yield will increase appreciably with increasing spatial variability. The effects of spatial variability can be reduced by selecting adjacent pairs of similar sampling units, one of which is measured at the beginning and the other at the end of a period. Studies in grazed swards may require the use of exclosures (p. 170). However, an assessment of spatial variability may be the objective of sampling (Chapter 5), which will require a different approach.

Positioning of sampling units

A first prerequisite of the positioning of sampling units is that all possible units have an equal chance of being selected (random sampling). To achieve this the field or plot to be sampled can be divided into sampling units by dividing the surface area by the size of the sampling unit and allocating a number to each unit. The required number of samples is then chosen from a list of randomized numbers. This can easily be done in small plots, where the number of possible sampling units is small. However, random sampling is very cumbersome in large areas, because an operator must consult this list for every sampling position. It is more efficient to use stratified random sampling by dividing the area into equal-sized strata that stretch from one border of the field to the opposite, e.g. marked by fence posts, selecting a transect at random within each stratum, and then positioning the quadrat or strip at equal distances at a given number of steps. The placement of the quadrat must be unbiased, which can be simply done by always placing it at the tip of the boot that lands at the selected position, though this can be difficult to do randomly in tall grasslands or shrublands. Throwing of quadrats is hardly ever unbiased, nor is selection of 'representative' sampling positions. Systematic sampling is the simplest. Sampling positions are selected at regular intervals along parallel transects at equal distances.

An area to be sampled may consist of easily recognizable sub-areas that have clear habitat differences but are reasonably homogeneous in themselves. These sub-areas can then be considered as strata, which are unlikely to be of the same size. Therefore, the number of sampling units to be taken from each stratum should be proportional to its surface area if a mean of the whole area is desired. Such a mean is often of little value, because it has no biological meaning.

A major form of bias that is often overlooked is associated with operators, who may have differences in quadrat placement, cutting technique, observational ability, or fatigue. To avoid operator bias, each one should deal with an equal number of sampling units in each treatment, or in replicated experiments each operator could do all the work in one replicate, so that operator differences are eliminated or confounded with block effects. Consultation between operators prior to sampling on matters such as cutting height will reduce differences between them.

A large proportion of sampling error arises from edge effects. There are two types of edge effects: those occurring at the edges of fields or plots and those of sampling units. Edges of fields or plots often have different conditions than the centres and should be avoided for sampling. Areas near gates into paddocks are usually highly atypical. Edge effects of sampling units may be due to difficulties of boundary definition or to disturbance of the vegetation by quadrat placement causing material to be pushed into or out of the sampling area. It has to be decided beforehand either to include only herbage that is rooted within the sampling area or else only material that is actually present within the vertical planes of the quadrat borders, irrespective of its point of origin. For very dense short vegetation, or with stoloniferous or creeping material, it is not possible to separate plant units and the only way is to include all material present within the quadrat boundaries. This method is more accurate and much quicker. For tall vegetation there are problems with vertical boundaries. Plants do not grow upwards in strictly vertical planes and material growing both within and outside the quadrat will cross the boundaries. Thus, especially with tall tussock grasses, it may be easiest to sample plants rooted within the quadrat rather than cut vertical planes. However, this is difficult to do with twining tropical legumes and it is easier to sample these by cutting vertical planes. With twining species, care must be taken that material is not pulled inside the quadrat, resulting in an overestimate of that species.

To reduce edge effects, the quadrat perimeter should be as small as possible in relation to the area of the sampling unit. This ratio is smallest for a circle and for this reason the use of circular quadrats has been recommended (e.g. Van Dyne *et al.*, 1963). However, circular quadrats are more difficult to place, except in short vegetation, or in the case of the 'sickledrat' (see next section). A special case of edge effects exists with power-driven harvesters due to inaccuracies of starting and stopping, which affects the area harvested (p. 157). Sampling units cut by machines should therefore have a large length : width ratio. In the case of twining legumes, sickle bar mowers will increase edge effects, because they tend to pull material in from outside the strip; flail-type cutters are likely to give a more precise vertical face.

Sampling units

Aspects to be considered when choosing sampling units are number, size, shape and the material from which they are made. Statistical, agronomic, ecological, practical and financial considerations determine the final choice. A non-statistical way to determine the optimal number and size of quadrats for a given vegetation type is to do a test sampling with different sized quadrats. The mean of the variable being estimated (e.g. DM yield) is plotted against the number of quadrats of the different sizes. The fluctuation of the mean will decrease with increasing quadrat numbers (cf. Greig-Smith, 1964). Taking into account the magnitude of the fluctuation of the mean and the time taken to harvest the quadrats, a decision can be made as to the optimum size and number of quadrats. The optimum number and size of quadrats are inversely related to the density and homogeneity of the vegetation. In very sparse vegetation a small quadrat will contain such a small amount of material that variability between quadrats will be very large and a very large number of quadrats will be needed to get a reliable estimate of the mean. Cutting and handling material from a very large number of small quadrats will also take more time than a smaller number of larger quadrats.

There are no exact rules for the best quadrat size. A rule of thumb is that each quadrat should be able to represent the vegetation, or parts of the vegetation in a field. The author has generally used *c.* 60–100 observations per treatment with quadrats of 50×50 cm whilst using the BOTANAL package (Tothill *et al.*, 1992) for botanical composition and DM yield estimations of paddocks ranging in size from 0.9 to 3.6 ha (Mannetje and Jones, 1990). Brocket (1996), using a pasture disc (p. 161) to estimate fuel loads in a rangeland in South Africa, found that the standard error of the mean did not decrease substantially as the number of readings exceeded 100, but at low DM yields (< 4 t ha^{-1}) more than 160 readings were required to achieve acceptable precision. When the samples are cut, the area sampled may range from 100% on small plots to $< 0.5\%$ on very extensive areas. The area sampled usually decreases as the area under study increases. However, with mechanized destructive and indirect non-destructive sampling it is possible for total sampling areas of 0.5% to be used in experiments of 100 ha or more.

Sample units may be rectangular, square or circular. Quadrat frames can be made of any material, but solid frames are best made of aluminium, because they are light and do not rust. In tall vegetation it is handy to leave one side of a four-sided quadrat open in order to slide the quadrat in place. Circular quadrats are difficult to place in any but short vegetation. To overcome this problem Kennedy (1972) developed a 'sickledrat', which consists of a stake pushed into the ground in the centre of the sampling position. An arm with a curved pointed crosspiece at the end is rotated around the stake as the material is cut. Circular turf corers are used in very short vegetation. In The Netherlands a tapered corer is used. It has a diameter of 56 mm at the bottom and 66 mm at the top, a depth of 10 cm, and is fitted with a cross handle. Hutchinson (1967) reported on the effects of core size and shape.

When the sampling area is longer than wide and the material is cut by machine, the sampling unit is usually called a *strip*. The advantages of strips are that they can easily be harvested by machine and that each strip covers more of the existing variation in the sward than a circle or a square. The width of a strip is determined by the width or diameter of the cutting mechanism and its length can be determined by any type of measuring device (e.g. tape, stick or piece of string), preferably before and after the cut has been taken, to reduce starting and stopping inaccuracies. However, the length of string or rope can expand with use, so its length should be checked occasionally. Using strips rather than quadrats may give a more precise estimate of the paddock mean, as a larger area can be sampled for no extra input, but less information is obtained about spatial variability.

Destructive Techniques

Cutting equipment

The simplest devices are hand-operated tools, such as scissors, shears, secateurs, sickles, knives and scythes. Small hand-held tools are useful for small quadrats when the material is to be divided into species or groups of species. Hand-held power-driven tools, such as sheep shears, clippers and lawn or hedge trimmers, may be connected to an engine or to electricity or may be battery operated. There are hand-held power scythes and self-propelled or tractor-driven harvesters. Engine-driven reciprocating cutter bar mowers and lawn mowers with a catcher can be used in short to medium tall swards. The hand-held and cutter bar devices have the disadvantage that they usually do not collect the cut material, although it is sometimes possible to add a collection tray. Van Dyne (1966) incorporated a vacuum cleaner with a sheep-shearing hand piece to collect the material. A commonly used Danish harvester[1] has a cutting width of 1.5 m, with adjustable stubble height (Fig. 7.1). The total fresh weight is automatically recorded for each plot. A sample of the cut material is taken by hand, or automatically in new models, for assessment of the percentage DM. After each plot the machine is emptied and the next plot cut and weighed. Normal forage harvesters with reduced cutting width can also be used.

---

[1] J. Haldrup A/S, Løgstør, Denmark

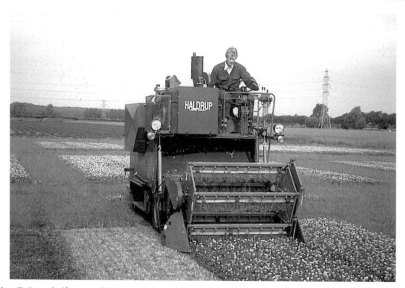

Fig. 7.1. Self-propelled weight recording plot harvester.

Height of cutting

It is essential with any type of cutting implement that cutting height above ground level can be controlled. Hand-held shears or secateurs can cut to near ground level. However, this may affect regrowth and sampling areas cut to ground level should be omitted from sampling again in the near future. Hand cutting may lead to personal bias when more than one person does the work. The easiest way to prevent this is to use a grid within the quadrat equipped with legs of the desired cutting height. Most mechanized cutting equipment cannot sample to ground level. When this is desirable, the amount of DM in the stubble could be sampled by hand afterwards. Hand-operated cutter bar equipment can be fitted with guide wheels to set the cutting height. Cutting heights will vary depending on the type of grassland, ranging from 1 cm in closely grazed pastures to 10–20 cm in tall swards. Low cutting heights and mechanized equipment can suck in extraneous material such as detached litter, twigs, gravel and dry faeces. Such equipment can generally not be used in stony areas.

Weighing and subsampling

Material from small quadrats can be dried and weighed without subsampling. However, with large amounts of material the fresh herbage must be weighed and a subsample taken immediately for drying and weighing to determine the DM%. When the subsample is not weighed immediately after taking, it must be kept in a moisture-tight container to avoid water loss before weighing.

Non-destructive Techniques

There has always been a demand for rapid methods, particularly for large-scale grazing experiments, and a number have been used in the past. Mannetje (1978) reviewed earlier methods, but most of these have been superseded by more accurate ones.

Destructive sampling requires high inputs of labour and/or equipment. This can be costly and may lead to insufficient sample numbers, resulting in low precision. Destructive sampling also prevents measuring changes of the sward in the sampling area. In small grazed plots the material removed by cutting may be a significant proportion of the feed available. For these reasons, non-destructive sampling techniques have been developed, which can be grouped into three categories: (i) visual estimation; (ii) height and density measurements; and (iii) measurement of non-vegetative attributes that can be related to DM yield.

Although non-destructive methods are less accurate on a per sample basis than cutting methods, they take less time per observation and involve less physical effort by the operators. Thus, when compared with destructive techniques, DM yields may be estimated more accurately even though the yield of each quadrat is measured less accurately. The larger number of quadrats also offers more opportunity for examining spatial heterogeneity (McDonald and Jones, 1997). The non-destructive methods in use are double sampling techniques, i.e. two overlapping methods are used. One is an accurate determination of DM yield in a few samples (standards) and the other is a visual estimate, height or capacitance reading of herbage in many samples, including the standards. Regression equations between the estimated non-yield parameter and DM yield of the standards provide the calibration of the technique. Therefore, non-destructive techniques still require some sample cutting, but the amount to be cut is small and, if necessary, cutting can be restricted to an area of the same sward that is outside the measurement or treatment area.

Direct visual estimation

Although experienced operators who are very familiar with the type of pasture under consideration may be able to estimate the amount of DM present in a field to within $c.$ 1 t ha^{-1}, without any calibration cuts, the procedure is of limited value in serious research. It is more likely to be successful if photographic standards of known yields are used when doing the estimations. This approach is probably best suited to pasture monitoring of commercial paddocks by farmers or graziers (Tothill and Partridge, 1998). It is less complicated for monospecific swards or very simple mixtures.

Comparative yield method (CYM)

Since its publication by Haydock and Shaw (1975) this method has been widely used, particularly in combination with the dry-weight-rank (DWR) method of Mannetje and Haydock (1963) or direct estimation of percentages, as outlined in the BOTANAL package (Tothill *et al.*, 1992). The combination has proved to be accurate, rapid and effective in dealing with large experimental areas, but also for small plots or exclosures (Waite, 1994). The combined use of the DWR or estimation of percentages and the CYM improves efficiency and also improves the accuracy of estimating percentages. Efficiency is increased because more parameters are dealt with in one quadrat at the same time and accuracy is increased because of a possible relation between DM yield and composition; for example, high-yielding quadrats may have a consistently different species composition to low-yielding quadrats (Jones and Hargreaves, 1979). Visual procedures for estimating botanical composition are described in Chapter 4.

With the CYM, standards are selected covering the range of DM yield usually on a scale of 1 (lowest) to 5 (highest). The area is then sampled using many quadrats, with yields estimated to 0.1 units on the same 1–5 scale. Within any one quadrat it is often easier to estimate DM yield in terms relative to a set of standards than to estimate DM yield in absolute terms. When sampling is completed, a new set of at least ten quadrats, spanning the range of yields, is set out. These are estimated independently by each operator and then cut, dried and weighed. The regression equations derived from the standards are then used to calculate the dry matter yields of the paddock samples. It is preferable to use computer programs, such as those of Hargreaves *et al.* (1992) and McDonald *et al.* (1996) in the BOTANAL package, to do these calculations. A hand-held computer can be used to enter data in the field (McDonald *et al.*, 1996) and save the time needed and risk of error associated with re-entering data. Although Haydock and Shaw (1975) reported correlation coefficients (r^2) of estimated values of DM obtained by CYM and by hand cutting of 0.98–1.00, it is more usual to find values between 0.90 and 0.98.

As an alternative, the actual yield of the standard and experimental quadrats can be estimated directly as kg ha^{-1}, following the same procedure for calibration. Although some operators find direct estimation more difficult than using scores as standards, it has proved to be well suited to experiments where there are pasture types with different plant structures within the one experiment. It is easier to switch between the pasture types if directly thinking in terms of yield rather than a single set of one to five standards based on one plant type. Alternatively, a new set of standards can be set up for each pasture type.

Height and density

The standing herbaceous biomass of an area of grassland is related to the density and height of its individual components. Brown (1954) and Mannetje (1978) reviewed earlier methods using this principle. The measuring of individual plant height, which is fraught with practical difficulties, is now not used to any extent, except in very sparse vegetation. Height and density measurements of a sward can be integrated using a 'weighted disc', 'rising plate', 'drop-disc', or 'pasture disc', of which there are many types in use. They consist of a round or square disc of light metal or of plastic foam of a given weight that can slide along a central rod, which is lowered or dropped from a fixed height on to the sward (Fig. 7.2). The height above ground level at which it rests is either noted from a scale on the rod, recorded on counters, or automatically recorded on an attached small computer, which also calculates the mean of a number of readings. In The Netherlands, a round plastic foam disc of 50 cm diameter, weighing 340 g, exerting a pressure of 1.7 kg m^{-2}, is commonly used.

A widely used implement in Europe is the HFRO sward stick (Barthram, 1986), which measures plant height rather than compressed sward height. It employs a 2×1 cm clear window that is lowered vertically on a shaft until its base touches the vegetation. The height contact above the ground is recorded in 0.5 cm bands. The operation of the sward stick is akin to that of the fresnel lens apparatus developed by Whitney (1974) for use on low-growing tropical grass swards.

In a study in Germany, Hoppe *et al.* (1995) found that sward height measured with a sward height meter made in New Zealand was more closely correlated with DM yield than average shoot height measured with a ruler. This can be expected, because the disc of a pasture meter is lowered on to the sward and the point where the disc stops depends on the resistance it gets from the sward, which depends on both height and density. This is less of a factor in very sparse vegetation as found in arid regions, in deserts and on sand dunes. Assaeed (1997), working on sand dunes in Saudi Arabia, found that DM yield of individual species was correlated with plant height, basal diameter and canopy diameter. He developed height–weight profiles for different species to assess utilization by grazing animals, based on estimates of the percentage height removed.

Bransby *et al.* (1977), working with a pasture of *Festuca arundinacea*, studied the effect of disc size and weight, using four discs of different sizes at a constant weight per unit area or discs of equal size but of different weights. They achieved correlation coefficients (r^2) ranging from 0.79 to 0.94 between meter readings and measured DM yield. Neither size nor weight of discs had a significant effect on the accuracy of calibration.

Douglas and Crawford (1994) reviewed disadvantages and problems with the drop-disc method. They found that disc estimates were most accurate ($r^2 = 0.83$) for *Lolium perenne* swards used for silage up to 4–5 t of vegetative growth per hectare. The presence of stems and lodging were detrimental to the accuracy of disc calibration. They found a linear relationship between the drop-disc meter and herbage DM, but warned for errors in estimating relatively small as well as large biomasses. E.A. Lantinga (Wageningen, 1996 personal communication) noted that the regression

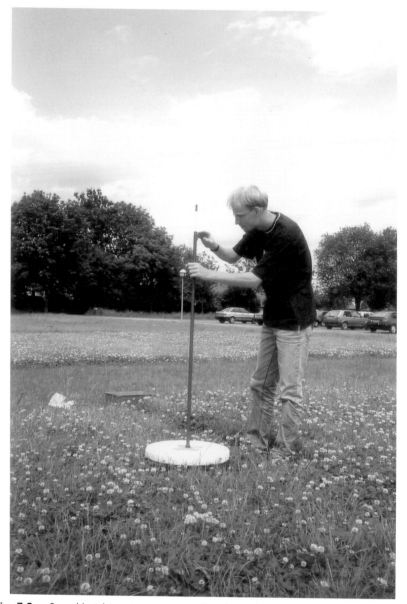

Fig. 7.2. Sward height meter consisting of a plastic disc that can move along a central rod with a height indicator at top.

coefficient (slope of the line) is determined by the density of the sward. Douglas and Crawford (1994) concluded that the drop-disc method is useful due to simplicity and rapidity with extremely low cost.

Michell (1982) in Tasmania and Michell and Large (1983) in England reported similar findings on *L. perenne* and *Trifolium repens* pastures. However, in Tasmania the relationship between meter readings and DM yield tended to become curvilinear in mid to late summer, when the grass became reproductive, but the addition of a quadratic term in the equation made little difference to DM yield estimates.

In conclusion, the weighted disc and the HFRO sward stick methods are very useful on short pastures, being frequently used on *L. perenne* and *T. repens* pastures. Neither method should be used in very tall or lodged grass, and they are less accurate with stemmy material. The calibration of height and DM yield needs to be established for each type of pasture under study, or before every sampling event when the structure of the herbage changes (e.g. when grass seed heads emerge).

Capacitance

The principle of capacitance meters is based on a signal produced by an oscillator in an electrical circuit, which changes as the capacitance under the measuring head changes. Herbage mass has a high capacitance whereas that of air and wood is very low. The difference in capacitance between a quadrat on bare ground and on a grass sward is an indirect method to measure DM yield.

Capacitance meters have been used since 1956 and although improved versions have been developed, their performance still leaves much to be desired, except under the special circumstances outlined below. The appearance and functioning have been modernized since the early days, when the equipment was heavy, consisting of two vertical plates or as many as 50 rods (Vickery *et al.*, 1980), requiring two people to carry it and which could not be easily manoeuvred in tall pasture. The first meters emitted a signal, which had to be captured by earphones, and values had to be recorded by hand. The present meters consist of a single lightweight probe and the data are automatically recorded for computer analysis, or they have an inbuilt calibration equation so that DM yields can be read off. The single rod probe as described by Vickery *et al.* (1980) and Vickery and Nicol (1982) weighs only 1.4 kg and it has a small box of electronic components attached to the rod, containing counting circuit, a loudspeaker, a liquid digital display and a switch for resetting. The loudspeaker emits a tone to indicate that a reading has been taken. The electronics look after storage of sequential readings and the calculation of the mean. The meters need to be calibrated before each sampling occasion, because the capacitance values depend on the species and the moisture content. However, Vickery *et al.*

(1980) and Vickery and Nicol (1982) have claimed that their single-probe meter, from which the New Zealand 'pasture probe' has been developed, is responsive to surface area of herbage DM and less sensitive to variation in moisture content of the sward. They adapted the calibration procedure by subtracting the mean plot reading from the measured mean air capacitance above the pasture in each plot, before calculating the regression of this corrected meter reading with herbage DM. The information provided by the firm[2] that markets the 'pasture probe' mentions that several calibration equations have been developed for different pasture species and seasons in New Zealand. The readings will be influenced by the factors that alter the relationship between surface area and dry matter. These can include species that have a different surface area to dry matter relationship, e.g. some C_4 species. Seasonal changes in pasture can also influence the relationship, such as changes from the vegetative to the reproductive growth stage.

Experience with capacitance meters in tropical pastures has been disappointing, at least with earlier versions (e.g. Jones *et al.*, 1977), the main problem being that the capacitance was strongly influenced by the DM content of the sward, moisture being a strong conductor. As the herbage became drier, the capacitance meter gave unreliable results.

Acceptable results have been obtained in temperate pastures with mostly green material, but better results were reported with CYM, weighted discs and the HFRO sward stick (p. 161).

Spectral analysis, remote sensing

Chapter 9 deals with the principles and Chapter 10 with the application of remote sensing in rangeland studies. Radiation reflectance is affected by leaf area index (LAI), which is related to vegetation cover, which in turn is related to DM yield, as long as LAI is below 1.0. As soon as the sward canopy becomes closed, LAI equals or exceeds 1 and the relationship no longer exists. Remote sensing can be very useful for qualitative studies and to estimate cover of open vegetation (Tucker, 1979; Foran, 1987; Wylie *et al.*, 1992, 1995; Pickup *et al.*, 1994). Remote sensing for vegetation studies is therefore useful for rangelands in dry climates. Examples of successful use of remote sensing techniques include the application of normalized difference vegetation index (NDVI) image data (see Chapter 9), which proved to be useful for monitoring seasonal growing conditions of Sahelian and Sudanian rangelands and for making long-term productivity comparisons between types of rangeland (Tappan *et al.*, 1992). Gabriel *et al.* (1996) successfully applied LANDSAT MSS images to estimate DM yield of open arid steppe in southern Patagonia, Argentina. Brown and Stephens (1995)

---

[2] Edwards and Williams Greenhouse Ltd, PO Box 22, Levin, New Zealand

could relate advanced very high-resolution radiometer-derived NDVI to milk fat production data collected daily from dairy farms in New Zealand. High-resolution visible multi-spectral data were used by Williamson (1990) to estimate biomass of improved pasture in South Australia with accuracy of 43–81% ($P = 0.95$).

Long-term vegetation changes are best monitored by repeated observations on permanent quadrats. Northup *et al.* (1999) applied near-ground remote sensing to describe plant canopy cover, bare ground and herbaceous yield at intervals in an open woodland. They fitted a quad bike with a camera gantry attached to a telescopic boom arm. Plot images were taken by a digital (or slide) camera and the data were automatically captured by an electronic theodolite. The data were then analysed by appropriate software. This method was compared with BOTANAL (Tothill *et al.*, 1992) and both with hand-measured standards. Northup *et al.* (1999) concluded that their imaging technique, combined with location and elevation data, allowed an 'explicit description of the spatial distribution of vegetative characteristics'. However, their method could not accurately define basal area and botanical composition, which are possible with BOTANAL. Therefore, they recommended combining the two methods.

Modelling

Many models for predicting grassland production have been developed in recent years. They are often based on growth, senescence, litter and standing biomass, using data on incoming radiation, temperature, soil moisture, day length and altitude (e.g. De Ridder and Van Keulen, 1995; Armstrong *et al.*, 1997; see also Chapter 3).

The simplest method of modelling primary production of grasslands is to relate DM yield to rainfall in arid regions, where soil moisture is the main limiting factor to growth (e.g. McCown, 1973; Le Houérou *et al.*, 1988; Wylie *et al.*, 1992).

A model for estimating DM yield of forage under plantation crops was proposed by Wilson and Ludlow (1991) and further developed by Wilson and Schwenke (1995). It uses a growth equation and data on incidental radiation above the tree canopy, intercepted radiation and light use efficiency of the pasture species.

Comparisons of methods

Murphy *et al.* (1995) compared cutting of quadrats, capacitance meter, a sward stick and rising plate for estimating DM yield on a pasture of *Poa pratensis* and *T. repens* in a rotational stocking experiment. Mean coefficients of variation, for pre- and post-grazing DM yields, were 28.8 and 20.2

for quadrat cutting, 15.5 and 10.1 for a capacitance meter, 27.2 and 21.4 for a sward stick and 27.9 and 18.4 for a rising plate, respectively. Correlation coefficients (r^2) between cut quadrats and pre- and post-grazing DM yield estimates were 0.65 and 0.36 for the capacitance meter, 0.70 and 0.31 for the sward stick and 0.72 and 0.05 for the rising plate, respectively. The authors concluded that the non-destructive methods were quick and provided a level of precision considered adequate for day-to-day grazing management decisions, although the accuracy quoted for post-grazing estimates is very low.

In a study in The Netherlands on *L. perenne* based pastures, Gabriëls and Van den Berg (1993) compared two rising plate methods (a 0.20 m^2 round aluminium disc, exerting a pressure of 8.5 Pa, and a 0.16 m^2 square plastic disc exerting a pressure of 17.0 Pa) and a single-probe capacitance meter (Vickery *et al.*, 1980). They validated the indirect estimates with cutting, weighing and subsampling of quadrats, followed by drying and weighing the subsamples. The correlation coefficients (r^2) of the estimated yields by the indirect methods with the cutting yields were lower for the capacitance probe (75.9–82.9) than for the rising plate methods (84.0–89.7). The lowest coefficient of variation was 26.1, which means that for an average DM yield of 1600 kg ha^{-1}, the residual standard error is about 450 kg ha^{-1}. However, the authors pointed out that spatial variability in density and height of the fields used in the comparison were high. They quoted other comparisons of similar methods with much smaller coefficients of variation (11.4–13.3).

Michell and Large (1983) compared a rising plate and a single-probe capacitance meter (Vickery *et al.*, 1980) on *L. perenne* and *T. repens* pastures. Correlation coefficients (r^2) between the meter readings and DM yield estimated by clipping were always > 0.9, but residual standard deviations were considerably higher for the capacitance than for the rising plate meter. Neither meter gave accurate results for tall herbage with senescent material.

Shrubs and Trees

Grasslands often contain native woody species ranging from small shrubs (e.g. *Calluna* spp.) to large shrubs (e.g. some *Acacia* spp.) or trees (e.g. *Eucalyptus* spp.), but fodder shrubs/trees may also be planted (e.g. *Stylosanthes scabra*, *Gliricidia* spp., *Leucaena* spp.). The approaches for estimating the DM yield of woody components in grassland differ according to the information that is desired. In ecological studies, e.g. for nutrient cycling, the total above-ground biomass may be the objective and in agronomic studies it may be the forage. Mannetje (1978) discussed methods in use before about 1975.

A sampling unit may be a single tree/shrub, a length of row or an area of land containing trees/shrubs.

Destructive techniques

For total DM yield the simplest way is to cut whole trees/shrubs at a certain height above ground level and to separate the material into wood (e.g. with a diameter > 5 mm), twigs (diameter < 5 mm), fruits and leaves, drying and weighing each component separately. Where only edible parts are of interest, the trees/shrubs can be stripped of leaves, fruit and twigs to a diameter of 5 mm, which are usually considered edible.

Non-destructive techniques

Several double sampling techniques to estimate forage DM yields have been developed for various species, based on stem measurements or photographic images.

Burrows and Beale (1970) developed a relationship ($r^2 = 0.98$) between stem circumference 30 cm above the ground and DM yield of leaves, expressed on logarithmic scales, of *Acacia aneura*, an important native forage tree in semiarid Australia. Bobek and Bergstrom (1978) found that tree diameter × height correlated well with total browse supply per tree. Although the intercept values were different for different woody species, the slope was similar. In other words, virtually the same regression could be used for different species. The authors measured diameter at 5–10 cm above the ground. The time required was 11 times less than the traditional harvest plot technique.

Uso *et al.* (1997) calculated non-linear regressions between height and diameter measurements and green biomass of each of several Mediterranean, mostly small shrub species. They also developed a simulation model for green and woody biomass growth based on the total volume of the shrubs and environmental parameters (air temperature, air humidity and rainfall).

In Italy, Piemontes *et al.* (1997) developed a method to estimate shrub biomass by a photographic technique. Pictures were taken from a given distance and the images were digitized. Computer image analysis gave reliable estimates of biomass with high precision when compared with destructive techniques.

The comparative yield method (CYM) can also be adapted to estimate edible biomass from shrubs. R.L. Roothaert and L. 't Mannetje (unpublished data) estimated the amount of edible DM of a protein bank in Kenya. They used individual shrubs as standards 1 (lowest) to 5 (highest) for edible

DM yield and scored all the shrubs in the protein bank. The edible DM yield of the standards was harvested and the mean yield calculated.

Composition of Yield and Percentage Green Material

DM yield of forage is usually of little use unless it is further qualified. The most important qualifying parameters are: (i) botanical composition (Chapter 4); (ii) sward structure (Chapter 5); (iii) nutritive value (Chapter 11); and (iv) chemical composition (Chapter 11). In addition to these parameters it can be useful to know the percentage of green material in the forage, as this has an important effect on animal production from pastures (Mannetje, 1974; Cowan and O'Grady, 1976; Mannetje and Ebersohn, 1980). Percentage green cover is also an important parameter for pasture production modelling (Chapter 3).

The percentage or DM yield of green material in the forage can be estimated by cutting and hand-sorting material, but that would mean that when leaf blades are part green and part dead they need to be cut into a green and a dead part. As this would be very laborious, it is better to use an indirect method. The following are available:

- Hunter and Grant (1961) applied the 'constituent differential' method, which was developed by Cooper et al. (1957) for the estimation of botanical composition of a two-component herbage mixture, where the components differ in the concentration of some constituent. The constituent concentration of a sample of the total herbage and that of each of the components is determined and the composition calculated as follows:

$$X = 100 \left[(C_t - C_1) / (C_2 - C_1) \right]$$

  where X is the percentage composition by weight of component 2, and C_t, C_1 and C_2 are the concentrations of the constituents of the total sample, of component 1 and of component 2, respectively. Hunter and Grant (1961) used either percentage DM or percentage crude protein as the distinguishing constituent of green and dead DM. Of these, the percentage DM gave acceptable results, but percentage crude protein did not.

- Hunter and Grant (1961) also described the 'pigmentation' method. Ground, oven-dried green and dead samples of the sward under study are mixed by weight to cover a full range from dead to green at 10% intervals. Methanol is added to each of these mixtures and the chlorophyll filtered off. Colour density, as measured by an absorptiometer, setting the 100% dead at 100% light transmission, is plotted against percentage green to give a calibration curve, which is nearly linear. Samples of unknown dead : green ratio are treated the same way and the percentage green can be read from the calibration curve.

- Grant (1971) introduced the 'chlorophyll extraction' method, which is similar to the pigmentation method, except for the preparation of the extract. This is done in subdued light with acetone and a trace of Na_2CO_3. Optical density of the standard and the unknown samples are read on a spectrophotometer. This method gave a correlation coefficient of 0.99 between percentage green material by extraction and by hand separation.

- Walker *et al.* (1997) used a 'green leaf' ranking scheme, developed by Walker (1976) in South Africa, to estimate the percentage of green biomass of a number of grass species at six sites in arid and semiarid Australia, ranging in long-term rainfall from 346 to 871 mm per annum. They estimated the percentage of green material in a tuft of grass of different species in classes 0–10, 11–25, 26–50, 51–75, 76–90, 91–99 and 100 and related it to soil moisture status.

- Waite and Kerr (1996) adapted the CYM of Haydock and Shaw (1975). Sites are selected containing very low (1) and high (5) apparent green leaf blade yields. Other sites (3, 2 and 4) are then selected with green leaf blade yields apparently halfway between 1 and 5 and similarly between 1 and 3 and between 3 and 5. At each site, two quadrats are placed with visually estimated similar leaf blade yields. One of each pair of quadrats is cut, and hand sorted into green leaf blade and other material, and the material is weighed fresh. If necessary, another site must be chosen if the earlier site 3 was not linearly between sites 1 and 5. After these preparations the sward under study is sampled, scoring quadrat sites in terms of the five standards, calculating the percentage green according to the CYM. The method was tested on several pastures. Correlation coefficients of 0.84 and 0.82 for two observers for green leaf material were slightly lower than for total DM yield (0.88 and 0.90).

- Curran and Williamson (1987) and Williamson (1990) estimated green leaf area index in northern England and South Australia, respectively, with reflectance in the red (0.6–0.7 µm) and near-infrared (0.8–1.1 µm) wavelength.

The use of the DWR multipliers of Mannetje and Haydock (1963) to estimate green and dead DM proportions, as recommended by Mannetje (1978), has been shown by Tothill *et al.* (1992) to be invalid.

Growth and Utilization

Pasture yield measurements are often used to calculate changes in vegetation mass due to growth or utilization by grazing animals. The standing vegetation mass at any one time is the end result of past growth minus removal by grazing or disappearance by decomposition. However, growth and utilization are not simply the difference between standing crop measurements on two occasions. In the time between measurements there may have been undetected changes in vegetation mass: material present at the first sampling and that produced since may have disappeared, by decomposition or by grazing by invertebrates or wildlife, before it could be measured.

Although several sampling techniques to estimate growth and utilization have been developed over the years, they all have severe limitations. The most limiting factor to sampling programmes for growth and utilization is the lack of precision that can be achieved due to the heterogeneity in most swards, particularly in grazed situations where there is selective defoliation, fouling and treading. Waddington and Cooke (1971) reported that, with four replicates, at least 32 caged sites were required in a field to estimate a 95% confidence interval for annual growth and consumption. Only in very homogeneous and near monospecific swards can growth and utilization over periods of a few days be measured reliably, even with a large number of sampling sites (Deenen and Lantinga, 1993).

Singh *et al.* (1975) reviewed and evaluated techniques for measuring herbage growth, ranging from measuring peak standing crop of current live material to the summation of increments in live, recent dead, old dead and litter. They found large and significant differences in estimated growth between different methods. Cacho (1993) reviewed methods and models for calculating growth under (continuous) grazing and presented a simple equation for herbage growth that can be used in models of sward dynamics.

The best approach now would be simulation modelling with inputs of vegetation mass, management options and environmental parameters. Several examples of such models are mentioned in Chapter 3.

Exclosures

Exclosures are used for the exclusion of grazing animals, either to measure the effects of grazing on the sward (e.g. Orr and Evenson, 1991) or to measure growth, utilization or decomposition over time. There are many types of exclosures, including movable cages or fences or loose panels erected on the spot. They are mostly made of wire, the mesh depending on the animal species and size to be excluded. Prendergast and Brady (1955) described a movable cage with electrified wires. The size of the exclosure depends on the animal species to be excluded, type of vegetation and the size of quadrat used in the study; it may vary from 1 to many square metres.

The main consideration regarding exclosures is their effect on herbage growth, which may be positive or negative (Mannetje, 1978). Positive effects may come from decreased wind velocity and increased relative humidity under the cage. Negative effects could be caused by reduced light intensity. Fences and hurdles cause higher temperatures, but the air temperature inside cages is usually lower than outside. Soil temperature and soil moisture are not affected (Williams, 1951; Dobb and Elliott, 1964). Positive effects of exclosures may also be due to the absence of grazing (defoliation, trampling, dung and urine patches) (Brown and Evans, 1973). However, considering the problems of sward heterogeneity and matching quadrat positions, temperature differences caused by exclosures are likely to be negligible.

To measure the vegetation within exclosures, use can be made of the normal methods for DM yield estimation, discussed above. However, the area is too small to apply the required number of observations in order to obtain the necessary precision when using standard visual estimation techniques such as BOTANAL. Waite (1994) adapted the BOTANAL method for use in exclosures by dividing the single 1 m² measuring area under 15 cages of 1.5 × 1.5 m into four areas of 50 × 50 cm. Within each of the 60 areas he carried out the usual ranking for botanical composition and DM yield using CYM. DM yield and botanical composition could thus be monitored without destroying the vegetation under the cages. This took only 10% of the time required for cutting the same 60 areas and the results were very similar. As this procedure was non-destructive, it enabled cumulative changes in yield over time to be followed.

Conclusion

The most appropriate method to use for an estimation of the herbage biomass present at any one time depends on the scale of operation, the purpose for which the data are required, the accuracy desired and the resources available. Three scales can be distinguished: small plot, paddock and regional.

Small scale

Plot size is measured in square metres and the purpose of the experiment may be preliminary testing of germplasm (Chapter 8) or measuring the response to fertilizer application. The most suitable method for measuring yield will depend on the accuracy required and whether the sward is a monoculture or a mixture. With preliminary testing of germplasm it may suffice to rate yield, even without calibration. If more accurate data are required, there is a choice between destructive and non-destructive methods. When samples are required for botanical and chemical analysis, hand cutting and simultaneous sorting may be the quickest, provided the components are easily distinguishable. In swards of short and medium height a capacitance or height meter may be suitable, taking into account the reservations pointed out previously. For all types of sward, CYM or its adaptation (Waite, 1994) can be used.

Paddock scale

Plot size is measured in hundreds of square metres or in hectares and plots may be part of a grazing experiment or a farm. Herbage biomass data may be needed to determine grazing pressure, the effect of management practices such as stocking rate or fertilizer applications. Double sampling or non-destructive methods, which are quicker and cheaper and need not be less accurate than destructive methods, are strongly recommended. BOTANAL (Tothill *et al.*, 1992) can be used under any condition and requires the least resources in terms of labour and equipment. The advantage of BOTANAL is that herbage biomass and botanical composition can be estimated on the same samples in a single operation.

In intensive systems on level ground, a double sampling method can be used, measuring height in many spots and cutting, say, 5–10% of the spots with a machine as described on p. 157. The machine data can then be used to calibrate the height measurements. A danger of destructive methods in which hand labour is used to cut samples is that not enough samples are taken, in order to save time and cost. In this case the accuracy of the data per sample may be high, but the precision of estimating the plot mean may be too low.

Researchers, extensionists and farmers use a weighted disc or HFRO sward stick for routine measurements. These implements are recommended for use in appropriate sward types because of their ease and simplicity of use, particularly when frequent estimates of DM yield are needed.

Regional scale

The area involved may be hundreds or thousands of hectares. Remote sensing to delineate vegetation types combined with ground surveys for rough biomass estimates by eye or more detailed methods (e.g. BOTANAL) may be appropriate (Chapters 9 and 10).

References

Armstrong, R.H., Grant, S.A., Common, T.G. and Beattie, M.M. (1997) Controlled grazing studies on *Nardus* grassland: effect of between-tussock sward height and species of grazer on diet selection and intake. *Grass and Forage Science* 52, 219–231.

Assaeed, A.M. (1997) Estimation of biomass and utilization of three perennial range grasses in Saudi Arabia. *Journal of Arid Environments* 36, 103–111.

Barthram, G.T. (1986) Experimental techniques: the HFRO sward stick. In: *Hill Farming Research Organisation Biennial Report 1984–85*. HFRO, Edinburgh, pp. 29–30.

Belsky, A.J. (1994) Influences of trees on savanna productivity: tests of shade, nutrients, and tree–grass competition. *Ecology* 75, 922–932.

Bobek, B. and Bergstrom, R. (1978) A rapid method of browse biomass estimation in a forest habitat. *Journal of Range Management* 31, 456–458.

Boyd, D.A. (1949) Experiments with leys and permanent grass. *Journal of the British Grassland Society* 4, 1–10.

Bransby, D.I., Matches, A.G. and Krause, G.F. (1977) Disk meter for rapid estimation of herbage yield in grazing trials. *Agricultural Journal* 69, 393–396.

Brocket, B.H. (1996) Research note: Calibrating a disc pasture meter to estimate grass fuel loads on the Zululand coastal plain. *African Journal of Range and Forage Science* 13, 39–41.

Brown, D. (1954) *Methods of Surveying and Measuring Vegetation.* Bulletin 42, Commonwealth Bureau of Pastures and Field Crops. CAB International, Farnham Royal, UK, 223 pp.

Brown, K.R. and Evans, P.S. (1973) Animal treading: a review of the work of the late D.B. Edmond. *New Zealand Journal of Experimental Agriculture* 1, 217–226.

Brown, L.J. and Stephens, P.R. (1995) Monitoring pasture productivity in New Zealand – an investigation using NOAA-11 AVHRR data and dairy farm milk fat production. *International Journal of Remote Sensing* 16, 967–972.

Burrows, W.H. and Beale, I.F. (1970) Dimension and production relations of mulga (*Acacia aneura* F. Muell) trees in semi-arid Queensland. In: *Proceedings of the 11th International Grassland Congress.* Surfers Paradise, Australia, pp. 33–35.

Cacho, O.J. (1993) A practical equation for pasture growth under grazing. *Grass and Forage Science* 48, 387–394.

Cooper, C.S., Hyder, D.N., Petersen, R.G. and Sneva, F.A. (1957) The constituent differential method of estimating species composition in mixed hay. *Agronomy Journal* 49, 190–193.

Cowan, R.T. and O'Grady, P. (1976) Effect of presentation yield of a tropical grass-legume pasture on grazing time and milk yield of Friesian cows. *Tropical Grasslands* 10, 213–218.

Curran, P.J. and Williamson, H.D. (1987) Airborne MSS data to estimate GLAI. *International Journal of Remote Sensing* 8, 87–94.

De Ridder, N. and Van Keulen, H. (1995) Estimating biomass through transfer functions based on simulation model results: a case study for the Sahel. *Agricultural Water Management* 28, 57–71.

Deenen, P.J.A.G. and Lantinga, E.A. (1993) Herbage and animal production responses to fertilizer nitrogen in perennial ryegrass swards. I. Continuous grazing and cutting. *Netherlands Journal of Agricultural Science* 41, 179–203.

Dobb, J.L. and Elliott, C.R. (1964) Effect of pasture sampling cages on seed and herbage yields of creeping red fescue. *Canadian Journal of Plant Science* 44, 96–99.

Douglas, J.T. and Crawford, C.E. (1994) An evaluation of the drop-disc technique for measurement of herbage production in ryegrass for silage. *Grass and Forage Science* 49, 252–255.

Foran, B.D. (1987) Detection of yearly cover change with Landsat MSS on pastoral landscapes in central Australia. *Remote Sensing of Environment* 23, 333–350.

Gabriel, O., Rial, P., Cibilis, A. and Borrelli, P. (1996) Evaluating carrying capacity using LANDSAT MSS images in south Patagonia. In: *Proceedings of the Fifth International Rangeland Congress.* Salt Lake City, Utah, 1, 408–409.

Gabriëls, P.C.J. and Van den Berg, J.V. (1993) Calibration of two techniques for estimating herbage mass. *Grass and Forage Science* 48, 329–335.

Grant, S.A. (1971) the measurement of primary production and utilization on heather moors. *Journal of the British Grassland Society* 26, 51–58.

Greig-Smith, P. (1964) *Quantitative Plant Ecology*, 2nd edn. Butterworths Scientific Publishers, London.

Hargreaves, J.N.G. and Kerr, J. (1992) *BOTANAL – a Comprehensive Sampling and Computing Procedure for Estimating Pasture Yield and Composition. 2. Computational package*, 2nd edn. Tropical Agronomy Technical Memorandum No. 79, Division of Tropical Crops and Pastures, CSIRO, St Lucia, Queensland.

Haydock, K.P. and Shaw, N.H. (1975) The comparative yield method for estimating dry matter yield of pasture. *Australian Journal of Experimental Agriculture and Animal Husbandry* 15, 663–667.

Hoppe, T., Weissbach, F. and Schmidt, L. (1995) Kontrolle des Weidemanagements durch Bestandshöhenmessung. In: *Kongressband 1995 Garmisch-Partenkirchen. Vorträge zum Generalthema des 107. VDLUFA-Kongresses von 18–23.9.1994 in Garmisch-Partenkirchen:Grünland als Produktionsstandort und Landschaftselement*, pp. 153–156.

Hunter, R.F. and Grant, S.A. (1961) The estimation of 'green dry matter' in a herbage sample by methanol-soluble pigments. *Journal of the British Grassland Society* 16, 43–45.

Hutchinson, K.J. (1967) A coring technique for the measurement of pasture of low availabilty to sheep. *Journal of the British Grassland Society* 22, 131–134.

Jones, R.M. and Hargreaves, J.N.G. (1979) Improvements to the dry-weight-rank method of measuring botanical composition. *Grass and Forage Science* 18, 181–189.

Jones, R.M., Sandland, R.L. and Bunch, G.A. (1977) Limitations of the electronic capacitance meter in measuring yields of grazed tropical pastures. *Journal of the British Grassland Society* 32, 105–113.

Kennedy, R.K. (1972) The sickledrat: a circular quadrat modification useful in grassland studies. *Journal of Range Management* 25, 312–313.

Le Houérou, H.N., Bingham, R.L. and Skerbek, W. (1988) Relationships between the variability of primary production and the variability of annual precipitation in world arid lands. *Journal of Arid Environments* 15, 1–18.

Mannetje, L. 't (1974) Relations between pasture attributes and liveweight gains on a subtropical pasture. *Proceedings of the 12th International Grassland Congress.* Moscow, vol. 3, pp. 299–304.

Mannetje, L. 't (ed.) (1978) *Measurement of Grassland Vegetation and Animal Production.* Bulletin 52, Commonwealth Bureau of Pastures and Field Crops. CAB International, Farnham Royal, UK.

Mannetje, L. 't and Ebersohn, J.P. (1980) Relations between sward characteristics and animal production. *Tropical Grasslands* 14, 273–280.

Mannetje, L. 't and Haydock, K.P. (1963) The dry-weight-rank method for the botanical analysis of pasture. *Journal of the British Grassland Society* 18, 268–275.

Mannetje, L. 't and Jones, R.M. (1990) Pasture and animal productivity of buffel grass with Siratro, lucerne or nitrogen fertilizer. *Tropical Grasslands* 24, 269–281.

McCown, R.L. (1973) An evaluation of the influence of available soil water storage capacity on growing season length and yield of tropical pastures using simple water balance models. *Agricultural Meteorology* 11, 53–63.

McDonald, C.K. and Jones, R.M. (1997) Measuring spatial variability within pastures. In: *Proceedings of the XVIII International Grasslands Congress.* Winnipeg and Saskatoon, Canada, Session 26, paper 26–1.

McDonald, C.K., Corfield, J.P., Hargreaves, J.N.G. and O'Toole, J.G. (1996) *BOTANAL – a Comprehensive Sampling and Computing Procedure for Estimating Pasture Yield and Composition. 3. Field Recording Direct to Computer,* 2nd edn. Tropical Agronomy Technical Memorandum No. 88, Division of Tropical Crops and Pastures, CSIRO, St Lucia, Queensland.

Michell, P. (1982) Value of a rising plate meter for estimating herbage mass of grazed perennial ryegrass–white clover swards. *Grass and Forage Science* 37, 81–87.

Michell, P. and Large, R.V. (1983) The estimation of herbage mass of perennial ryegrass swards: a comparative evaluation of a rising-plate and a single probe capacitance meter calibrated at and above ground level. *Grass and Forage Science* 38, 295–299.

Murphy, W.M., Silam, J.P. and Barreto, A.D.M. (1995) A comparison of quadrat, capacitance meter, HFRO sward stick, and rising plate for estimating herbage mass in a smooth-stalked, meadowgrass-dominant white clover sward. *Grass and Forage Science* 50, 452–455.

Northup, B.K., Brown, J.R., Dias, C.D., Skelly, W.C. and Radford, B. (1999) A technique for near-ground remote sensing of herbaceous vegetation in tropical woodlands. *Rangeland Journal* 21, 229–243.

Orr, D.M. and Evenson, C.J. (1991) Effects of sheep grazing *Astrebla* grasslands in central western Queensland. III. Dynamics of *Astrebla* spp. under grazing and exclosure between 1975 and 1986. *Rangeland Journal* 13, 36–46.

Pickup, G., Bastin, G.N. and Chewings, V.H. (1994) Remote-sensing-based condition assessment for nonequilibrium rangelands under large-scale commercial grazing. *Ecological Applications* 4, 497–517.

Piemontese, S., Stagliano, N., Pardini, A. and Argenti, G. (1997) Modello geometrico par la stima della fitomassa di arbusti di rove (*Rubus* sp.) mediante analisi informatica di immagini fotografiche.[Geometric mathematical model to estimate the biomass of *Rubus* sp. using image analysis.] *Revista di Agronomia* 31, 1027–1033.

Prendergast, J.J. and Brady, J.J. (1955) Improved movable cage for use in grassland research. *Journal of the British Grassland Society* 10, 189–190.

Samarakoon, S.P., Wilson, J.R. and Shelton, H.M. (1990) Growth, morphology and nutritive quality of shaded *Stenotaphrum secundatum, Axonopus compressus* and *Pennisetum clandestinum. Journal of Agricultural Science* 114, 161–169.

Singh, J.S., Lauenroth, W. and Steinhorst, R.K. (1975) Review and assessment of various techniques for estimating net aerial primary production in grasslands from harvest data. *Botanical Review* 41, 181–232.

Tappan, G.G., Tyler, D.J., Wehde, M.E. and Moore, D.G. (1992) Monitoring rangeland dynamics in Senegal with Advanced Very High Resolution Radiometer data. *Geocarto International* 7, 87–98.

Tothill, J.C. and Partridge, I.J. (eds) (1998) *Monitoring Grazing Lands in Northern Australia.* Occasional Publication No. 9, Tropical Grasslands Society of Australia, Brisbane.

Tothill, J.C., Hargreaves, J.N.G., Jones, R.M. and McDonald, C.K. (1992) *BOTANAL – a Comprehensive Sampling and Computing Procedure for Estimating Pasture Yield and Composition. 1. Field Sampling.* Tropical Agronomy Technical Memorandum No. 78, Division of Tropical Crops and Pastures, CSIRO, St Lucia, Queensland.

Tucker, C.J. (1979) Red and photographic infrared linear combinations for monitoring vegetation. *Remote Sensing of Environment* 8, 127–150.

Uso, J.L., Mateu, J., Karjalainen, T. and Salvador, P. (1997) Allometric regression equations to determine aerial biomasses of Mediterranean shrubs. *Plant Ecology* 132, 59–69.

Van der Honing, Y. and Alderman, G. (1988) Feed evaluation and nutrient requirements. 2. Ruminants. *Livestock Production Systems* 19, 217–278.

Van Dyne, G.M. (1966) Use of a vacuum-clipper for harvesting herbage. *Ecology* 47, 624–626.

Van Dyne, G.M., Vogel, W.G. and Fisser, H.G. (1963) Influence of small plot size and shape on range herbage production estimates. *Ecology* 44, 746–759.

Vickery, P.J. and Nicol, G.R. (1982) *An Improved Electronic Capacitance Meter for Estimating Pasture Yield: Construction and Performance tests.* Animal Research Laboratories Technical Paper No. 9, CSIRO, Armidale, Australia.

Vickery, P.J., Bennett, I.L. and Nicol, G.R. (1980) An improved electronic capacitance meter for estimating herbage mass. *Grass and Forage Science* 35, 247–252.

Waddington, J. and Cooke, D.A. (1971) The influence of sample size and number on the precision of estimates of herbage production and consumption in grazing experiments. *Journal of the British Grassland Society* 26, 95–101.

Waite, R.B. (1994) The application of visual estimation procedures for monitoring pasture yield and composition in exclosures and small plots. *Tropical Grasslands* 28, 38–42.

Waite, R.B. and Kerr, J.D. (1996) Measuring yields of green leaf blade in pastures by visual estimation techniques. *Tropical Grasslands* 30, 314–318.

Walker, B.H. (1976) An approach to the monitoring of changes in the composition and utilization of woodland and savanna vegetation. *South African Journal of Wildlife Research* 6, 1–32.

Walker, B.H., McFarlane, F.R. and Langridge, J.L. (1997) Grass growth in response to time of rainfall and season along a climate gradient in Australian rangelands. *Rangeland Journal* 19, 95–108.

Whitney, A.S. (1974) Measurement of foliage height and its relationship to yields of two tropical forage grasses. *Agronomy Journal* 66, 334–336.

Williams, S.S. (1951) Microenvironment in relation to experimental techniques. *Journal of the British Grassland Society* 6, 207–217.

Williamson, H.D. (1990) Estimating biomass of an improved pasture using SPOT HRV data. *Grass and Forage Science* 45, 235–241.

Wilson, J.R. and Ludlow, M.M. (1991) The environment and potential growth of herbage under plantations. In: Shelton, H.M. and Stür, W.W. (eds) *Forages for Plantation Crops.* Australian Centre for International Agriculture Research Proceedings No. 32, Canberra, pp. 10–24.

Wilson, J.R. and Schwenke, T. (1995) Estimating potential yield of forage under plantations. In: Mullen, B.F. and Shelton, H.M. (eds) *Integration of Ruminants into Plantation Systems in South-east Asia. Proceedings of a Workshop at Lake Toba, North Sumatra, Indonesia, 9–13 September 1994.* Australian Centre for International Agricultural Research, Canberra, pp. 32–36.

Wilson, J.R., Catchpoole, V.R. and Weier, K.L. (1986) Stimulation of growth and nitrogen uptake by shading a rundown green panic pasture on Brigalow clay soil. *Tropical Grasslands* 20, 134–143.

Wylie, B.K., Pieper, R.D. and Southward, G.M. (1992) Estimating herbage standing crop from rainfall data in Niger. *Journal of Range Management* 45, 277–284.

Wylie, B.K., Denda, I., Pieper, R.D., Harrington, J.A. Jr, Reed, B.C. and Southward, G.M. (1995) Satellite-based herbaceous biomass estimates in the pastoral zone of Niger. *Journal of Range Management* 48, 159–164.

Evaluation of Species and Cultivars

R. Schultze-Kraft[1] and L. 't Mannetje[2]

[1]Institute of Plant Production and Agroecology in the Tropics and Subtropics, University of Hohenheim, Stuttgart, Germany; [2]Department of Plant Sciences, Wageningen University, Wageningen, The Netherlands

Introduction

Grassland and forage production improvement requires continuing inputs of new species and cultivars in order to meet the ever-changing needs of efficient and sustainable forage production. New species or cultivars may be sought because of new developments (as is the case in many tropical regions), because existing species and cultivars are being threatened by pests or diseases, or because new material, becoming available through collection or from breeding programmes, offers higher production or better nutritive value.

In this chapter, evaluation of tropical forages is separated from that of temperate ones because of fundamental differences between the two groups, including the following:

- Most new tropical forages represent essentially undomesticated species selected from wild populations, about which usually only little is known regarding taxonomy, ecology, reproductive biology, etc.
- Farming systems in the tropics often combine livestock with cropping or tree plantations; these require adapted forage species.
- Low soil fertility is a major limitation in the tropics and very little fertilizer is applied to forages. Consequently, not only are species often required to have low fertility requirements, but they may have to maintain or enhance soil fertility.

- In the tropics, woody forage species (mainly leguminous trees and shrubs) are important. They require different evaluation procedures than herbaceous plants.
- Lastly, tropical species pose particular nutritive-value challenges. The crude protein concentration and dry matter (DM) digestibility of C_4 grasses are not only inherently low but also decrease rapidly with increasing plant age. Also many legumes have anti-nutritive factors.

This chapter is mainly concerned with the evaluation of germplasm for forage production; evaluation for social/amenity aspects (landscaping, ornamental, lawn, etc.) is not considered. For soil conservation and soil fertility improvement refer to Sarrantonio (1991) and Anderson and Ingram (1993).

Evaluating Tropical Forages

There are, in principle, four approaches to commencing an evaluation project with tropical forages:

- To test cultivars that are commercial elsewhere. There are many of these, mainly in Australia. A substantial amount of knowledge that has been generated during the past 30–40 years about the environments and farming systems where they are adapted is summarized in books (Skerman et al., 1988; Skerman and Riveros, 1990; Mannetje and Jones, 1992; Humphreys and Partridge, 1995). Information on some Australian cultivars is available on the Internet[1]. The advantage of this approach is that evaluation results can be readily related to results from studies elsewhere, and, if the cultivars are commercial in the respective country, there will be no seed supply constraints and no or reduced delays because of quarantine. Evaluation will start at the 'preliminary evaluation' level (p. 189).
- To introduce experimental lines that have been identified as promising under similar agroecological conditions elsewhere. An example is the material used in the West and Central African Forage Network (RABAOC, its acronym in French) (CIAT, 1995). This approach can usually build upon information generated elsewhere and it is widely applied in tropical countries. Evaluation will again start at the 'preliminary evaluation' level.
- To introduce germplasm (accessions, experimental lines) from a gene bank for evaluation of larger collections. The objective is usually to find better lines within a species already showing promise. Depending on knowledge about the species and on the researcher's interest,

---

[1] http://www.dpi.qld.gov.au/pastures/

evaluation may start at the 'characterization' (p. 186) or 'preliminary evaluation' level and can be linked to subsequent breeding programmes.

• To collect germplasm (populations, genotypes, ecotypes) in the wild for subsequent evaluation and/or storage in gene banks for future studies. This approach provides the chance to find new variability but is usually restricted to research institutions with major responsibilities for conservation of genetic resources.

In the tropics, most commercial varieties and cultivars have been developed by evaluating and selecting within populations of wild, as yet undomesticated, species. Only in few instances have cultivars been bred, as with *Macroptilium atropurpureum* cv. Siratro (Hutton, 1962) and *Centrosema pascuorum* cv. Cavalcade (Clements *et al.*, 1986). Examples of present breeding efforts are the *Brachiaria* and *Stylosanthes* improvement projects at the Centro Internacional de Agricultura Tropical (CIAT) in Colombia (Miles and do Valle, 1996) and at the Commonwealth Scientific and Industrial Research Organization (CSIRO) in Australia (Cameron *et al.*, 1997), respectively.

The full research sequence leading to a commercial variety, involving a step-by-step reduction of the number of accessions under study, is:

• Germplasm acquisition: collection and/or introduction of genetic material with a subsequent quarantine phase.
• Germplasm characterization: description and primary evaluation of genetic material for classification, seed increase and selection of representative lines.
• Preliminary evaluation: agronomic evaluation of selected germplasm in small plots, usually under cutting.
• Production evaluation: evaluation of selected germplasm in larger plots or paddocks under grazing (pasture species) or cutting (cut-and-carry species).
• Pre-release: testing of selected, promising material under practical conditions by farmers and seed increase for eventual release.
• Cultivar release: the moment of release to the seed industry and farmers for commercial use.

Although this scheme is conceptually common to most forage cultivar development programmes in the tropics (Jones and Walker, 1983; Peters and Tothill, 1988; Toledo *et al.*, 1989), some of the phases may be omitted or combined.

The evaluations may be carried out on-station or on-farm. The latter can apply even at the preliminary evaluation level if, for example, the intention is to expose the new germplasm to farmers at an early stage, or when an on-farm phase is to complement the main on-station phase. Practical guidelines for early on-farm testing, with special reference to smallholder systems in Southeast Asia, are given by Cheng and Horne (1997). The convenience of doing large-scale evaluation with livestock on-farm will depend on the level of sophistication required and the availability of the necessary cooperation capability. For discussion of participatory on-farm research, see Ashby (1990) and Chapter 16. It should be recognized, however, that the success of such on-farm trials can be at risk if there is no appropriate security of treatments or control of animals. Concrete on-farm evaluation experiences within the International Tropical Pastures Evaluation Network (RIEPT, its acronym in Spanish) in tropical America, including methodological details, can be found in Argel *et al.* (1993) and CIAT (1993).

Germplasm acquisition

Plant collection

Germplasm collection must be preceded by thorough consideration and definition of the objectives, which can be according to plant species (collections can be broadly targeted, or restricted to particular genera or species) or according to target regions. The latter can be an administrative region, such as the collections made by the Instituto de Zootecnia in the state of São Paulo, Brazil (da Rocha *et al.*, 1979), or regions with soil or climate conditions of particular interest, such as the CIAT collections on acid soils (Schultze-Kraft and Giacometti, 1978) and the CSIRO homologous-climate concept for germplasm collections (Reid, 1980).

In all cases, the collection should be carried out where genetic diversity is greatest and must therefore be based on a thorough analysis of information from botanical literature and herbaria. Such information also reveals the most appropriate season for collection – that is, when plants are seeding. The threat of genetic erosion in a region should also be considered. There is increasing evidence that, due to habitat destruction, genetic erosion of species with potential as forage plants is occurring (Schultze-Kraft *et al.*, 1993). Collection and conservation in germplasm banks (in addition to *in situ* conservation) may contribute to the maintenance of species.

Collection procedures for tropical forage germplasm have been extensively described in Shaw and Bryan (1976), Mott (1979), Clements and Cameron (1980), McIvor and Bray (1983), Lazier (1985) and Guarino *et al.* (1995).

An optimum collection strategy implies that seed from up to 100 plants in a population should be collected (Marshall and Brown, 1983). In practice, however, there are often only a few individuals at a given site. Instead of time-consuming searches for further plants, the resulting lack of variability should be compensated by more collection sites in the area. For practical purposes, a general guideline would be to collect as many seeds from as many plants in a particular population as is possible within given time limitations.

Genetic variability becomes particularly critical when the species of interest is apomictic or does not produce viable seed, or when no seed can be found. The consequent need to collect vegetative material (stolons, rhizomes, seedlings) will result in a very narrow variability, which should be compensated by more collection sites (Sackville Hamilton and Chorlton, 1995).

Herbarium voucher specimens should be collected for future reference (Womersley, 1981; Miller and Nyberg, 1995). Although such material may not be relevant for describing genetic variability, it will greatly assist in the solution of possible taxonomic problems.

The collection of *Rhizobium/Bradyrhizobium* is most desirable for legumes. However, such a collection is useless unless there are facilities for receiving, isolating and maintaining the material (Date, 1995).

Points to be stressed with the description of collection sites and with the documentation of the collected samples are as follows:

- The need to identify the collection site accurately. In the past, this was usually done by means of vehicle kilometre readings and a road map for subsequent estimation of geographical coordinates. Modern GPS (global positioning system) technology, however, renders such record-keeping unnecessary. It is very precise, is becoming increasingly inexpensive and should be a standard tool in collecting missions. The identification of a collection site is also important for application of GIS (geographical information system) technology.
- A hand-held computer is the most convenient way of recording information while collecting. Alternatively, a portable tape recorder could be used; this is more appropriate than taking notes in a field book. However, the most essential information should also be written on paper just in case modern technology fails.
- Essential details for the site description comprise: associated vegetation, land use, relevant soil information and evidence of stresses such as drought, waterlogging, shade, fire, etc. Essential details for the sample description are: sample size, evidence of outcrossing, grazing and biotic stresses (damage by diseases or insects), outstanding population and individual plant characteristics, and nodulation (legumes).

Seed collection involves drying and cleaning of samples, dehulling of seeds and subsequent disinfection with a pesticide. For vegetative material, preservation refers to maintaining adequate moisture in plastic bags containing stolons, rhizomes or uprooted plants. The 'passport' (site and collection) data should be as complete as possible (Guarino *et al.*, 1995).

Germplasm introduction
The introduction of genetic material from gene banks or other sources is more common than collection. It offers the advantage that information on

the origin, characterization and even evaluation of the material may enable some preselection at the beginning of the evaluation process. However, such preselection should not be based on information about the original collection site alone as this could underestimate species adaptability. An example is *Leucaena leucocephala*, which is a successful species in the humid and subhumid tropics but originates from a semiarid zone.

The gene banks holding the major collections of tropical forage germplasm are the Australian Tropical Forages Genetic Resource Centre at CSIRO[2] in Brisbane, Australia, CIAT[3] in Cali, Colombia, and ILRI[4] (formerly ILCA) in Addis Ababa, Ethiopia (Schultze-Kraft *et al.*, 1993). Passport data of accessions in the CIAT and ILRI collections can be accessed on the Internet[5] in the SINGER (System-wide Information Network for Genetic Resources) database maintained by IPGRI[6]. Two further important collections of tropical forage germplasm are those of EMBRAPA Recursos Genéticos y Biotecnologia[7] in Brasília, Brazil, and of the University of Florida's Indian River Research and Education Center in Fort Pierce[8], USA. Generally, only small seed quantities per accession can be provided. Requests from abroad have to abide by national quarantine regulations that usually require an import permit and a phytosanitary certificate accompanying the seed. For legumes with known *Rhizobium/Bradyrhizobium* specificity, importation of appropriate inoculum – usually available from the same source – is strongly recommended.

Quarantine and glasshouse phase

The final stage of the introduction phase – and at the same time the transition to characterization – is concerned with quarantine and growing the new material in a glasshouse. The main objective of quarantine regulations is to ensure that potential plant health hazards are not introduced along with the genetic material. This is particularly important when germplasm is brought in from a different continent. Independent of any specific quarantine regulations, there are four fundamental phyto-sanitary rules: (i) the transfer of vegetative material should be avoided as

---

[2] Commonwealth Scientific and Industrial Research Organization (CSIRO) Tropical Agriculture, 306 Carmody Road, St Lucia, Queensland 4067, Australia
[3] Centro Internacional de Agricultura Tropical (CIAT), Apartado Aéreo 6713, Cali, Colombia, S.A.
[4] International Livestock Research Institute (ILRI), PO Box 5689, Addis Ababa, Ethiopia
[5] http://noc1.cgiar.org/seartype.htm
[6] International Plant Genetic Resources Institute (IPGRI), Via delle Sete Chiese 142, 00145 Rome, Italy, http://www.singer.cgiar.org
[7] Empresa Brasileira de Pesquisa Agropecuária Recursos Genéticos e Biotecnologia (formerly EMBRAPA-CENARGEN), Caixa Postal 02372, 70770–900 Brasília, DF, Brazil
[8] University of Florida, Institute of Food and Agricultural Sciences (IFAS), Indian River Research and Education Center Fort Pierce, 2199 South Rock Road, Fort Pierce, FL 34945–3138, USA

much as possible; (ii) seed samples must be free of any non-seed material, particularly plant debris and soil particles; (iii) seeds should undergo a surface disinfection (e.g. with concentrated sulphuric acid) in order to destroy any pathogens on the seed surface; and (iv) particular attention should be paid to symptoms of possible seed-borne diseases, mainly viruses, during the first grow-out in the glasshouse. Close cooperation with plant pathologists is necessary.

During the glasshouse/quarantine phase, species identification can be confirmed, accessions partially characterized and seed collected. Species identity can be checked by preparing specimens and consulting with national herbaria or international specialists, e.g. at the Royal Botanic Gardens, Kew[9]. Accession characterization during this phase can refer to attributes such as growth habit, flowering behaviour and life cycle (annual, or living longer than one year); it will be complemented in field trials (see next section). Information on reproductive biology can also be collected; for example, flowering but no fruiting of legumes indicates dependence on insects for pollination.

Seed increase and/or vegetative propagation is very important in the evaluation process and should start as soon as an accession is released from quarantine. The amount of seed or propagules to be produced will depend on future research and gene bank requirements, but also on the necessary turnover rate in a glasshouse, and is a matter of the availability of space and labour. The potential for cross-pollination of different accessions in a species should be recognized and steps taken to avoid it.

Some practical procedures in the first grow-out in the glasshouse (for details, see Mott, 1979; Clements and Cameron, 1980) are as follows.

- Seed scarification in the case of hardseeded legumes. This is mainly by mechanical scarification such as hand-rubbing the seed surface with fine emery paper or nicking the testa with a razor blade.
- Pre-germinating the seeds (e.g. in petri dishes). This includes their protection with a wettable fungicide and, if necessary, breaking physiological dormancy with appropriate chemicals (legumes: 1% thiourea solution; grasses: 0.2% KNO_3 solution).
- Transferring the pre-germinated seeds into appropriate-sized pots (one or two seeds per pot) containing a free-draining but water-retentive soil such as a loam : sand : peat mixture of 50 : 25 : 25 vol.%. Appropriate watering, fertilizing and pest control are particularly necessary in this glasshouse stage. The need for an accurate, double-check labelling system throughout the entire glasshouse process is also stressed.
- Seed collecting. This is usually done by handpicking ripe seeds (pods) two or three times per week.

---

[9] The Herbarium, Royal Botanic Gardens, Kew, Richmond, Surrey TW9 3AB, UK

Germplasm characterization

Objectives

In most cases, characterization is concerned with one species or genus and aims to assess the variability in a collection and to reduce collections to a manageable size for subsequent evaluations. Furthermore, it enables the identification of duplicates. In some instances germplasm characterization is done in combination with 'preliminary evaluation' (see below). Pure germplasm characterization, i.e. not carried out under conditions relevant to any production system, is largely restricted to major genetic resources institutions. An example is *Panicum maximum* in EMBRAPA Gado de Corte (formerly EMBRAPA-CNPGC) in Campo Grande, Brazil (Jank *et al.*, 1997). An important classification goal may consist of forming 'core' collections which represent the variability in an entire collection (Hodgkin *et al.*, 1995).

There are several sources of data for the characterization of germplasm: (i) original collection sites; (ii) the glasshouse during the quarantine phase; (iii) laboratory research; and (iv) the field nursery. The eventual germplasm classification can be based on data from each of these sources independently, or combined. A recent example using a combination of morphological data with isozyme electrophoresis is the classification of a 60-accession collection of *Pennisetum purpureum* in Brazil (Daher *et al.*, 1997).

Laboratory studies

Molecular markers are used to assess variability within a collection and to aid in identification of duplicates. Until recently, this was done using isozymes, e.g. in the classification of an *Arachis glabrata* collection (Maass and Ocampo, 1995). Currently, DNA markers such as RAPD are mostly used – for example, by Liu (1996), who assessed variation in *Lablab purpureus*. Detailed protocol descriptions for the use of molecular markers are given by Ferreira and Grattapaglia (1996).

Nursery trials

Nursery trials are mostly established with spaced plants, using seedlings raised under greenhouse conditions and transplanted into plots consisting of single rows usually with 8–15 plants (Fig. 8.1). The distance between plants will depend on the species and whether observations are based on single plants, or if eventual development of a sward is intended. The distance between rows will depend on plant vigour and growth habit, and must be large enough to avoid, or easily control, invasion of plants from neighbouring rows. The number of replications will depend on available resources and should be at least two. When the nursery is established with accessions of contrasting growth habits, blocks of accessions of similar

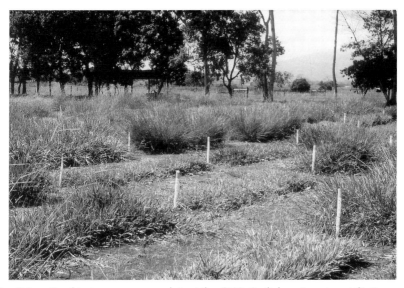

Fig. 8.1. *Brachiaria* spp. nursery plots at the CIAT-Quilichao Experiment Station, Colombia. (Photograph by R. Schultze-Kraft.)

growth habit should be established separately. In species where outcrossing can occur and seed is to be harvested, distances between plots and replications should be as large as feasible to reduce cross-pollination.

Adequate fertilizer to ensure near-optimum growth should be applied, using N for legumes unless appropriate *Rhizobium/Bradyrhizobium* strains are available. Irrigation can be considered. Further nursery management includes regular weeding and, if necessary, the use of pesticides. To avoid weeding, woven black polyethylene cloth or 'weedmat' can be used as a ground cover into which holes are cut and seedlings transplanted. Weedmat also facilitates collection of fallen seed but does not allow observations on seedling recruitment and sward formation via stolons.

The duration of the characterization-phase nursery will depend on the objectives and often comprises one vegetative and one reproductive cycle. Thereafter, plants can be cut to obtain information on regrowth characteristics. Cutting height of such adult plants will vary according to plant type and growth habit. Once the characterization phase is concluded, the nursery can be used for seed increase.

Observations and measurements in a characterization nursery concentrate on plant attributes that are regarded as largely environment independent but may be relevant to the use as forage. Such characteristics will vary according to the target species or species group, and to any details required. Consequently, the number of descriptors used in characterization can vary considerably.

Suggested descriptors that are largely environment independent and useful for a forage-related characterization of germplasm, are:

- Growth habit. Grasses – tussock-forming (erect, decumbent, or adscendent) or creeping; presence of stolons and/or rhizomes. Legumes – twining, creeping, stoloniferous; herbaceous, shrub, sub-shrub; erect, decumbent, adscendent.
- Life cycle. Grasses are generally annual or perennial; legumes can be annual, short-lived or true perennial.
- Length of vegetative phase (number of days to first flower).
- Relative leafiness at a predetermined stage, such as at first flower.
- Mating system. Indication of cross-pollination or self-pollination/ apomixis (based on segregations observed and seed-setting dependence on visiting insects).
- Regeneration mechanism. Seedling recruitment (if plants were allowed to set seed), stolon-borne new plants; regrowth, after a cut, from tiller meristems (grasses); for legumes, localization of regrowth meristems on the stubble (underground, basal, apical, evenly distributed).
- Unusual and/or remarkable morphological particularities.

Forage shrubs and trees can, in addition, be characterized in terms of plant height and width, and branching capacity (number of branches up to a predetermined stem height) at a predetermined age (e.g. 6 months after transplanting).

An important attribute, but difficult to assess, is the potential of new, introduced material to become an undesirable noxious weed. There has always been concern about introduced plants becoming weeds in cropping areas and there is increasing concern in some countries about the potential for introduced plants to invade native plant communities and reduce biodiversity.

Because of (i) the lack of knowledge about the heritability of descriptors that can be used for germplasm characterization and (ii) the labour need in small-plot research, the plant nursery phase is frequently combined with the 'preliminary evaluation' phase. By this, the objectives extend to environment-dependent attributes and the characterization may become more site specific and, therefore, of less value for other environments.

Recording of observations; statistical tools

Recording of observations is done numerically by (i) measuring or counting (e.g. number of days); (ii) rating on a 0–5 scale, where 0 = nil and 5 = very high (e.g. leafiness); and (iii) assigning number codes to different expressions of a morphological characteristic (e.g. localization of regrowth meristems on the legume stubble: 1 = underground; 2 = basal; 3 = apical; 4 = evenly distributed). The presence or absence of a particular characteristic can be coded by using '1' or '0', respectively.

Analysis of variance or presentation of frequency distributions is appropriate for analysing the data and describing the variability of single characteristics. Multivariate methods such as principal component or cluster (= pattern) analysis are required for classifying and grouping of accessions using data from several attributes. Cluster analysis results are conveniently presented in the form of dendrograms, and diversity within a group can then be described using a minimum spanning tree (see Chapter 2).

Preliminary evaluation

Objectives and general considerations

The objective is to identify new suitable species for a given environment or new accessions that are superior to known material (e.g. regarding DM production, edaphic or climatic adaptation) and overcome any particular constraint (e.g. pests or diseases). Evaluation should, as far as possible, be under realistic site and production system conditions. Methodology depends on the target production system and final use, which might be cut-and-carry, grazed pastures, or other uses (e.g. soil cover, protein bank, ley farming). Seed increase is a particularly important component of this phase as all subsequent evaluation steps require an adequate supply of experimental seed.

Experimental details

There are several guidelines available for the evaluation of herbaceous forages (e.g. Toledo, 1982; Tarawali *et al.*, 1995), woody species (Maass *et al.*, 1996) and multi-purpose trees (Briscoe, 1989).

Suggested plot sizes range from 4 m^2 to 25 m^2 and there should be a minimum of two and preferably three or more replications, arranged in conventional experimental designs such as randomized complete blocks. For new groups of accessions it is recommended to use a fresh plot of land to avoid contamination from regrowth of the previous group and also to lower the weed potential. To assess the extent of the latter, sowing could conveniently be delayed until the first rainfall events. Areas no longer used for experimental observations can be left to be grazed for observations on relative palatability and/or persistence, or to produce seed.

Plots can be established by seeding into rows or by broadcasting, or by using spaced plants, directly sown or transplanted as seedlings. When using vegetatively propagated legumes it should be recognized that such material does not form proper taproots and so dry-season evaluation may be affected. This may also hold for plants established from seed but later transplanted as big plants. Planting distance will depend on growth habit and may range between 0.25 m and > 1 m. At this evaluation stage, mostly single-species plots are established, but it is also possible to sow legume accessions with a common grass and vice versa (Shaw and Bryan, 1976).

Plot management, which includes fertilization, inoculation of legumes with *Rhizobium/Bradyrhizobium*, weeding, cutting regime, etc., will depend on particular evaluation objectives. Fertilization, in most cases with emphasis on P for legumes and N for grasses, may follow prevailing recommendations for commercial improved-pasture establishment in the region, which are usually low levels. However, for germplasm of particular interest or best-bet accessions, an additional fertilization treatment (such as without vs. with, or low vs. high) may give some useful first information on fertility requirements of new germplasm.

Preliminary evaluation is mostly done under cutting but grazing (which can be complementary to cutting) is also possible when appropriate facilities and skills are available (e.g. Shaw and Bryan, 1976). It should be recognized, however, that evaluation under common grazing may be affected by palatability differences among species or accessions. For prostrate-growing species, it should be recognized that low DM yields when evaluating under cutting can lead to an underestimation of the species' potential to produce and persist under grazing.

Evaluation parameters

Screening that focuses on a specific constraint (e.g. disease resistance) is not considered here. Suggested general evaluation parameters, related mainly to environmental adaptation (soil, climate, biotic stresses) and seasonal productivity, are:

- Establishment vigour: at regular intervals, estimating percentage soil cover and/or rating of plant vigour; for woody plants, additional measurements of height and width are optional.
- Biotic and edaphic constraints: at regular intervals, assessment of incidence and severity of diseases and insect pests, and of mineral deficiency symptoms (Toledo, 1982).
- Climatic constraints: resistance to drought ratings, or percentage estimates, of green leaf during the dry season.
- Seasonal (wet and dry season) DM production (g m^{-2} or g per plant; cutting height can be 10–25 cm for herbaceous plants and 30–100 cm for woody legumes), e.g. 8 weeks after a standardization cut, based on sufficiently large samples (1–2 m^2 or minimum of four plants per plot). DM production can also be assessed by rating.
- Regrowth vigour after cutting (rating).

When a large morphological variation among accessions is obvious, leaf : stem ratio (based on a representative sample of separated leaf and stem, or by rating of leafiness) can also be assessed. Furthermore, nutritive-value analyses (crude protein concentration and *in vitro* DM digestibility) of both wet- and dry-season leaf material can be considered, mainly for accessions showing promise towards the end of the trial. Representative accessions of new species may also warrant mineral content analysis (Chapter 11) and tests for anti-nutritive factors (e.g. tannins, alkaloids, saponins).

In addition, it may be worth having separate plots on which plants are allowed to mature so as to enable better assessment of the length of the vegetative phase (number of days to first flower), flowering intensity (rating) and the seed production potential (rating or seed weight per plant or per square metre). The seed production potential of promising accessions can also be assessed using the evaluation plots once the trial has finished.

The above list should not be considered a prescription but rather a guideline. Depending on particular objectives and the researcher's skill and experience, successful identification of superior accessions may well be possible based on fewer evaluation parameters and using ratings rather than measurements. It must also be pointed out that, although there is a need for quantitative data, there is still an 'art' in selecting promising accessions. This is because conditions during testing can never fully reproduce the demands that will be made on the species in practice. Furthermore, the importance of different attributes will vary with different production conditions and no set of parameters is fully indicative of likely success in the field.

The evaluation parameters mentioned refer to both grasses and legumes. Legumes, in addition, can be evaluated for nodulation (rating of root nodule abundance and effectiveness) and the presence of anti-nutritive compounds (based on acceptability observations with livestock or on laboratory analyses, or known occurrences in certain genera). Additional evaluation aspects specific to forage trees and shrubs are discussed by Borel (1992) and Maass *et al.* (1996).

The duration of this type of trial will depend on specific objectives. Often, the desired information may be obtained after two rainy and two dry seasons. If grazing is involved, the trial should last longer. This is particularly so if persistence is an important selection criterion.

Regional trials

The objective of regional trials is to assess the adaptability of species or experimental lines to a broader range of environments. An important side effect is the promotion of promising material. To optimize data comparison and network analysis, a uniform methodology such as that described in Toledo (1982) and used in tropical America in the RIEPT network is required. A modified version of this methodology was subsequently adopted by the RABAOC network in Africa (Schultze-Kraft and Toledo, 1990). Its key elements consist of an establishment phase with measurements for up to 6 months, followed by a 1–2-year production phase with measurements, based on season-specific cutting regimes, during periods of maximum and minimum rainfall ('wet' and 'dry' seasons, respectively). Another relevant multi-locational evaluation example is the OFI (Oxford Forestry Institute) *Gliricidia sepium* provenance trial network (Dunsdon and Simons, 1996).

Statistical tools

Unless there are specific objectives, and depending on the number of treatments, analysis of variance and multivariate analyses (principal component, cluster) are appropriate (Chapter 2). For multi-locational trials, analysis of adaptability based on Eberhart and Russell (1966) has been useful (e.g. Amézquita *et al.*, 1991).

Production evaluation (grazing, cut-and-carry)

Objectives and general considerations

The objective of this evaluation stage is to assess the potential of an accession in terms of its behaviour, productivity and persistence under grazing or cutting management.

Animal species used in the evaluation of experimental lines for pastures should be those used in the relevant production systems. The existence of palatability differences between animal species should be recognized (Cárdenas and Lascano, 1988). Grazing evaluation consists of two parts: the agronomic evaluation of an accession in reaction to grazing by livestock in small paddocks; and the larger-scale evaluation in terms of the accession's effect on livestock performance.

Agronomic pasture evaluation

This refers to assessment of the reaction of a sward, in terms of persistence and stability, to defoliation and trampling by the grazing animal. In cultivar development, this is usually done as a separate step prior to the phase of livestock performance evaluation. Performance under grazing is a selection criterion to reduce the number of accessions under evaluation, or when dealing with species/experimental lines under advanced testing.

The evaluation subject can be monospecific swards, i.e. one species only, or swards composed of species mixtures (usually grass/legume mixtures, but species mixtures within the grass or legume family are possible). With mixtures, possible palatability differences between components, leading to selective grazing, should be recognized. Such differences, which can exist among accessions within one species, may be known prior to designing the experiment. An indication of relative selectivity can be obtained in small-plot 'cafeteria' grazing trials which, prior to the measurement phase, should include an adjustment period (Schultze-Kraft *et al.*, 1989), or even by grazing preliminary evaluation trials. If no fertilization treatments are intended, trials at this stage may be fertilized at standard rates for local pasture establishment.

Paddock size will depend on animal species and size, and on pasture productivity. It may be constrained by land or seed availability, and by fencing costs. A minimum size of 500 m^2 has been suggested (Paladines and Lascano, 1993). Small individually fenced and rotationally grazed paddocks, where each species or species mixture is in a separate paddock, avoids the problem of selective grazing biasing the results (Jones and Mannetje, 1986). One paddock, however, can also contain more than one forage treatment, e.g. when a number of equally palatable accessions or mixtures are to be compared. Then, the minimum plot size/treatment should be 25–50 m^2, depending on growth habit. The participation of a biometrician in the planning of cost-intensive grazing experiments is strongly recommended, especially as factorial designs may not be suitable. The experiment should last a minimum of 2 years of grazing (Paladines and Lascano, 1993). For legumes it should preferably last longer in order to obtain adequate information on plant persistence, ideally until the original plants have died (see Chapter 6).

Grazing management options relevant to this evaluation stage have been discussed in Shaw and Bryan (1976) and in Paladines and Lascano (1993). They range from common or 'mob' stocking, using a large number of animals during a short period of time, to continuous stocking with a flexible or set number of animals. An alternate grazing scheme can also be used with, say, 1 week grazing and 3–4 weeks resting, with seasonal adjustments (e.g. Maldonado *et al.*, 1995). When a multi-accession collection is being evaluated, it is recommended that at least two different grazing intensities or frequencies be considered (Shaw and Bryan, 1976; Paladines and Lascano, 1993).

There is considerable scope for flexible grazing regimes in later-stage evaluation, but this flexibility must be based on understanding of the species involved in the trial. For example, when comparing Peru and Cunningham leucaena, Jones and Jones (1984) increased stocking rates over the summer months to avoid leucaena growing beyond the reach of grazing cattle, which could well have occurred if fixed stocking rates had been used year-long. Spain *et al.* (1985) developed a very interesting and useful concept for evaluation under flexible grazing, although the actual grazing management practices they recommend for applying this flexibility may not be appropriate in all situations.

Agronomic measurements

In both stages of grazing evaluation, sward measurements aim at assessing species productivity and persistence. This usually includes: (i) seasonal DM production or presentation yields at intervals (Chapter 7); (ii) botanical composition, e.g. on a DM weight basis (Chapter 4); and, less often: (iii) percentage ground cover (Chapter 4); and (iv) soil seed reserve and seedling recruitment (Chapter 6). Monitoring of pests and diseases and of nutrient deficiencies is also recommended. In long-term experiments where soil characteristics are likely to be affected by livestock and pasture species, relevant soil physical and chemical characteristics (e.g. water infiltration rate and top soil organic matter and nutrient contents, respectively) should also be monitored (Chapter 12).

Evaluation for cut-and-carry

This does not refer to annual fodder crops but to perennial grasses and legumes, mainly shrubs, for smallholder production systems (e.g. *P. purpureum* and *L. leucocephala*). At this stage, the comparison of accessions can be combined with cutting (height, frequency) or fertilization treatments. Considering that plants used for cutting are usually tall, plots should be large enough to allow for sample sizes of 4 m^2 or, in the case of space-planted legumes, four to eight plants per cut. Measurements of interest are mainly yield, DM percentage, leafiness, plant survival (legumes) and regrowth vigour, and nutritive value (Chapter 11).

Animal performance

In the final evaluation stage, the effect of forage on livestock production is assessed. Grazing experiments are usually long term and large paddocks are used. Chapter 14 considers experimental design and Chapter 15 looks at methodology. Comments particularly relevant to the tropics are given in Shaw and Bryan (1976) and in Lascano and Pizarro (1986). The importance of accompanying animal production measurements by the agronomic measurements, as outlined above, is stressed. In addition, seasonal pasture DM production measurements could be complemented by selective nutritive value analyses.

Pre-release

This phase consists of essentially two activities. Firstly, promising material, of which sufficiently large quantities of seed must be produced during the previous evaluation phase, is issued to farmers for testing under practical conditions and exposed to their management decisions (possibly with some guidance from researchers). This on-farm validation phase could be concurrent with large-scale grazing evaluation (see preceding section). Secondly, promising material is issued to the seed industry or to experienced contract farmers, for producing basic seed for eventual cultivar release and for studying seed production problems (Loch and Ferguson, 1999).

Cultivar release and adoption

Cultivar release consists of the official delivery of a variety (after successful evaluation) and of relevant information to farmers, extensionists and the seed industry. Successful adoption is intimately linked to the availability of seed and the previous exposure of the new material to farmers during evaluation, particularly in the pre-release phase. Thus effective seed production should be under way before the time of cultivar release, unless seed is commercially available from elsewhere. Organizational and technical aspects of the release of tropical forage cultivars and issues related to the multiplication of basic seed are discussed by Ferguson (1985). Seed production research issues related to cultivar release and the importance of developing locally successful seed supply systems which may involve smallholders, such as in northeast Thailand, are addressed in Loch and Ferguson (1999). Additional points to be stressed are, firstly, the need for an adequate, unambiguous description of the genetic material to be released (e.g. the descriptions of Australian cultivars in Oram, 1990) and, secondly, the need to accompany the release process with extension, press and advertising campaigns. In some countries new cultivars are released under 'plant variety rights', to secure intellectual property (p. 196).

Supporting research

Depending on the manpower, infrastructure and responsibilities of the respective research institutions, the evaluation process as described in the preceding sections is often accompanied by supporting research (Shaw and Bryan, 1976; CIAT, 1987). The resulting information represents essential components of the whole improved-forage technology package, of which the released cultivar is only one part. Such support research deals mainly with the usage optimization of the new cultivar and can comprise plant nutrition and fertilization aspects, rhizobiology (legumes), pasture establishment and management, population dynamics, cutting management (frequency, height) of cut-and-carry varieties, nutritive-value aspects (including palatability and anti-nutritive compounds), pest and disease evaluation and management, seed production, and others.

Methodology problems for future research

Consideration of the above evaluation methodologies reveals where some further research is needed to improve available tools and optimize the evaluation process, mainly at the germplasm characterization and preliminary evaluation levels. Suggested areas for the development of low-cost procedures and corresponding concrete guidelines are: (i) early identification of genetic duplicates; (ii) mating system assessment and optimum management of cross-pollinated populations; (iii) heritability assessments (including genotype × environment interaction studies) for important plant descriptors; (iv) illustrated diagnostic help for the identification of disease problems; and (v) rapid assessment of soil-improving effects of forage plants.

Cultivar Evaluation for Temperate Grasslands and Fodder Crops

Unlike tropical grasslands and fodder crops, new cultivars of temperate grasses and legumes in western European countries are obtained by plant breeding and subsequent selection. There are still some instances where cultivars in other temperate areas, such as New Zealand and southern Australia, are derived from direct introductions or selections within farmers' paddocks. In western Europe, wild representatives of established species are used for the enhancement or improvement of desirable properties, such as disease resistance or better persistence, the latter particularly in white clover (*Trifolium repens*) (Rhodes *et al.*, 1989). There are generally two steps before a new variety or cultivar can be released for use in practice: (i) it needs to be registered for plant variety rights (PVR); and (ii) it needs to be approved and put on the recommended list before it can be traded. In general terms, these steps would apply to all areas where temperate forage cultivars are being developed, but in some countries it may not be an obligatory requirement.

Variety registration

Variety registration takes place according to the Convention of the International Union for the Protection of New Varieties of Plants (UPOV), which has so far been signed by about 40 (mostly temperate) countries in the world (UPOV, 1995). For the purpose of the UPOV convention a variety is a 'plant grouping within a single botanical taxon of the lowest known rank'. PVR can be given for all botanical genera and species, including hybrids between genera or species. PVR can be granted by National Councils for Plant Variety Rights for varieties that are: (i) distinct; (ii) uniform; (iii) stable and (iv) novel.

The tests for these properties are carried out by testing organizations appointed by the government of a country. Such testing organizations need not be in the country in which the variety rights have been applied for. The granting of PVR is not related to agronomic value. PVR apply only to the 'variety constituents', i.e. whole plants or parts of plants that are capable of producing entire plants. In most cases this will be seed:

- *Distinctness* of a variety is shown by comparing a proposed variety with all other known varieties of that species in the expression of the characteristics resulting from the genotype. The new variety must have some characteristics that make it readily distinguishable from all other varieties of the same species.
- *Uniformity* of a variety means that, subject to the natural variation that may be expected from its form of propagation, it is sufficiently uniform

in those characteristics that are included in the examination of distinctness as well as those used for its description.

- *Stability* means that the expression of characteristics used in the examination of distinctness, as well as those used for its description, remain unchanged after repeated propagation.
- *Novelty* means that variety constituents or harvested material have not been sold or otherwise disposed of to others by or with the consent of the breeder for purposes of exploitation of the variety.

The sale or use of registered varieties is only allowed if the holder of the PVR gives his permission in return for payment of royalties. However, farmers may use propagation material they have harvested themselves from registered varieties ('Farmers' Privilege') of certain species, including the forages *Cicer arietinum* (chickpea milkvetch), *Lupinus luteus* (yellow lupin), *Medicago sativa* (lucerne), *Pisum sativum* (field pea), *Trifolium alexandrinum* (berseem/Egyptian clover), *Trifolium resupinatum* (Persian clover), *Vicia faba* (field bean) and *Vicia sativa* (common vetch).

Cultivar evaluation

In the European Union, cultivars can only be traded after they have been added to a National List or to the European Union Common Catalogue. Only cultivars registered under PVR can be listed and then only after testing for 'value for cultivation and use' by an approved institution.

Protocols for evaluation

For the UK, Frame (1992) has outlined the evaluation process for cultivars that are intended for the National List of the common grass and legume species in use in the region, viz. *Lolium perenne*, *Lolium multiflorum*, *Phleum pratense* (timothy) and *T. repens*. Cultivars of *L. perenne* are sown in 2 consecutive years and harvested for 2 full years under conditions of simulated grazing, i.e. seven to nine cuts per year and also under a silage regime (four to five cuts). Plots are fertilized to ensure that nutrition is not limiting, with N at 360 and 350 kg ha^{-1} per year for the simulated grazing and silage regimes, respectively. For *P. pratense* only the silage regime is applied. *L. multiflorum* and hybrid ryegrass are cut five times during the establishment year and five to seven cuts are taken during the following 2 years, viz. an 'early bite' harvest (c. 1.1 t ha^{-1}), two conservation cuts and then monthly cuts until the end of the season. For each cut 50 kg N ha^{-1} is applied.

T. repens material is tested in mixture with a cultivar of *L. perenne*, which is sown in two successive years and is cut five to seven times per year, with the yields measured in the second and third harvest years at target DM yields of 1.5 t ha^{-1}. The plots are fertilized with 200 kg N ha^{-1} and adequate P and K. Sowings of the clover are also made in plots that are infected with

Sclerotinia to test resistance and in plots that are subjected to very frequent cutting (every 10–15 days) to observe persistence under simulated intensive grazing, but without taking measurements. The basis for addition to the National List are persistence (measured by survival and ground cover), digestibility and crude protein concentration.

A non-statuary Recommended List of the best varieties for use in seed mixtures is compiled from the National List in the UK (Frame, 1992). In addition to data from the National List, information is collected from supplementary testing on farms, including acceptability to grazing stock, spring growth, ground cover, disease resistance and other practical information. The Recommended List gives descriptive information along the lines of: 'Very good mid-season digestibility and good ground cover combined with good resistance to crown rust' for a variety of perennial ryegrass. Varieties are removed from the Recommended List when they have come to the bottom of the list of best cultivars.

In The Netherlands new cultivars of perennial species proposed for inclusion in the National and Recommended Lists are tested for 5 years and annual Italian ryegrass for 4 years. Testing procedures vary for different species and maturity types of grasses. Late and mid-season cultivars of perennial ryegrass are sown in the first year in two grazing trials with dairy cattle and one cutting trial. In the second year, sowing takes place for another grazing trial and an observation trial. The grazing trials are situated on clay and sandy soil, the cutting trial on sandy soil and the observation trial, mainly under grazing, on peat soil. Yield measurements (six to eight cuts per year) are taken in the second, third and fourth year, so that after 4 years there will have been eight data sets for DM yield from grazing and three from cutting trials, respectively. White clover cultivars are tested by growing them with perennial ryegrass under grazing. Competition trials are established and are maintained for 4 years for cultivars of white clover, *P. pratense*, *Festuca pratensis* (meadow fescue) and *Poa pratensis* (smooth-stalked meadow grass; Kentucky bluegrass), the treatments consisting of a monoculture and a mixture with perennial ryegrass[10].

These very rigid requirements for evaluation are only given as examples, as many countries outside western Europe would not have such detailed requirements.

Measurements and observations

In the UK the main evaluation parameters are: seasonal and annual DM yields; digestible organic matter as a percentage of DM (D value); crude

---

[10] Official Protocol for the Dutch Recommended List of Varieties (unpublished); H. Bonthuis, Plant Research International, Wageningen University and Research Centre, Wageningen, The Netherlands (personal communication)

protein and water soluble carbohydrate contents of the first two silage cuts in the first year of harvest (Frame, 1992). The Target D value for first silage cuts is 67, which is estimated by monitoring heading date of a reference variety, whose ear emergence/digestibility relationship is known. Other parameters evaluated are survival or persistence (judged by ground cover), drought tolerance and susceptibility to pests and diseases. Artificial infections are carried out to test resistance for the very common crown rust infection, *Drechslera*, *Rhynchosporium* and ryegrass mosaic virus. Winter hardiness is a very important property for ryegrass in northwestern Europe and this is tested *in situ* in the UK at 300 m above sea level and in The Netherlands in growth chambers.

In The Netherlands, the following parameters are measured or noted:

- Emergence is noted a few weeks after sowing on a scale of 1–9.
- Cover is estimated three times a year as a percentage, in early spring, end of summer and autumn. The data are translated into persistence.
- Winter hardiness is observed and related to death of plants or the sward. Damage by snow fungus is separately observed.
- Heading is estimated at every cut or grazing as the percentage of flower heads present.
- Dry matter yields in grazing and cutting trials are usually done with a self-propelled harvester (see Chapter 7). In grazing trials a strip is cut when 90% of the cultivars under test have an estimated DM yield of 1.5–1.8 t ha^{-1} and a silage cut is taken from cutting trials at an estimated DM yield of 2.5–3.5 t ha^{-1}. Autumn cuts may be taken at somewhat lower yields.
- Competitive ability is expressed as the proportion (%) of cover of the relevant species in mixture with perennial ryegrass in early spring, end of summer and autumn.
- Resistance against prevailing diseases is scored visually on a scale of 1–9 and usually repeated after 1 week.

Conclusions

Many different procedures are being followed in the development and release of new cultivars. In general, development of tropical cultivars is different from that of temperate cultivars. Tropical forage cultivars are still usually developed from direct introductions, do not have to undergo rigid systems of evaluation or variety testing, and are often released without PVR. In contrast, almost all temperate cultivars are derived from breeding programmes and, particularly in western Europe, are released under PVR following detailed procedures for varietal testing.

References

Amézquita, M.C., Toledo, J.M. and Keller-Grein, G. (1991) Agronomic performance of *Stylosanthes guianensis* cv. Pucallpa in the American tropical rainforest ecosystem. *Tropical Grasslands* 25, 262–267.

Anderson, J.M. and Ingram, J.S.I. (1993) *Tropical Soil Biology and Fertility. A Handbook of Methods*, 2nd edn. CAB International, Wallingford, UK, 221 pp.

Argel, P.J., Durán, C.V. and Franco, L.H. (1993) *Planeación y Conducción de Ensayos de Evaluación de Gramíneas y Leguminosas Forrajeras en Fincas*. RIEPT-CAC. Memorias, Taller realizado en Costa Rica y Panamá, 7–17 Junio 1993. Documento de Trabajo No. 133, Centro Internacional de Agricultura Tropical (CIAT), Cali, Colombia, 338 pp.

Ashby, J.A. (1990) *Evaluating Technology with Farmers: a Handbook*. Centro Internacional de Agricultura Tropical (CIAT), Cali, Colombia, 95 pp.

Borel, R. (1992) Critical aspects of methodologies for the nutritional evaluation of forage trees and shrubs. In: Ruiz, M.E. and Ruiz, S.E. (eds) *Ruminant Nutrition Research: Methodological Guidelines*. Inter-American Institute for Cooperation on Agriculture (IICA), San José, Costa Rica, pp. 35–45.

Briscoe, C.B. (1989) *Field Trials Manual for Multipurpose Tree Species*. Multipurpose Tree Species Network Technical Series, Manual No. 3. Winrock International Institute for Agricultural Development, Morrilton, Arkansas, 163 pp.

Cameron, D.F., Trevorrow, R.M. and Liu, C.J. (1997) Recent advances in studies of anthracnose in *Stylosanthes*. II. Approaches to breeding for anthracnose resistance in *Stylosanthes* in Australia. *Tropical Grasslands* 31, 424–429.

Cárdenas, E.A. and Lascano, C.E. (1988) Utilización de ovinos y bovinos en la evaluación de pasturas asociadas. *Pasturas Tropicales* 10(2), 2–10.

Cheng, Y. and Horne, P. (1997) *Field Experiments with Forages and Crops: Practical Tips for Getting it Right the First Time*. Australian Centre for International Agricultural Research (ACIAR) and Australian Agency for International Development (AusAID), Canberra, 48 pp.

CIAT (1987) *Investigaciones de Apoyo para la Evaluación de Pasturas*. Memorias de la 3a. reunión de trabajo del Comité Asesor de la RIEPT, 15–18 de octubre de 1985, Red Internacional de Evaluación de Pastos Tropicales. Centro Internacional de Agricultura Tropical (CIAT), Cali, Colombia, 195 pp.

CIAT (1993) *Investigación con Pasturas en Fincas*. Memorias, VII Reunión del Comité Asesor de la Red Internacional de Evaluación de Pastos Tropicales (RIEPT) en CIAT, Palmira, Colombia, 27–29 Agosto 1990. Documento de Trabajo No. 124. Programa de Forrajes Tropicales, Centro Internacional de Agricultura Tropical (CIAT), Cali, Colombia, 277 pp.

CIAT (1995) *Réseau de Recherche en Alimentation du Bétail en Afrique Occidentale et Centrale RABAOC-AFRNET. SNRA-CIRAD/EMVT-CIAT-ILCA. Résultats 1990–1994*. 5ème Réunion Annuelle, Lomé, Togo, 3–9 Avril 1995. Document de Travail No. 145. Centro Internacional de Agricultura Tropical (CIAT), Cali, Colombia, 258 pp.

Clements, R.J. and Cameron, D.G. (eds) (1980) *Collecting and Testing Tropical Forage Plants*. Commonwealth Scientific and Industrial Research Organization (CSIRO), Melbourne, 154 pp.

Clements, R.J., Winter, W.H. and Thomson, C.J. (1986) Breeding *Centrosema pascuorum* for northern Australia. *Tropical Grasslands* 20, 59–65.

da Rocha, G.L. and 19 co-authors (1979) Coleta, identificação e distribuição de leguminosas forrageiras tropicais brasileiras – Brasil Central – Fase I. *Boletim de Indústria Animal (Nova Odessa, SP)* 36, 255–324.

Daher, R.F., Moraes, C.F., Cruz, C.D., Pereira, A.V. and Xavier, D.F. (1997) Diversidade morfológica e isozimática em capim-elefante (*Pennisetum purpureum* Schum.). *Revista Brasileira de Zootecnia* 26, 255–264.

Date, R.A. (1995) Collecting *Rhizobium, Frankia* and mycorrhizal fungi. In: Guarino, L., Ramanatha Rao, V. and Reid, R. (eds) *Collecting Plant Genetic Diversity: Technical Guidelines.* CAB International, Wallingford, UK, and International Plant Genetic Resources Institute (IPGRI), Rome, pp. 551–560.

Dunsdon, A.J. and Simons, A.J. (1996) Provenance and progeny trials. In: Steward, J.L., Allison, G.E. and Simons, A.J. (eds) *Gliricidia sepium – Genetic Resources for Farmers.* Oxford Forestry Institute (OFI), University of Oxford, Oxford, pp. 93–97.

Eberhart, S.A. and Russell, W.A. (1966) Stability parameters for comparing varieties. *Crop Science* 6, 36–40.

Ferguson, J.E. (1985) An overview of the release process for new cultivars of tropical forages. *Seed Science and Technology* 13, 741–757.

Ferreira, M.E. and Grattapaglia, D. (1996) *Introdução ao Uso de Marcadores Moleculares em Análise Genética.* Empresa Brasileira de Pesquisa Agropecuária (EMBRAPA) – Centro Nacional de Pesquisa de Recursos Genéticos e Biotecnologia (CENARGEN), Brasília, DF, 220 pp.

Frame, J. (1992) *Improved Grassland Management.* Farming Press, Ipswich, UK, 351 pp.

Guarino, L., Ramanatha Rao, V. and Reid, R. (eds) (1995) *Collecting Plant Genetic Diversity: Technical Guidelines.* CAB International, Wallingford, UK, and International Plant Genetic Resources Institute (IPGRI), Rome, 748 pp.

Hodgkin, T., Brown, A.H.D., Hintum, Th.J.L. van and Morales, E.A.V. (eds) (1995) *Core Collections of Plant Genetic Resources.* J. Wiley & Sons, Chichester, UK, 269 pp.

Humphreys, L.R. and Partridge, I.J. (1995). *A Guide to Better Pastures for the Tropics and Subtropics,* revised 5th edn. New South Wales Agriculture, Paterson, New South Wales, 86 pp.

Hutton, E.M. (1962) Siratro – a tropical pasture legume bred from *Phaseolus atropurpureus. Australian Journal of Experimental Agriculture and Animal Husbandry* 2, 117–125.

Jank, L., Calixto, S., Costa, J.C.G., Savidan, Y. and Curvo, J.B.E. (1997) *Catálogo de Caracterização e Avaliação de Germoplasma de* Panicum maximum*: Descrição Morfológica e Comportamento Agronômico.* Empresa Brasileira de Pesquisa Agropecuária (EMBRAPA) – Centro Nacional de Pesquisa de Gado de Corte (CNPGC), Campo Grande, MS, Brazil, 53 pp.

Jones, R.J. and Walker, B. (1983) Strategies for evaluating forage plants. In: McIvor, J.G. and Bray, R.A. (eds) *Genetic Resources of Forage Plants.* Commonwealth Scientific and Industrial Research Organization (CSIRO), East Melbourne, pp. 185–201.

Jones, R.M. and Jones, R.J. (1984) The effect of *Leucaena leucocephala* on liveweight gain, thyroid size and thyroxine levels of steers in south-eastern Queensland. *Australian Journal of Experimental Agriculture and Animal Husbandry* 24, 4–9.

Jones, R.M. and Mannetje, L. 't (1986) *A Comparison of Bred* Macroptilium *Lines and cv. Siratro in Subcoastal Southeast Queensland with Special Reference to Legume*

Persistence. Tropical Agronomy Technical Memorandum No. 47, Commonwealth Scientific and Industrial Research Organization (CSIRO), Division of Tropical Crops and Pastures, St. Lucia, Queensland, 11 pp.

Lascano, C. and Pizarro, E. (eds) (1986) *Evaluación de Pasturas con Animales. Alternativas Metodológicas.* Memorias de una reunión de trabajo celebrada en Perú, 1–5 de octubre, 1984, Red Internacional de Evaluación de Pastos Tropicales. Centro Internacional de Agricultura Tropical (CIAT), Cali, Colombia, 290 pp.

Lazier, J.R. (1985) Theory and practice in forage germ-plasm collection. In: Kategile, J.A. (ed.) *Pasture Improvement Research in Eastern and Southern Africa. Proceedings of a workshop held in Harare, Zimbabwe, 17–21 September 1984.* International Development Research Centre (IDRC), Ottawa, pp. 260–295.

Liu, C.J. (1996) Genetic diversity and relationships among *Lablab purpureus* genotypes evaluated using RAPD as markers. *Euphytica* 90, 115–119.

Loch, D.S. and Ferguson, J.E. (eds) (1999) *Forage Seed Production, Vol. 2: Tropical and Subtropical Species.* CAB International, Wallingford, UK, 479 pp.

Maass, B.L. and Ocampo, C.H. (1995) Isozyme polymorphism provides fingerprints for germplasm of *Arachis glabrata* Bentham. *Genetic Resources and Crop Evolution* 42, 77–82.

Maass, B.L., Schultze-Kraft, R. and Argel, P.J. (1996) Revisión de la evaluación agronómica de especies arbustivas. In: Pizarro, E.A. and Coradin, L. (eds) *Potencial del Género* Cratylia *como Leguminosa Forrajera.* Memorias del taller de trabajo sobre *Cratylia* realizado 19–20 de Julio de 1995, Brasília, D.F., Brasil. Centro Internacional de Agricultura Tropical (CIAT), Cali, Colombia, pp. 107–114.

Mannetje, L. 't and Jones, R.M. (eds) (1992) *Plant Resources of South-East Asia No. 4, Forages.* Pudoc Scientific Publishers, Wageningen, The Netherlands, 300 pp.

Maldonado, H., Keller-Grein, G., do Nascimento, D. Jr and Regazzi, A.J. (1995) Produção de pastagens associadas sob três taxas de lotação. *Pasturas Tropicales* 17(3), 23–26.

Marshall, D.R. and Brown, A.H.D. (1983) Theory of forage plant collection. In: McIvor, J.G. and Bray, R.A. (eds) *Genetic Resources of Forage Plants.* Commonwealth Scientific and Industrial Research Organization (CSIRO), East Melbourne, pp. 135–148.

McIvor, J.G. and Bray, R.A. (eds) (1983) *Genetic Resources of Forage Plants.* Commonwealth Scientific and Industrial Research Organization (CSIRO), East Melbourne, 337 pp.

Miles, J.W. and do Valle, C.B. (1996) Manipulation of apomixis in *Brachiaria* breeding. In: Miles, J.W., Maass, B.L. and do Valle, C.B. (eds) Brachiaria: *Biology, Agronomy, and Improvement.* Centro Internacional de Agricultura Tropical (CIAT), Cali, Colombia, and Empresa Brasileira de Pesquisa Agropecuária (EMBRAPA) – Centro Nacional de Pesquisa de Gado de Corte (CNPGC), Campo Grande, MS, Brazil, pp. 164–177.

Miller, A.G. and Nyberg, J.A. (1995) Collecting herbarium vouchers. In: Guarino, L., Ramanatha Rao, V. and Reid, R. (eds) *Collecting Plant Genetic Diversity: Technical Guidelines.* CAB International, Wallingford, UK, and International Plant Genetic Resources Institute (IPGRI), Rome, pp. 561–573.

Mott, G.O. (ed.) (1979) *Handbook for the Collection, Preservation and Characterization of Tropical Forage Germplasm Resources.* Centro Internacional de Agricultura Tropical (CIAT), Cali, Colombia, 95 pp.

Oram, R.N. (comp.) (1990) *Register of Australian Herbage Plant Cultivars*, 3rd edn. Commonwealth Scientific and Industrial Research Organization (CSIRO), East Melbourne, 304 pp.

Paladines, O. and Lascano, C.E. (eds) (1993) *Forage Germplasm under Small-Plot Grazing: Evaluation Methodologies. Proceedings of a workshop held in Cali, Colombia, 22–24 September 1982.* International Tropical Pastures Evaluation Network (RIEPT), Centro Internacional de Agricultura Tropical (CIAT), Cali, Colombia, 249 pp.

Peters, K.J. and Tothill, J.C. (1988) Strategy of ILCA to improve productivity of pasture and forage resources in Africa. *Giessener Beiträge zur Entwicklungsforschung, Reihe I*, 17, 35–49.

Reid, R. (1980) Collection and use of climatic data in pasture plant introduction. In: Clements, R.J. and Cameron, D.G. (eds) *Collecting and Testing Tropical Forage Plants.* Commonwealth Scientific and Industrial Research Organization (CSIRO), Melbourne, pp. 1–10.

Rhodes, I., Collins, R.P., Evans, D.R. and Glendining, M.J. (1989) Breeding reliable white clover for low input pastures. In: *Proceedings, XVI International Grassland Congress.* Nice, France, Vol. 1, pp. 315–316.

Sackville Hamilton, N.R. and Chorlton, K.H. (1995) Collecting vegetative material of forage grasses and legumes. In: Guarino, L., Ramanatha Rao, V. and Reid, R. (eds) *Collecting Plant Genetic Diversity: Technical Guidelines.* CAB International, Wallingford, UK, and International Plant Genetic Resources Institute (IPGRI), Rome, Italy, pp. 467–484.

Sarrantonio, M. (1991) *Methodologies for Screening Soil-Improving Legumes.* Rodale Institute, Kutztown, Pennsylvania, 310 pp.

Schultze-Kraft, R. and Giacometti, D.C. (1978) Genetic resources of forage legumes for the acid, infertile savannas of tropical America. In: Sanchez, P.A. and Tergas, L.E. (eds) *Pasture Production in Acid Soils of the Tropics.* Centro Internacional de Agricultura Tropical (CIAT), Cali, Colombia, pp. 55–64.

Schultze-Kraft, R. and Toledo, J.M. (1990) *Methodology for the Agronomic Evaluation of Forage Plants in Regional Trials of the West and Central African Forage Evaluation Network (WECAFNET).* Second WECAFNET Workshop, Avétonou, Togo, 16–21 April 1990; revised document June 1990. Centro Internacional de Agricultura Tropical (CIAT), Cali, Colombia, 19 pp.

Schultze-Kraft, R., Lascano, C., Benavides, G. and Gómez, J.M. (1989) Relative palatability of some little-known tropical forage legumes. In: *Proceedings, XVI International Grassland Congress.* Nice, France, Vol. 2, pp. 785–786.

Schultze-Kraft, R., Williams, W.M. and Keoghan, J.M. (1993) Searching for new germplasm for the year 2000 and beyond. In: *Proceedings, XVII International Grassland Congress.* New Zealand and Australia, Vol. 1, pp. 181–187.

Shaw, N.H. and Bryan, W.W. (eds) (1976) *Tropical Pasture Research: Principles and Methods.* Commonwealth Bureau of Pastures and Field Crops Bulletin 51, Commonwealth Agricultural Bureaux (CAB), Farnham Royal, UK, 454 pp.

Skerman, P.J. and Riveros, F. (1990) *Tropical Grasses.* FAO Plant Production and Protection Series No. 23. Food and Agriculture Organization of the United Nations, Rome, Italy, 832 pp.

Skerman, P.J., Cameron, D.G. and Riveros, F. (1988) *Tropical Forage Legumes.* FAO Plant Production and Protection Series No. 2, 2nd edn. Food and Agriculture Organization of the United Nations, Rome, Italy, 692 pp.

Spain, J.M., Pereira, J.M. and Gualdrón, R. (1985) A flexible grazing management system proposed for the advanced evaluation of associations of tropical grasses and legumes. In: *Proceedings, XV International Grassland Congress.* Kyoto, Japan, pp. 1153–1155.

Tarawali, S.A., Tarawali, G., Larbi, A. and Hanson, J. (1995) *Methods for the Evaluation of Forage Legumes, Grasses and Fodder Trees for Use as Livestock Feed.* ILRI Manual 1. International Livestock Research Institute (ILRI), Nairobi, Kenya, 31 pp.

Toledo, J.M. (ed.) (1982) *Manual para la Evaluación Agronómica, Red Internacional de Evaluación de Pastos Tropicales.* Centro Internacional de Agricultura Tropical (CIAT), Cali, Colombia, 168 pp.

Toledo, J.M., Lenné, J.M. and Schultze-Kraft, R. (1989) Effective utilization of tropical pasture germplasm. In: FAO (ed.) *Utilization of Genetic Resources: Suitable Approaches, Agronomical Evaluation and Use.* FAO Plant Production and Protection Paper 94. Food and Agriculture Organization of the United Nations, Rome, Italy, pp. 27–57.

UPOV (1995) Plant Variety Protection. Publication No. 438. *Gazette and Newsletter of the International Union for the Protection of New Varieties of Plants*, No. 77, Geneva, Switzerland.

Womersley, J.S. (1981) *Plant Collecting and Herbarium Development: A Manual.* FAO Plant Production and Protection Paper 33. Food and Agriculture Organization of the United Nations, Rome, Italy, 137 pp.

Remote Sensing in Vegetation and Animal Studies

M.L. Roderick[1], V. Chewings[2] and R.C.G. Smith[3]

[1]Ecosystem Dynamics, Research School of Biological Sciences, Australian National University, Canberra, Australia; [2]Centre for Arid Zone Research, CSIRO, Division of Wildlife and Ecology, Alice Springs, Australia; [3]Remote Sensing Services, Department of Land Administration, Perth, Australia

Introduction

Instruments based on the principles of remote sensing are widely used in both science and society. Examples include neutron moisture probes and instruments based on time domain reflectometry (TDR) for measuring soil moisture, temperature measurement by infra-red radiometers, determination of chemical composition by mass spectrometers, X-rays and ultrasound imaging systems used in medical science, depth sounders used by hydrographers and fishermen, light meters on cameras, and so on.

Despite the everyday nature of many of the above devices, there has often been a tendency to view the use of satellite imagery as a (costly) 'high tech' solution in agricultural and environmental sciences. Certainly the design, construction, launch and subsequent operation of satellites is 'high tech'. However, the images produced by many of these satellites are essentially photographs and as such are based on some relatively simple physical principles. When viewed in this context, the application of (space) photography to grasslands cannot be considered 'high tech' at all.

Rather than describe and list the various applications of remote sensing, we have deliberately chosen to describe the physical principles underlying the acquisition of remotely sensed images and to use those principles as a basis for understanding how the technology can be applied in grassland environments. We have limited the chapter to the use of images that are based on recording reflected solar radiation, though there are comments and references to other remote sensing systems. Most of the major earth resource satellite missions such as Landsat, SPOT and

NOAA-AVHRR carry sensors that record reflected solar radiation. The first of these satellites, Landsat, was launched in 1972 so there is now considerable experience in the use of such images for a variety of resource management problems. There is also a large archive of historical data covering most parts of the earth, offering an unparalleled opportunity to monitor longer-term changes in grasslands. Further applications of remotely sensed imagery in monitoring and land degradation studies are discussed in Chapter 10.

We begin by describing some basic physical principles and then propose a very simple model of vegetation canopy reflectance. Using this model as a guide we list the various methods available for extracting information from satellite images, with particular emphasis on grasslands. Finally, we take a brief look at future developments in remote sensing.

Physical Principles

The electromagnetic spectrum

Remote sensing in the most general sense is based on measuring the interaction between electromagnetic (EM) radiation and a target such as the surface of the earth and using those measurements to infer properties of the target, such as its size and composition. Under this definition, human vision is a classic example of remote sensing. There are two basic system types: passive and active. Passive remote sensing systems use an external energy source such as solar radiation whilst active systems, such as the radar imaging devices used to track aircraft at airports, provide their own energy source. Satellite remote sensing is restricted to regions in the EM spectrum in which the atmosphere is relatively transparent (Fig. 9.1) whilst airborne and hand-held sensors can be used over a much larger range.

All objects whose temperature is above absolute zero emit EM radiation over a particular wavelength range at rates that are dependent on the temperature of the object. Thus the sun emits a characteristic spectrum largely confined to the 0.3–3 μm range with a peak in the visible spectrum at 0.6 μm (Monteith and Unsworth, 1990). Most of the solar radiation is in the visible (VIS) (see Fig. 9.1 for abbreviations) and near infrared (NIR) and some small amounts of ultra-violet (UV) and mid infrared (MIR). At typical surface temperatures (e.g. 15–25°C) the earth emits thermal infrared (TIR) centred at approximately 10 μm (Monteith and Unsworth, 1990). Since this emission coincides with an atmospheric window, it can be sensed from outside the atmosphere using TIR sensors and can be used to estimate the temperature of the land surface (Price, 1989; Kerr et al., 1992). For example, forest and grassland fires can be detected in MIR–TIR regions (Belward et al., 1994; Pereira and Setzer, 1997).

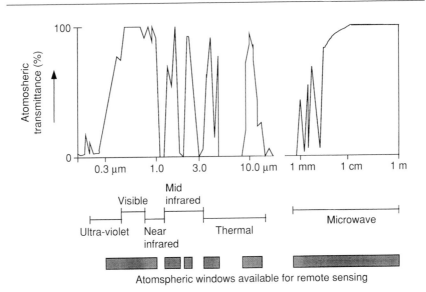

Fig. 9.1. Transmittance of electromagnetic (EM) radiation through the earth's atmosphere and resultant atmospheric windows useful for remote sensing. EM radiation is commonly classified according to wavelength as follows: UV (ultraviolet) 0.1–0.4 μm; VIS (visible) 0.4–0.7 μm; NIR (near infrared) 0.7–1.1 μm; MIR (mid infrared) 1.1–3.0 μm; and TIR (thermal infrared) 3.0–12 μm. The VIS range can be further subdivided as: B (blue) 0.4–0.5 μm; G (green) 0.5–0.6 μm; and R (red) 0.6–0.7 μm. (Reproduced from Smith, 1997, with permission of Royal Society of Western Australia.)

Radar (acronym for radio detection and ranging) systems generate microwaves which have the useful property that they travel through clouds. Accordingly, they are widely used in mission-critical applications such as aircraft tracking, ice detection in shipping lanes and military operations. Radar systems can also be used for general topographic mapping (Zebker *et al.*, 1994) and there are civilian satellites that can provide imagery that is ideal for mapping in heavily cloud covered areas such as the tropics. It has recently been shown that space-borne radar systems can be used to measure the very small changes in elevation (approximately 1 cm) that often occur after an earthquake (Massonnet *et al.*, 1994). This suggests that it may be possible to use such systems to measure rates of soil erosion, although as far as we are aware this has not been attempted. The all-weather capability of radar has also attracted the interest of grassland researchers (Smith *et al.*, 1995).

Further discussions on radar, thermal and other systems are available in textbooks (Curran, 1985; Lillesand and Kiefer, 1994). The physics of thermal radiation are covered by Monteith and Unsworth (1990) while Price (1989) provides specific details on the use of satellite-based thermal imagery. The remainder of this chapter focuses on remote sensing in the VIS–NIR regions of the solar spectrum.

Spectral reflectance

When energy interacts with a target it can be either absorbed, transmitted or reflected. Satellite remote sensing in the solar spectrum is based on measuring the reflected component, which varies with wavelength and the surface type (Fig. 9.2). The reflectance spectra of healthy green vegetation is very different from virtually all other land surface features, having low VIS and high NIR reflectance. The low visible reflectance is due to absorption in these wavelengths by chlorophyll for photosynthesis (Nobel, 1991). The slight increase in reflectance at green wavelengths (compared with blue and red) results in plants appearing green. The high reflectance of healthy leaves in the NIR is due to enhanced scattering by the internal structure of leaves and it appears to be largely related to the water content and turgor of cells within the leaf (Gausman and Allen, 1973).

In contrast, senesced and nitrogen- or water-stressed leaves often appear bright yellow and have a corresponding higher VIS and lower NIR reflectance than healthy green leaves. Reflectance from water bodies largely depends on the depth and turbidity of the water column, and the colour of the bottom in shallow waters. Hence water is generally blue (or blue-green) since it reflects more light at those wavelengths. Virtually all of the NIR is absorbed by water. Fortunately, soil reflectance spectra are quite different from both water and vegetation in that the reflectance is highly

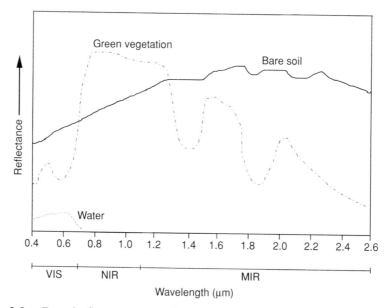

Fig. 9.2. Typical reflectance spectra for green vegetation, soil and water in the VIS–NIR–MIR. (Reproduced from Smith, 1997, with permission of Royal Society of Western Australia.)

correlated across all wavelengths. Thus a black soil has a low VIS reflectance and a correspondingly low NIR reflectance, whilst bright soils (e.g. white/red) in the VIS also tend to be bright in the NIR. The reflectance from soil also varies depending on the moisture content and soils tend to darken when wet. The highly correlated nature of soil reflectance is the basis for virtually all remote sensing studies interested in vegetation.

The continuous spectra depicted in Fig. 9.2 can be measured using laboratory and field spectrometers, which can now also be mounted in aircraft (e.g. Wessman *et al.*, 1997). However, current satellite sensors (known as radiometers) measure the reflectance for relatively broad spectral regions which are known as bands. The exact location and width of each spectral band varies between both satellites and instruments (see Table 9.1) although most earth resource satellites include at least a red (R) and NIR band, which makes them very useful for vegetation studies. In theory at least, it would seem that remote sensing should be able to determine the composition of any target based on reflectance spectra. However, under field situations it is virtually impossible to sample the 'pure' targets which are carefully prepared in laboratories. The consequences are demonstrated in the following section.

Canopy reflectance

Individual satellite measurements are approximately, but not exactly (Wilson, 1988), averaged over a ground area known as a pixel and images are composed of pixels in a regular rectangular grid pattern. Pixel sizes vary depending on the sensor but mostly range from 5 to 100 m for sensors designed for landscape-scale work. Thus the measurement recorded for each pixel must be a composite measure, which is determined by the mixture of surface types within the pixel (Price, 1994). Also, there may be shadows, which are determined by the vertical structure of objects such as trees, shrubs, surface stones, etc. and the position of the sun (Graetz and Gentle, 1982). When in a shadow, an object such as a leaf receives light scattered from other sunlit surfaces and also receives diffuse radiation. Since the amount of diffuse radiation is minimal on sunny days during the middle hours of the day (Spitters *et al.*, 1986; Monteith and Unsworth, 1990), we can assume that for most practical purposes objects that are in shadows make a relatively small contribution to the overall pixel reflectance (Franklin and Hiernaux, 1991; Leblon *et al.*, 1996). The fraction of the pixel that is apparently covered by shadows will also change depending on the direction from which the pixel is viewed.

A number of models have been developed that exploit the presence of shadows to infer the vegetation structure and biomass in forest and woodland environments (Jupp *et al.*, 1986; Li and Strahler, 1986). The basic philosophy of these models is that the shadows also contain information.

Table 9.1. Characteristics of some common earth resource satellite sensors. The SPOT and IRS satellites can change the viewing angle of the sensor and can acquire images of the same ground area more frequently than Landsat. For off-nadir viewing, the pixel and image sizes are larger. The NOAA-AVHRR sensor views ± 55° either side of nadir, giving a swathe width of 2700 km. Bands are: V = visible, with subscripts (b, g, r) to signify which part of the visible spectrum; NIR = near infrared; MIR = mid infrared; TIR = thermal infrared; SIR = shortwave infrared (0.7–3.0 μm).

Name	Pixel size (m)	Image size (km)	Spectral and radiometric resolution	Interval between nadir observations (days)	Interval between off-nadir observations (days)	Overpass time (local solar time, h)	Lifetime
Landsat MSS	80	185	4 bands Vg, Vr, NIR, NIR [6 or 7 bit]	16	16	0935–1000	1972–1997
Landsat TM	30[a]	185	7 bands Vb, Vg, Vr, NIR, MIR, MIR, TIR [8 bit]	16	16	0935–1000	1984–present
SPOT XS	20	60[c]	3 bands Vg, Vr, NIR [8 bit]	26	3 or 5[d]	1000–1030	1986–present
SPOT PAN	10	60[c]	1 band V [8 bit]	26	3 or 5[d]	1000–1030	1986–present
NOAA AVHRR	1100[b]	2700	5 bands Vr, NIR, MIR, TIR, TIR [10 bit]	9	1/4[e]	0800–0900[f] 1500–1700[g]	1978–present
IRS LISS	25, 36, 72	142	4 bands Vb,Vg,Vr,NIR [7 bit]	24	5	1030	1988–present
IRS WiFS	180	774	3 bands Vr, NIR, SIR [7 bit]	24	5	1030	1995–present
IRS PAN	5	70	1 band V [6 bit]	24	5	1030	1995–present

[a]TIR band is 120 m; [b]1100 m at nadir. Can be up to 8 km at edge of scan; [c]60 km for nadir view but up to 120 km for off-nadir viewing; [d]Depends on latitude; [e]Four overpasses per day; [f]Morning overpass; [g]Afternoon overpass.

These so-called geometric–optical models are based on generalizing the scene in terms of the vegetation stand structure (e.g. height, average crown spacing, overall shape, etc.) in a mathematical framework. When the position of the sun and sensor are specified, it is possible to calculate the position of shadows, and satellite observations can then be used to invert the model and estimate the various parameters. While the basic approach appears quite general (Hall *et al.*, 1995), the major problem is that it is necessary to define a set of mathematical equations for each different vegetation structure, though this does not pose severe problems in a grassland environment.

A much simpler approach, known as a linear mixture model, is to assume that the pixel reflectance is the sum of the reflectance from the various surface types normalized for their relative areal cover in the pixel (Fig. 9.3). Whilst this figure depicts the shadow as being cast by a tree, it should be noted that grass, litter, surface stones, etc. may also cast shadows and it is assumed that S includes all shadows within the pixel. The total reflectance (ρ) for the pixel in a given band is then (Pech *et al.*, 1986):

$$\rho = S\rho(S) + T\rho(T) + G\rho(G) + L\rho(L) + B\rho(B) \tag{9.1}$$

where $\rho()$ is the reflectance of the respective elements as defined in Fig. 9.3. Whilst this model ignores multiple reflections, such as when light is reflected by tree or grass leaves on to the soil surface, it is a reasonable approximation for grassland and savanna environments when the sensor is

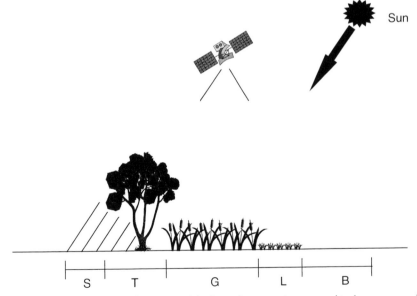

Fig. 9.3. A simplified landscape model where the scene is assumed to be composed of shadow (S), tree and/or shrub (T), green grass (G), litter (L) and bare soil (B).

located directly above the target (Pech *et al.*, 1986; Graetz *et al.*, 1988; Hanan *et al.*, 1991). The basic model can be modified as necessary to include features such as soil crusts, which may have distinct spectra (O'Neill, 1994; Karnieli, 1997). Equation 9.1 is used as a basis for evaluating various information extraction techniques in the section 'Information Extraction from Satellite Images' below.

Satellite Remote Sensing Systems

Satellite systems can be characterized by their spatial, spectral, temporal and radiometric resolution (Table 9.1). Spatial resolution refers to the size of each pixel on the ground and the total ground area covered by the image. Spectral resolution is the number and location of the spectral bands of the sensor. Temporal resolution is the time between images (assuming no clouds) for a given location and radiometric resolution is the precision with which the satellite measurement is recorded.

It is essential to match the characteristics of the satellite sensor with those of the proposed application (Graetz, 1987; see also Chapter 10). For example, with 1100 m pixels and a daily repeat cycle, NOAA-AVHRR is ideally placed to support continental and very large-scale regional applications such as drought monitoring (Hutchinson, 1991; Peters *et al.*, 1991) and estimation of primary productivity across large regions (Tucker *et al.*, 1985; Prince, 1991a, b). However, for mapping the extent and severity of land degradation at landscape and paddock scales (e.g. 100 km^2), the pixel size of NOAA-AVHRR is inappropriate and another satellite sensor should be used (Bastin *et al.*, 1995).

Whilst largely ignored in this chapter, it is noted that various airborne remote sensing systems are also available. The most common are black-and-white, colour and NIR aerial photographs, which have been widely used since the 1950s. An alternative to aerial photography is airborne video systems, which can capture digital images in the VIS and NIR (King, 1995; Everitt *et al.*, 1996). The pixel and image size of photographs and video images is governed by the focal length of the sensor and the distance from the target; each pixel can be as small as a few centimetres, depending on flying height restrictions.

It is also possible to mount imaging spectrometers (so-called hyper-spectral scanners) in aircraft and these have been used in grassland applications (Wessman *et al.*, 1997). Typical scanners include the AVIRIS, Daedelus and CASI systems. Whilst the operational details of these systems vary, the overall concept is that they can measure reflectance in a number (often as many as 256) of very narrow wavelength intervals. These very narrow bands have been used most extensively by geologists to detect specific minerals based on known libraries of atomic absorption spectra. Field- and laboratory-based instruments have also been used to infer the nutritional status of grasslands (e.g. Garciaciudad *et al.*, 1993; Clifton *et al.*, 1994; Dealdana *et al.*, 1995). However, as noted above in the section on canopy reflectance, the use of more bands and smaller pixels does not necessarily change the basic concept that under most field conditions pixels are really mixels (Price, 1994) and that shadows can be a large fraction of each mixel.

Information Extraction from Satellite Images

Up to now this chapter has concentrated on understanding the basic principles underlying satellite remote sensing, which are essential to apply the technology successfully. In this section, those basic concepts are used to describe several methods of extracting information from remotely sensed images.

Visual interpretation

So far the focus has been on each pixel as an independent entity character-ized by its reflectance. However, humans primarily use context, pattern and texture to interpret images visually. For example, most people are able to distinguish roads, rivers, mountains and forests on satellite images without knowing anything about how those images were made. Accordingly, much information can be gleaned from images using photo-interpretation skills (Lillesand and Kiefer, 1994). Modern software systems make it relatively easy to combine these interpretative skills with image processing tech-niques in a hybrid manner that is now commonly used to classify images. Digital image processing techniques can also be used to enhance image features locally as a further aid to image interpretation (Harrison and Jupp, 1990; Lillesand and Kiefer, 1994). A little used but potentially powerful technique is to examine the texture in an image using digital image pro-cessing techniques. For example, Pickup (1989) proposed that as a land-scape becomes more degraded the variance of the landscape in terms of the cover components increases, leading to an increasingly patchy structure. Models such as these are ideal for use with satellite imagery, though they have rarely been used, and this is an area where research could well focus.

Image classification

The basic idea of classification is to allocate each pixel in an image to a land cover class using the reflectance of the pixel in one or more bands (Fig. 9.4). Many different classification techniques are available, ranging from relatively simple if-then rules (e.g. if reflectance is within these limits,

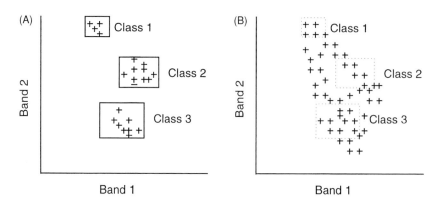

Fig. 9.4. Simplified concept of image classification where the reflectance of a pixel is uniquely related to a particular land cover class. Two bands have been used for illustration purposes, but the concept is equally applicable to *n* bands, which define an *n* dimensional space. (A) The classical concept is that each land cover class has a unique spectral signature and can thus be identified; (B) The reality is that classification is an attempt to subdivide a 'blur' of points. (See main text for discussion.)

then pixel = Class 1, etc.) to sophisticated multivariate analysis routines (Richards, 1986; Harrison and Jupp, 1990; Lillesand and Kiefer, 1994) that may incorporate additional features such as soil types and slopes (Richards, 1986; Skidmore, 1989). In principle, the classification methodology appears to violate the mixture model concept since the classification model implicitly assumes a relatively homogeneous reflectance for each type of land cover. In reality, land cover types such as forest and grassland contain a distinctive mixture of elements, which allows them to be considered approximately homogeneous at broad scales. For example, closed forests are characterized by relatively high proportions of T and S (see Fig. 9.3), whilst grasslands are characterized by relatively high proportions of G, L and B. When used at this level of detail, image classification is a powerful technique and is widely used.

Direct estimation of landscape components

If the aim of a particular study is to look at differences in cover within a particular grassland landscape rather than to separate the grassland from forest or woodland, then the situation becomes more complex and the mixture model approach must be used. The direct estimation of the underlying landscape components in the mixture model for each pixel in an image represents the holy grail for remote sensing technologists. This section describes how the mixture modelling approach can be adapted for use in grassland studies.

The typical structure of an R–NIR scattergram is shown in Fig. 9.5. The high degree of correlation between the bands is a characteristic feature of most remotely sensed data sets from earth resource satellites. The overall structure of this space was described by Kauth and Thomas (1976) as the 'tasselled cap' in which the major features were a plane of soils (i.e. the soil line) and a plane of green vegetation. Different coloured soils plot along the soil line, as do the shadows and litter (Huete *et al.*, 1984; Pech *et al.*, 1986; Frank and Aase, 1994). For the example shown, it is not possible to distinguish between changes in shadows, litter or soil reflectance. However, in the R–NIR space, it is possible to separate the green from the non-green component of the vegetation based on the distance from the soil line and this is generally used when the prime interest is the amount of green cover (Tucker and Miller, 1977; Smith *et al.*, 1990). In an analogous manner, the G–R space has been shown to discriminate the total (rather than green) cover from a variable soil background (Pickup *et al.*, 1993) and is an alternative if the total is of more interest than the green cover.

Since the bands are often highly correlated, the inversion of mixture models tends to be an ill-posed statistical problem (Pech *et al.*, 1986; Graetz *et al.*, 1988). One solution to this problem is to include more bands in the

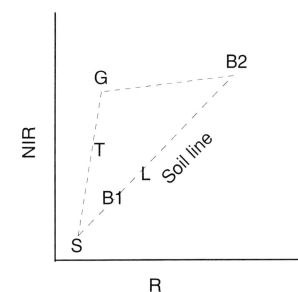

Fig. 9.5. A typical red–near infrared (R–NIR) scattergram of a grassland/rangeland scene showing the typical reflectance for each of the scene elements described in Equation 9.1 and Fig. 9.3. Here B1 represents a dark (e.g. black) soil; B2 is a bright (e.g. red) soil. In most cases, soil colour is more likely to vary continuously along the soil line (Williamson, 1989). (Based on data in Graetz and Gentle, 1982; Pech *et al.* 1986.)

analysis, which is an area where hyperspectral scanners can be used effectively (Wessman et al., 1997) and is one of the reasons that remote sensing scientists are keen for sensors to include more bands.

There are also many ways in which the basic model can be simplified. For example, if the soil background is assumed to be uniformly bright, such as the red soils typical of many arid areas, then an estimate of cover is simply the R reflectance on the assumption that most other surface elements are darker than the soil (Foran, 1987; Ringrose and Matheson, 1987; Graetz et al., 1988). In cases where the soil background is not homogeneous, it is virtually impossible to separate the litter, shadow and soil components and one pragmatic solution is to use a vegetation index.

Vegetation indices

The basic idea of a vegetation index is to collapse the multi-band imagery to a single measure which is related to some characteristic (normally vegetation cover or green cover) of the target. Most indices have been based on the R–NIR space and some of the more widely used include the simple ratio (SR) and normalized difference vegetation index (NDVI) (Tucker, 1979), perpendicular vegetation index (PVI) (Richardson and Wiegand, 1977) and soil adjusted vegetation index (SAVI) (Huete, 1988; Qi et al., 1994). All of the above essentially seek a measure of the green cover, and hence a measure of the interception of light by the photosynthetically active fraction of the canopy. If total cover is of more interest than the green fraction, the G–R space can be used to derive the PD54 index (Pickup et al., 1993). The geometric interpretation of these indices is shown in Fig. 9.6.

It is evident from Fig. 9.6 that the vegetation indices are essentially trying to mimic the structure of the R–NIR space (cf. Figs 9.5 and 9.6). Each uses a soil line and measures the (green or total) cover as some, often non-linear, distance from the soil line. The NDVI, SR and SAVI are not orthogonal indices since the isolines are not parallel. It is evident that the NDVI and SR both assume that the soil reflectance is equal in both bands, which is a reasonable approximation for most soils (Huete et al., 1984, 1985; Williamson, 1989; Ben-Dor and Banin, 1994). The SAVI was designed using a simple two-stream radiative transfer model to account for first-order scattering between the soil and vegetation (Huete, 1988) and in its simplest form also assumes that the R and NIR reflectance from the soil is equal. Rather than just assume a soil line, it is also possible to identify the soil line on an R–NIR plot and then use that as a basis for the calculations. This latter approach has been adopted by Baret and Guyot (1991), who modified the SAVI, and is also the basis of the PVI and PD54. So which index is the best?

In hilly terrain the ratio indices (SR, NDVI) partially compensate for changes induced by the topography (Holben and Justice, 1981; Burgess

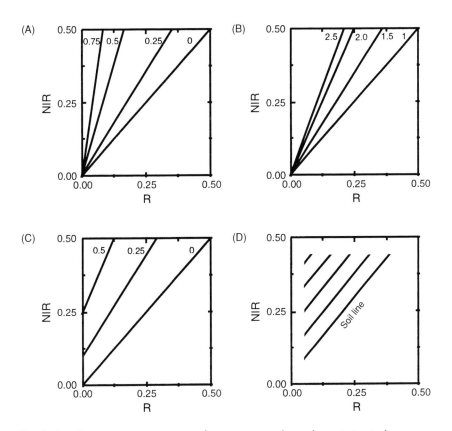

Fig. 9.6. Geometric interpretation of some commonly used vegetation indices (note that, in formulae, N = NIR; R = red). (A) Normalized difference vegetation index (NDVI) = (N − R) / (N + R). The NDVI ranges from −1 to 1 and has a nominal soil line at 0. (B) Simple ratio (SR) = N / R. The simple ratio ranges from $-y^{-\infty}$ to y^{∞} and has a nominal soil line at 1. (C) Soil adjusted vegetation index (SAVI) = (1 + L)(N − R) / (N + R + L), and L = 0.5 was used. The range and soil line are as for NDVI. (D) The perpendicular vegetation index (PVI) is based on the image analyst identifying the soil line; contours are then computed parallel to this soil line (see Richardson and Weigand, 1977, for details).

et al., 1995). The SR and NDVI also compensate for changes in the shadow fraction, since the point of full shadow is near the origin of the R–NIR space (Graetz and Gentle, 1982; Pech *et al.*, 1986; Hall *et al.*, 1995). Since the PVI and PD54 isolines do not go through the origin, these indices do not compensate for the topographic effect and should only be used on flat landscapes where shadows are minimal. The major disadvantage of the NDVI and SR is that differences between the actual and assumed (i.e. R = NIR) soil line can cause large errors, particularly over dark soil backgrounds (Huete and Tucker, 1991; Roderick *et al.*, 1996a), whereas the SAVI is much less sensitive to variations in the soil background colour. The NDVI is generally regarded as a measure of the fraction of PAR (photosynthetically active radiation) intercepted by green vegetation and hence is related to the potential productivity of the vegetation (Tucker, 1979; Asrar et al., 1984; Paruelo et al., 1997). In contrast the SR is more closely related to the green leaf area index of the canopy (Sellers, 1985; Sellers et al., 1994).

All of the indices are essentially empirical solutions to the mixture model described in Equation 9.1 and rely on the observation that soil reflectance is approximately equal in the R and NIR bands. In studies based on the analysis of relatively few images, the identification of a unique soil line for each image is the obvious option. One could then define a unique index based on that soil line (Pech et al., 1986) or use one of the indices that have the facility to incorporate a user-defined soil line. Where many hundreds of images are involved, such as with NOAA-AVHRR time series, this approach becomes difficult and either NDVI, SR or SAVI is commonly used.

Field data to support remote sensing studies

It should be apparent that a single satellite measurement taken from above is mostly related to horizontal ground cover, although the image can contain some information on height depending on the sun-sensor geometry and vertical structure of the scene elements. Thus, field measures of cover are necessary for testing. In contrast, many studies try to relate satellite measurements to the mass of dry matter per unit area. Since species have different morphologies (e.g. Scanlan et al., 1996), correlations between a satellite-derived measure of cover and a field measure of dry matter will depend on the species morphology and cannot be transferred to a different group of species. In addition, cover is generally only a good estimate of the amount of dry matter at lower levels of cover (Tucker, 1979; Foran, 1987).

Multi-temporal studies

Perhaps the most exciting opportunity for using remotely sensed data is the ability to map and monitor changes over time. This potential has attracted much interest and it is also the most technically demanding application. The major issues in multi-temporal work include the acquisition of cloud-free imagery, calibration of the images in the sequence, and the measurement precision necessary for change detection.

In grassland ecosystems, persistent cloud cover does not tend to pose the same problem for image acquisition as it does over forests. In this context, it is assumed that cloud-free imagery is available and the focus will be on the creation of calibrated sequences of imagery. Satellite measurements are converted to an integer format for transmission to a ground station. Unfortunately, the calibration of many satellite radiometers appears to drift over time (Frouin and Gautier, 1987; Slater *et al.*, 1987; Kaufman and Holben, 1993). It is also often difficult to get the actual original satellite measurements, since many organizations modify the data using image processing techniques to enhance the contrast in the image for viewing purposes (Pickup *et al.*, 1993). Whilst it is possible to determine the appropriate calibration corrections, this normally requires substantial skills in radiative transfer physics (e.g. Kaufman and Holben, 1993). An alternative approach is to use invariant targets, such as salt flats, that appear in the imagery. Variations in the reflectance (or appropriate vegetation index) of these targets is then assumed to be due to changes in calibration and/or atmospheric conditions (Hall *et al.*, 1991; Yool *et al.*, 1997) and the images are subsequently adjusted so that the measure being calibrated is constant for the chosen targets. In the case of the NDVI data derived from NOAA-AVHRR, this approach has been shown to be at least as good as those from highly detailed physical models (Roderick *et al.*, 1996b). The second factor to be considered is variation in the viewing geometry and the associated change in shadows through time. One approach is to select images from the same time of the year to minimize this effect (Graetz *et al.*, 1988). If continuous coverage is required, or the images were acquired with different sun-sensor geometry, then a vegetation index is the next best pragmatic solution. For example, data from NOAA-AVHRR is almost exclusively processed to either NDVI or SR to account partially for the large range of viewing angles experienced, as described above.

Perhaps one of the most important but often overlooked issues is how much change is necessary before it can be detected by satellite. It is relatively easy to show that the precision of a satellite measurement in a single band is a function of the sensor analogue-to-digital conversion characteristics and the solar zenith angle (Tucker, 1980; Roderick *et al.*, 1996a). For example, Graetz and Gentle (1982) concluded that there was not enough dynamic range in the Landsat MSS sensor to detect ecologically significant change in areas of southern Australia (latitude approximately 30°) in winter, due to low sun angles. Since satellite measurements are ultimately converted to integers before transmission to a ground station, then there must be some rounding-off error in the measurement. Table 9.2 assumes a best-case scenario that this conversion is the only source of error and computes the minimum change in green cover that can be detected over black and red soils using a single measurement from the Landsat MSS, TM and NOAA-AVHRR satellites in the R band. The results show that, since the contrast between green vegetation and soil is greatest over red soils, then smaller changes in green vegetation can be detected over those soils. They also show that on a red soil (B2), Landsat MSS could detect a change in green cover of 5% whilst on a black soil a change of 20% in green cover is necessary before it can be detected. This basic analysis can also be extended

Table 9.2. (a) The total reflectance in the red (R) band for two landscapes having different soil colours (B1, black soil; B2, red soil) that have varying fractional green cover of vegetation (G). Reflectance values for 'pure' materials are assumed to be 0.10 for G, 0.05 for B1 and 0.30 for B2. (b) Sensitivity analysis: dR is the typical precision of a reflectance measurement for each sensor, based on a solar zenith angle of 60° (Roderick et al., 1996a); dG is the minimum change in G that can be measured based on the landscape characteristics and dR.

	B1	B2
(a) Green cover (G)		
0.0	0.05	0.3
0.2	0.06	0.26
0.4	0.07	0.22
0.6	0.08	0.18
0.8	0.09	0.14
1.0	0.1	0.1
(b) Sensitivity analysis		
Landsat MSS		
dR	0.01	0.01
dG	0.2	0.05
Landsat TM, SPOT		
dR	0.005	0.005
dG	0.1	0.025
NOAA-AVHRR		
dR	0.002	0.002
dG	0.04	0.01

to the use of two or more bands, which in most cases is a more realistic situation.

Future Developments

This section is a brief review of several current and future developments in remote sensing. The development of airborne spectrometers that can measure what are essentially continuous spectra will lead to the development of more sophisticated mixture models (Wessman et al., 1997). There is also continuing interest in measuring spectra using field (Clifton et al., 1994) and laboratory-based instruments (Garciaciudad et al., 1993; Dealdana et al., 1995) to infer the nutritional status of grasslands. There are also several satellites planned for the near future with pixels in the 1–5 m range offering vastly improved spatial resolution, though the image coverage will decrease accordingly (Aplin et al., 1997).

However, perhaps the biggest change will come from a different source: the development of global and national scale broad-band communication networks. The widespread acceptance of the Internet has encouraged vendors and other suppliers of satellite imagery to make their archives available electronically. These archives can be searched and orders placed immediately for the supply of imagery. In some cases the images can now be delivered over the network, or alternatively they can be supplied on CD-ROMs. Such facilities will greatly improve the accessibility of satellite imagery.

Summary

Remotely sensed images are not magical – they are essentially photographs, though they are very special in a number of ways. Firstly, they cover large areas and hence users can rapidly develop landscape overviews. Secondly, they can sense in other parts of the EM spectrum, and hence see many features of the world quite differently from the human eye. Thirdly, they are routinely acquired and archived by many agencies around the world and are readily available at reasonable costs. As a consequence they are a practical cost-effective resource for covering the large areas that are typical of grassland ecosystems. We trust that this chapter has established the basic theoretical framework for using satellite imagery in a productive manner. The application of these principles for monitoring purposes is discussed in Chapter 10.

References

Aplin, P., Atkinson, P.M. and Curran, P.J. (1997) Fine spatial resolution satellite sensors for the next decade. *International Journal of Remote Sensing* 18, 3873–3881.

Asrar, G., Fuchs, M., Kanemasu, E.T. and Hatfield, J.L. (1984) Estimating absorbed photosynthetic radiation and leaf area index from spectral reflectance in wheat. *Agronomy Journal* 76, 300–306.

Baret, F. and Guyot, G. (1991) Potentials and limits of vegetation indices for LAI and APAR assessment. *Remote Sensing of Environment* 35, 161–173.

Bastin, G., Pickup, G. and Pearce, G. (1995) Utility of AVHRR data for land degradation assessment: a case study. *International Journal of Remote Sensing* 16, 651–672.

Belward, A.S., Kennedy, P.J. and Gregoire, J.M. (1994) The limitations and potential of Avhrr gac data for continental scale fire studies. *International Journal of Remote Sensing* 15, 2215–2234.

Ben-Dor, E. and Banin, A. (1994) Visible and near-infrared (0.4–1.1 μm) analysis of arid and semi-arid soils. *Remote Sensing of Environment* 48, 261–274.

Burgess, D.W., Lewis, P. and Muller, J.-P.A.L. (1995) Topographic effects in AVHRR NDVI data. *Remote Sensing of Environment* 54, 223–232.

Clifton, K.E., Bradbury, J.W. and Vehrencamp, S.L. (1994) The fine-scale mapping of grassland protein densities. *Grass and Forage Science* 49, 1–8.

Curran, P.J. (1985) *Principles of Remote Sensing*. Longman, London, 282 pp.

Dealdana, B.R.V., Criado, B.G., Ciudad, A.G. and Corona, M.E.P. (1995) Estimation of mineral content in natural grasslands by near infrared reflectance spectroscopy. *Communications in Soil Science and Plant Analysis* 26, 1383–1396.

Everitt, J.H., Escobar, D.E., Alaniz, M.A. and Davis, M.R. (1996) Comparison of ground reflectance measurements, airborne video, and SPOT satellite data for estimating phytomass and cover on rangelands. *Geocarta International* 11, 69–86.

Foran, B.D. (1987) Detection of yearly cover change with Landsat MSS on pastoral landscapes in central Australia. *Remote Sensing of Environment* 23, 333–350.

Frank, A.B. and Aase, J.K. (1994) Residue effects on radiometric reflectance measurements of northern great plains rangelands. *Remote Sensing of Environment* 49, 195–199.

Franklin, J. and Hiernaux, P.H.Y. (1991) Estimating foliage and woody biomass in Sahelian and Sudanian woodlands using a remote sensing model. *International Journal of Remote Sensing* 12, 1387–1404.

Frouin, R. and Gautier, C. (1987) Calibration of NOAA-7 AVHRR, GOES-5, and GOES-6 VISSR/VAS solar channels. *Remote Sensing of Environment* 22, 73–101.

Garciaciudad, A., Garciacriado, B., Perezcorona, M.E., Dealdana, B.R.V. and Ruanoramos, A.M. (1993) Application of near-infrared reflectance spectroscopy to chemical analysis of heterogeneous and botanically complex grassland samples. *Journal of the Science of Food and Agriculture* 63, 419–426.

Gausman, H.W. and Allen, W.A. (1973) Optical parameters of leaves of 30 plant species. *Plant Physiology* 52, 57–62.

Graetz, R.D. (1987) Satellite remote sensing of Australian rangelands. *Remote Sensing of Environment* 23, 313–331.

Graetz, R.D. and Gentle, M.R. (1982) The relationships between reflectance in the Landsat wavebands and the composition of an Australian semi-arid shrub rangeland. *Photogrammetric Engineering and Remote Sensing* 48, 1721–1730.

Graetz, R.D., Pech, R.P. and Davis, A.W. (1988) The assessment and monitoring of sparsely vegetated rangelands using calibrated Landsat data. *International Journal of Remote Sensing* 9, 1201–1222.

Hall, F.G., Strebel, D.E., Nickeson, J.E. and Goetz, S.J. (1991) Radiometric rectification: toward a common radiometric response among multidate, multisensor images. *Remote Sensing of Environment* 35, 11–27.

Hall, F.G., Shimabukuro, Y.E. and Huemmrich, K.F. (1995) Remote sensing of forest biophysical structure using mixture decomposition and geometric reflectance models. *Ecological Applications* 5, 993–1013.

Hanan, N.P., Prince, S.D. and Hiernaux, P.H.Y. (1991) Spectral modelling of multicomponent landscapes in the Sahel. *International Journal of Remote Sensing* 12, 1243–1258.

Harrison, B.A. and Jupp, D.L.B. (1990) *Introduction to Image Processing.* CSIRO, Canberra, 256 pp.

Holben, B.N. and Justice, C.O. (1981) An examination of spectral band ratioing to reduce the topographic effect on remotely sensed data. *International Journal of Remote Sensing* 2, 115–133.

Huete, A.R. (1988) A soil-adjusted vegetation index (SAVI). *Remote Sensing of Environment* 25, 295–309.

Huete, A.R. and Tucker, C.J. (1991) Investigation of soil influences in AVHRR red and near-infra-red vegetation index imagery. *International Journal of Remote Sensing* 12, 1223–1242.

Huete, A.R., Post, D.F. and Jackson, R.D. (1984) Soil spectral effects on 4-space vegetation discrimination. *Remote Sensing of Environment* 15, 155–165.

Huete, A.R., Jackson, R.D. and Post, D.F. (1985) Spectral response of a plant canopy with different soil backgrounds. *Remote Sensing of Environment* 17, 37–53.

Hutchinson, C.F. (1991) Uses of satellite data for famine early warning in sub-Saharan Africa. *International Journal of Remote Sensing* 12, 1405–1421.

Jupp, D.L.B., Walker, J. and Penridge, L.K. (1986) Interpretation of vegetation structure in Landsat MSS imagery: a case study in disturbed semi-arid eucalypt woodlands. 2. Model-based analysis. *Journal of Environmental Management* 23, 35–57.

Karnieli, A. (1997) Development and implementation of spectral crust index over dune sands. *International Journal of Remote Sensing* 18, 1207–1220.

Kaufman, Y.J. and Holben, B.N. (1993) Calibration of the AVHRR visible and near-IR bands by atmospheric scattering, ocean glint and desert reflection. *International Journal of Remote Sensing* 14, 21–52.

Kauth, R.G. and Thomas, G.S. (1976) The tasseled cap, a graphic description of the spectral–temporal development of agricultural crops as seen by Landsat. In: *Proceedings of the Symposium on Machine Processing of Remotely Sensed Data.* University of Purdue, Indiana, pp. 6.23–7.20.

Kerr, Y.H., Lagouarde, J.P. and Imbernon, J. (1992) Accurate land surface temperature retrieval from AVHRR data with use of an improved split window algorithm. *Remote Sensing of Environment* 41, 197–209.

King, D.J. (1995) Airborne multispectral digital camera and video sensors: a critical review of system designs and applications. *Canadian Journal of Remote Sensing* 21, 245–273.

Leblon, B., Gallant, L. and Granberg, H. (1996) Effects of shadowing types on ground-measured visible and near-infrared shadow reflectances. *Remote Sensing of Environment* 58, 322–328.

Li, X. and Strahler, A.H. (1986) Geometric-optical bidirectional reflectance modeling of a conifer forest canopy. *IEEE Transactions Geoscience and Remote Sensing* GE-24, 906–919.

Lillesand, T.M. and Kiefer, R.W. (1994) *Remote Sensing and Image Interpretation*, 2nd edn. John Wiley & Sons, New York, 750 pp.

Massonnet, D., Feigl, K., Rossi, M. and Adragna, F. (1994) Rada interferometric mapping of deformation in the year after the landers earthquake. *Nature* 369, 227–230.

Monteith, J.L. and Unsworth, M. (1990) *Principles of Environmental Physics*, 2nd edn. Arnold, London, 291 pp.

Nobel, P.S. (1991) *Physiochemical and Environmental Plant Physiology.* Academic Press, San Diego, California, 635 pp.

O'Neill, A.L. (1994) Reflectance spectra of microphytic soil crusts in semi-arid Australia. *International Journal of Remote Sensing* 15, 675–681.

Paruelo, J.M., Epstein, H.E., Lauenroth, W.K. and Burke, I.C. (1997) ANPP estimates from NDVI for the central grassland region of the United States. *Ecology* 78, 953–958.

Pech, R.P., Graetz, R.D. and Davis, A.W. (1986) Reflectance modelling and the derivation of vegetation indices for an Australian semi-arid shrubland. *International Journal of Remote Sensing* 7, 389–403.

Pereira, A.C. and Setzer, A.W. (1997) Comparison of fire detection in savannas using Avhrrs channel 3 and TM images. *International Journal of Remote Sensing* 17, 1925–1937.

Peters, A.J., Rundquist, D.C. and Wilhite, D.A. (1991) Satellite detection of the geographic core of the 1988 Nebraska drought. *Agricultural and Forest Meteorology* 57, 35–47.

Pickup, G. (1989) New land degradation survey techniques for arid Australia – problems and prospects. *Australian Rangeland Journal* 11, 74–82.

Pickup, G., Chewings, V.H. and Nelson, D.J. (1993) Estimating changes in vegetation cover over time in arid rangelands using Landsat MSS data. *Remote Sensing of Environment* 43, 243–263.

Price, J.C. (1989) Quantitative aspects of remote sensing in the thermal infrared. In: Asrar, G. (ed.) *Theory and Applications of Optical Remote Sensing.* John Wiley & Sons, New York, pp. 578–603.

Price, J.C. (1994) How unique are spectral signatures? *Remote Sensing of Environment* 49, 181–186.

Prince, S.D. (1991a) A model of regional primary production for use with coarse resolution satellite data. *International Journal of Remote Sensing* 12, 1313–1330.

Prince, S.D. (1991b) Satellite remote sensing of primary production: comparison of results for Sahelian grasslands 1981–1988. *International Journal of Remote Sensing* 12, 1301–1311.

Qi, J., Chehbouni, A., Huete, A.R., Kerr, Y.H. and Sorooshian, S. (1994) A modified soil adjusted vegetation index. *Remote Sensing of Environment* 48, 119–126.

Richards, J.A. (1986) *Remote Sensing Digital Image Analysis: An Introduction.* Springer-Verlag, Berlin, 281 pp.

Richardson, A.J. and Wiegand, C.L. (1977) Distinguishing vegetation from soil background information. *Photogrammetric Engineering and Remote Sensing* 43, 1541–1552.

Ringrose, S. and Matheson, W. (1987) Spectral assessment of indicators of range degradation in the Botswana hardveld environment. *Remote Sensing of Environment* 23, 379–396.

Roderick, M.L., Smith, R.C.G. and Cridland, S.W. (1996a) The precision of the NDVI derived from AVHRR observations. *Remote Sensing of Environment* 56, 57–65.

Roderick, M.L., Smith, R.C.G. and Lodwick, G.D. (1996b) Calibrating long term AVHRR derived NDVI imagery. *Remote Sensing of Environment* 58, 1–12.

Scanlan, J.C., Pressland, A.J. and Myles, D.J. (1996) Grazing modifies woody and herbaceous components of North Queensland woodlands. *Rangeland Journal* 18, 47–57.

Sellers, P.J. (1985) Canopy reflectance, photosynthesis and transpiration. *International Journal of Remote Sensing* 6, 1335–1372.

Sellers, P.J., Tucker, C.J., Collatz, G.J., Los, S.O., Justice, C.O., Dazlich, D.A. and Randall, D.A. (1994) A global 1° × 1° NDVI data set for climate studies. 2. The generation of global fields of terrestrial biophysical parameters from the NDVI. *International Journal of Remote Sensing* 15, 3519–3545.

Skidmore, A.K. (1989) An expert system classifies eucalypt forest types using thematic mapper data and a digital terrain model. *Photogrammetric Engineering and Remote Sensing* 55, 1449–1464.

Slater, P.N., Biggar, S.F., Holm, R.G., Jackson, R.D., Mao, Y., Moran, M.S., Palmer, J.M. and Yuan, B. (1987) Reflectance and radiance-based methods for the in-flight absolute calibration of multi-spectral sensors. *Remote Sensing of Environment* 22, 11–37.

Smith, A.M., Major, D.J., McNeil, R.L., Williams, W.D., Brisco, B. and Brown, R.J. (1995) Complementarity of radar and visible-infrared sensors in assessing rangeland condition. *Remote Sensing of Environment* 52, 173–180.

Smith, M.O., Ustin, S.L., Adams, J.B. and Gillespie, A.R. (1990) Vegetation in deserts. II. Environmental influences on regional abundance. *Remote Sensing of Environment* 29, 27–52.

Smith, R.C.G. (1997) Applications of satellite remote sensing for mapping and monitoring land surface processes in Western Australia. *Journal of the Royal Society of Western Australia* 80, 15–28.

Spitters, C.J.T., Toussaint, H.A.J.M. and Goudriaan, J. (1986) Separating the diffuse and direct component of global radiation and its implication for modelling canopy photosynthesis. I. Components of incoming radiation. *Agricultural and Forest Meteorology* 38, 217–229.

Tucker, C.J. (1979) Red and photographic infrared linear combinations for monitoring vegetation. *Remote Sensing of Environment* 8, 127–150.

Tucker, C.J. (1980) Radiometric resolution for monitoring vegetation. How many bits are needed? *International Journal of Remote Sensing* 1, 241–254.

Tucker, C.J. and Miller, L.D. (1977) Soil spectra contributions to grass canopy spectral reflectance. *Photogrammetric Engineering and Remote Sensing* 43, 721–726.

Tucker, C.J., Vanpraet, C.L., Sharman, J. and Van Ittersum, G. (1985) Satellite remote sensing of total herbaceous biomass production in the Senegalese Sahel: 1980–1984. *Remote Sensing of Environment* 17, 233–249.

Wessman, C.A., Bateson, C.A. and Benning, T.I. (1997) Detecting fire and grazing patterns in tallgrass prairie using spectral mixture analysis. *Ecological Applications* 7, 493–511.

Williamson, H.D. (1989) Reflectance from shrubs and under-shrub soil in a semi-arid environment. *Remote Sensing of Environment* 29, 263–271.

Wilson, A.K. (1988) The effective resolution of Landsat thematic mapper. *International Journal of Remote Sensing* 9, 1303–1314.

Yool, S.R., Makaio, M.J. and Watts, J.M. (1997) Techniques for computer-assisted mapping of rangeland change. *Journal of Range Management* 50, 307–314.

Zebker, H.A., Werner, C.L., Rosen, P.A. and Hensley, S. (1994) Accuracy of topographic maps derived from ERS-1 interferometric radar. *IEEE Transactions Geoscience and Remote Sensing* 32, 823–836.

Assessing Rangeland Condition and Trend

10

M.H. Friedel[1], W.A. Laycock[2] and G.N. Bastin[1]

[1]CSIRO, Department of Wildlife and Ecology, Alice Springs, Northern Territory, Australia; [2]Department of Rangeland Ecology and Watershed Management, College of Agriculture, University of Wyoming, Laramie, Wyoming, USA

Introduction

Once, it was simple to define rangelands. They were semi-natural ecosystems which were used for livestock production because the climate or terrain was too harsh for intensive agriculture (Stoddart *et al.*, 1975; Harrington *et al.*, 1984). Now, rangelands are no longer defined by a single use throughout the world, although traditional pastoralism still prevails in many areas. Rangeland is now more commonly defined as a kind of land with specific vegetation and climate (e.g. Society for Range Management, 1989; Heady and Child, 1994; National Rangeland Management Working Group (Australia), 1994) and the value of rangelands is no longer determined by their diverse economic outputs alone.

About half the earth's land surface is rangeland (Williams *et al.*, 1968; World Resources Institute, 1986), though estimates of the proportion vary with the way rangelands are defined. Since there has been no comprehensive global assessment of the extent of rangelands, the most common approximation is the area of the world's arid and semiarid lands. The best estimate by the World Resources Institute (1986) is provided in Table 10.1.

Most commonly, rangelands are characterized by aridity with extremes of heat or cold, but they also include land that is too rocky, steep, saline or seasonally wet for cultivating crops or timber. Grasslands, shrublands, savannas and deserts provide the majority of range ecosystems, with wetlands, forests, alpine grasslands and tundra (arctic grasslands) making up the remainder. As a consequence, rangelands can vary from tropical to desert grasslands, and from desert shrublands to arctic grasslands.

Table 10.1. Distribution of the world's rangelands, adapted from World Resources Institute (1986).

Region	Estimated total area (million hectares)	Per cent of total land area
North America	913	50
Europe	153	33
Former USSR	861	39
Central America	145	46
South America	819	47
Africa	1945	65
Asia (except China)	721	41
China	538	58
Oceania	627	75
World total	6722	51

Economically, production has been limited by difficult climate or topography, so that communal pastoralism or extensive commercial grazing has been the norm in many countries. Ownership of commercial grazing land has tended to be more in public hands when compared with temperate cropping and pasture regions, due to lower and riskier economic returns. Rangelands also provide traditional living areas for non-pastoral people and can support a diversity of wildlife, which offers both a source of food and an attraction for tourists and recreational hunters. Watershed maintenance and conservation of biodiversity are increasingly important roles for rangelands too.

While the human population of arid rangelands remains fairly static at about 15% of the world's total, absolute numbers continue to grow. Seventy per cent of drylands under agriculture are affected by land degradation in some degree (Tolba, 1992). In developing countries, moister margins of the rangelands are commonly under pressure from the expansion of demand for cropping land, while more and more people are attempting to wrest a living from pastoralism in the inner core. Political boundaries and policies prevent the traditional seasonal migrations of animals being herded, so that grazed rangelands are subject to increased stocking pressure and may no longer have the opportunity for recovery that they once had. In developed countries, commercial pastoralism is declining in importance, as costs outpace financial returns and demands for other commercial and non-commercial uses grow. Because of this increased interest in rangelands, there are increasing calls for accountability on publicly owned lands.

In order to understand what causes rangelands to change and what the impacts of different uses are, some sort of record must be kept of the current status of land, the influences that cause change, and the direction of change. The current status of land is often called range condition, and is sometimes equated with 'health', in that there is no single measure of absolute condition but, rather, a series of indicators – not one of them sufficient on their own. We will use the term 'range condition' in a generic sense, although in the US in particular, it is identified with a specific underlying model of change.

The essence of range monitoring is to detect change over time as measured by indicators of condition or health, and to identify causes, whether environmental variability or management. In rangelands, the necessary record might be as simple as a photograph or it might involve detailed measurements.

In this chapter, we will briefly outline the nature of change in rangelands, the different ways in which change is conceptualized and the consequent debate about what range condition actually is. We will provide a basic framework within which range monitoring should occur, and detail the diversity of methods available and in what circumstances they should be applied.

Understanding Change in Rangelands

Rangeland environments often experience climatic extremes, low and erratic rainfall, severe cold or high temperatures, resulting in high season-to-season variability. Changes in the vegetation and soil may follow in the short or long term. Other powerful causes of change are grazing of domestic stock or wildlife, fire, cultivation for cropping and harvesting of resources like firewood, foods and building materials.

When a use is imposed on the variability inherent in range environments, separating the effect of the use from the background variation may not be simple. For example, rainfall may vary within years, from year to year and on longer-term cycles. This variability may result in year-to-year fluctuations in forage production that may be greater than any change caused by improper grazing management. Moreover, a particular rangeland use may cover extensive areas of land and considerable environmental variation. Heterogeneity across the landscape on scales from metres to kilometres tends to cause differential use, which the pattern of water availability, shade and fence placement will further influence. With two or more uses or the occurrence of fire in addition, identifying the effect of a single use may not be possible.

Fundamental to assessing current status of rangeland and/or directions of change under a particular use is recognizing the scale of key spatial and temporal processes (Smith, 1990; Brown and Smith, 1993). Measuring density of a species may be appropriate to understanding a population, but not necessarily a community or a collection of communities within a management unit. Detecting erosional surfaces on soils at a 5 m scale may not indicate degradation if the erosion patches are embedded in a matrix of stable surfaces at a 100 m scale. Natural patterns and processes of production and resource movement have to be understood before management effects can be distinguished.

Concepts of Change

In order to decide how, what, when and where to measure, we need models of how rangelands change in response to use, even if the models are simply conceptual. Different models have been proposed over the years as the complexities of rangeland dynamics have been recognized.

Clementsian succession vs. the state-and-transition model

The range succession model in use in many parts of the world was first proposed as a method to evaluate range condition in the US by Dyksterhuis (1949). However, it was strongly based on the ideas of Clements (1916) and Sampson (1919). In the successional model all possible states of vegetation can be arrayed on a continuum and condition is the term for the vegetation's position on this continuum. Trend describes the vegetation's travel along the continuum.

A number of authors have concluded that the succession model does not fit observed community dynamics for many rangeland communities throughout the world (Smith, 1989; Westoby *et al.*, 1989; Laycock, 1991), particularly the more arid shrub-dominated systems. It may be that the succession model is more applicable in moister environments, while arid environments are better described by a more discontinuous model (Dankwerts and Adams, 1991; Laycock, 1994).

Although many have essentially abandoned the successional concept, others have kept and modified it to fit specific circumstances. Bosch and Kellner (1991) described a 'degradation gradient' in southern Africa, which used aspects of the successional model. They fitted their degradation gradient into different 'domains of attraction' (p. 232) with irreversible transitions between them.

Westoby *et al.* (1989) proposed that dynamics of many rangelands might be described by a set of discrete 'states' and 'transitions' between these states. They defined a 'state' in terms of a recognizable assemblage of species, encompassing a certain amount of variation in space and time. 'Transitions' between states may be triggered by natural events (weather, fire, etc.) or by management actions or a combination of both (Fig. 10.1).

A state-and-transition model should contain catalogues of possible alternative states, possible transitions from one state to another, and 'opportunities and hazards'. The latter catalogue lists climatic conditions under which management actions can produce a favourable transition and

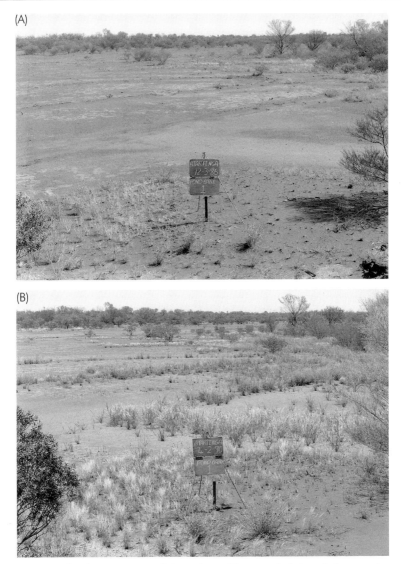

Fig. 10.1. A landscape in central Australia in (A) an eroded, largely bare and unproductive state has been changed by management action to (B) a vegetated and much more productive state. This change in state is a consequence of building large earthen ponding banks to intercept water, sediment and organic matter, thus improving soil moisture and nutrient status and the soil seed bank.

those that could produce an unfavourable transition. The value of a state-and-transition model is that it displays all that is known about a specific community or vegetation type and how it behaves in response to climate and management. In contrast to the succession model, it does not assume predictable succession or reversibility along a continuum. A state-and-transition model can also incorporate aspects such as the soil condition and landscape functional analyses of Ludwig and Tongway (1995) and Tongway (1995).

Thresholds

Friedel (1991) introduced the concept of 'thresholds of environmental change' into the determination of condition of rangelands, though the concept was well recognized in ecological literature. She described a threshold as: 'first, it is the boundary in space and time between two states, e.g. grassland and shrub-invaded grassland; and second, the initial shift across the boundary is not reversible on a practical time scale without substantial intervention by the range manager' (Friedel, 1991). The latter characteristic implies that a community that has crossed a threshold has moved into another 'domain' (see next section) and simple management actions such as stocking rate reductions are not enough to cause a reversion to the former state. Critical losses of topsoil or of palatable shrubs are further examples. The concept is compatible with the state-and-transition model, focusing on those transitions that are not readily reversed, and is appropriate for environments where temporal variation in shorter-lived plant species is high.

Stability vs. resilience

Holling (1973) defined the stability of a system by its ability to return to an equilibrium state after a temporary disturbance: 'the more rapidly it returns and the less it fluctuates, the more stable it would be'. Resilience, on the other hand, is 'a measure of the persistence of systems and their ability to absorb change and disturbance and still maintain the same relationships between populations or state variables'. True stability is probably never achieved in reality. Exploring the theoretical behaviour of interacting populations in the absence of external events, Holling (1973) concluded that there is a 'domain of attraction' for populations within which there is a stable equilibrium, and beyond that, the population becomes extinct. With the occurrence of random events such as major rainfall or fire or the introduction of grazing, systems can shift from one domain to another. Links to the state-and-transition model are clear.

In rangelands, which often fit the resilience model best, assessing the boundaries of domains of attraction, or whether the system persists or not, might be more useful than focusing on equilibrium states. While the theoretical models applied largely to species and populations, these concepts have direct relevance to some measures obtained from remote sensing (pp. 250–254).

Equilibrium vs. non-equilibrium

Concepts of equilibrium and non-equilibrium also appear in rangeland literature, e.g. Ellis and Swift (1988), and they are often used in reference to range management systems. Where the succession model of vegetation change underpins management systems, it is assumed that the task of the range manager is to maintain a stable sub-climax, in order to achieve a steady flow of animal products (Behnke and Scoones, 1993). The stocking density at which the balance is achieved is the carrying capacity. On the other hand, a non-equilibrium model assumes a limit set by the *ecological* carrying capacity, at which births and deaths of animals are in balance, and neither animals nor vegetation are in top condition. Any stocking level below this is possible, depending on the desired outcomes. Rangeland ecosystems are frequently 'event-driven' (by rainfall or fire) and there are lags in response, so that livestock and vegetation rarely fluctuate in unison. In low production systems it is unrealistic to match vegetation condition with a particular carrying capacity, since the potential for rapid stocking rate adjustments is low. Conservative set stocking may be the best option in commercial farming operations. Most of the terminology associated with range condition in fact relates to the *economic* carrying capacity of commercial farming systems, and not to the long-term stocking densities possible in management systems with other goals.

Limitations

The limitation of most of these concepts or models is that they have insufficient spatial or temporal context. In a patchy environment shaped by patterns of run-on and runoff, attributes such as species composition will vary independently of grazing, on several scales. In turn, certain types of patches may be preferentially grazed, from local scale to whole vegetation communities. If the scale of disturbance is large, where should measurements be made and over what area? When Petraitis *et al.* (1989) explored the effects of disturbance on species diversity, they compared the outcomes of equilibrium and non-equilibrium models and concluded that they embodied the same types of processes although the spatial and temporal scales were different. If disturbances cover areas larger than the sampling unit, the system appears to be a non-equilibrium one. If the time frame is extended, event-driven changes become continuous.

Without some understanding of the processes that drive change, the scales of landscape variation and the scale of the assessment to be undertaken, the most appropriate model may be hard to identify. Moreover, since models such as Clementsian and state-and-transition are simplifications of reality, they should only be used where they apply and not asserted to be universally applicable.

What are Range 'Condition' and 'Trend'?

Defining range condition

'Range condition' is a value-laden term, often associated with particular models of rangeland change or particular modes of measurement. Sometimes, it is assumed to exist in some absolute form and assessments are designed to capture it, or at least to approximate it as closely as possible. The differences amongst definitions are significant, and reflect the perceptions of how and why change occurs under use, and the objectives of assessment.

The term is simply a concept, comparing the level of specific indicators such as vegetation cover, production or composition or soil erosion at a particular location with the assumed potential for that attribute within that vegetation type or compared with other locations. Since the term is used worldwide, we shall use it in this sense, although in the US in particular, it is identified with the succession model.

Two approaches that prevailed in the US for decades, and that influenced approaches elsewhere, represent the different perceptions that still exist. One was the site potential approach (Humphrey, 1949) based on primary productivity, which rated productive potential separately for each use, in relation to the maximum potential for that use. The other was the ecological or successional approach of Dyksterhuis (1949), which held climax vegetation to be the yardstick and was assumed subsequently by some to be appropriate for any kind of use, not just grazing. Nevertheless, both depended on the assessment of the 'forage' layer and hence implicitly the presumptive use was grazing.

Of course, not all the diverse uses of range that are now established depend solely on the forage layer, nor do they depend on its compositional climax for their optimal functioning. Density of different wildlife species can peak at levels below climax (e.g. Pieper and Beck, 1990; Nelson *et al.*, 1997 for New Mexico). Landsberg *et al.* (1997) found that there was no consistent pattern in total species numbers for a variety of taxonomic groups along extended gradients of grazing, representing successional gradients, in Australian rangelands. Water yield, firewood supplies or tourism values may be optimal at some level very different than climax. Even cattle numbers may be optimal at a level somewhat below climax (Pieper and Beck, 1990). Hence, an 'excellent' condition rating may be meaningless, in terms of both production and non-production values.

The Unity in Concepts and Terminology Task Group (1995) concluded that range condition in the US, as assessed by successional status of the vegetation, was not a reliable indicator of biodiversity, erosion potential, nutrient cycling, value for wildlife species, or productivity. In addition, the relationships between 'condition' scores and productivity or erosion rate have never been established and would be different for every vegetation type, if they ever could be established (Smith, 1989; Wilson, 1989).

Soil is likely to be an important indicator of the 'condition' of the resource. A major limitation to including soil in assessments has been the absence, until recently, of process-based methods for rating soil and landscape function (Ludwig and Tongway, 1995; Tongway, 1995), and relevant models of geomorphic processes. Subjective estimates of soil erosion have been used since the 1940s (Moir, 1989) but it has been assumed generally that the state of the vegetation provides an adequate surrogate for soil (e.g. Wilson *et al.*, 1984). However, accelerated erosion can be initiated well before vegetation change can be detected (Kinloch and Friedel, 1996). As far as we know, a holistic view of erosion has not been part of earlier soil assessments; that is, the phases of transfer and deposition have been ignored. Depending on the scale at which observations are made, loss of soil from one location may enhance plant production at another, arguably causing spatial rearrangement of resources without overall loss of condition. For a discussion of physical, chemical and biological soil parameters, see Chapter 12.

Veld assessment in South Africa (Tainton, 1981) and range assessment in Australia (Lendon and Lamacraft, 1976) and Argentina (Bonvissutto and Somlo, 1995) were initially based on the US model of comparing the composition of the forage layer with a benchmark. However, each country subsequently modified their approaches to suit their own particular circumstances. The South African system recognized a fire/grazing climax and departure from climax due to under- and over-grazing. This climax was not an end-point but a balance point in the midst of bidirectional change, in humid regions. In the absence of fire and grazing, succession continued beyond this climax, whereas in arid regions it did not. In Australia, a unified methodology never developed. Land management was a State rather than a Federal responsibility and there were major regional differences in climate and vegetation. Depending on whether key forage species were grasses or shrubs, whether shrub encroachment and fire were significant, whether grasses were predominantly perennial or short lived, different attributes were assessed. Soil assessment was incorporated into some systems where nutrient-rich soil veneers were at risk, and where ground-layer vegetation was in short supply during dry years. The availability of multivariate analysis later enhanced the possibilities of comparing assessments with one another across space and time, and notional benchmarks became less important. Range 'condition' was much less closely identified with succession and climax than it was in the US, and the development of the state-and-transition model was in part a response to the discontinuous nature of both environment and change in Australian rangelands. The state-and-transition approach has also proved useful elsewhere (e.g. Paruelo *et al.*, 1993; Milton and Hoffman, 1994).

With the development of satellite-based technologies, indices of cover could be mapped over large areas but, even after stratification into vegetation types, they still reflect short-term, local variation in rainfall, if they are estimated at single points in time. Pickup *et al.* (1994) developed a method that estimated the potential for rangeland to recover after rain, along gradients of grazing within individual paddocks, using the difference between dry and wet period images. 'Condition' in this case was the recovery potential for vegetation cover throughout a paddock, as compared with its least grazed areas.

Range health

Recognizing the limitations of earlier approaches, the US Committee on Rangeland Classification (1994) proposed the concept of 'range health', which inferred a more global index of ecological status, rather than an index such as range condition relating to a particular use. The US Committee defined range health as the degree to which the integrity of the soil and ecological processes are sustained. They recommended that the 'minimum standard for rangeland management should be to prevent human-induced loss of rangeland health'. They proposed categories of *healthy*, *at risk* and *unhealthy*, to be assessed on the basis of soil and watershed stability, ecosystem function (nutrient cycling, energy flow and recovery mechanisms) and productive capacity. While they recommended that there should be a minimum set of multiple indicators, the parallel with the 'climax' approach is apparent. There is still an implication that 'healthy' is the desirable goal, although it may be less than optimum for different uses.

The 'health' metaphor is now widely used in the US but West *et al.* (1994) have recommended against the use of the word 'health'. They said: '"Condition" and "health" have become value-laden terms. Because societal views and values can change, so does our interpretation of their meaning.' They further pointed out that the 'health' metaphor comparing a rangeland community to a sick person with various symptoms returns to an early ecological notion of a plant community as an 'organism' rather than as an amalgamation of species.

Indicators for assessing soil and watershed stability, ecosystem function and productive capacity are potentially very complex, and yet need to be quantifiable, if they are to be comparable across vegetation types or over time. Standardized indicators and methods suggested by the Committee on Rangeland Classification (1994) would enhance repeatability and comparability, but also increase the likelihood of assessments without an ecological understanding of the context. Such standardized approaches for determining rangeland 'health' are being translated into checklists by the public land management agencies in the US. Broad questions on these checklists require 'yes' or 'no' answers based on one-time observations in the field; they provide no quantitative data to determine trend over time, and underlying causes of change may not be detectable at all.

The Unity in Concepts and Terminology Task Group (1995) proposed some significantly different concepts, which they determined should not be tied to a specific model of succession. They proposed that conservation of the soil should be the key indicator for sustainability of range management, based on attributes of vegetation and soil. More than one vegetation state might occupy a given area of a given vegetation type or 'ecological site' (a US term denoting a kind of land which can be distinguished from others by its physical features, vegetation attributes and response to management). The Desired Plant Community could be selected for a specific management goal, provided it maintained the 'ecological site' below the Site Conservation Threshold (SCT). Thus, the goal of a single 'climax' vegetation type could be avoided. However, methodologies to identify the SCT for erosion on a given 'ecological site' are not presently identified.

Trend

Trend is the direction of change in condition or state of rangeland. In other words it is the component of change that can be ascribed to use, as distinct from external influences like rain or snowfall. However, a true representation of trend has rarely been measured successfully by comparing data over time. Commonly, methodologies change over time (Wagner, 1989) so that data are not comparable. More importantly, there has been a great deal of emphasis on the detection of condition at a point in time, but few serious attempts at testing whether methods that assess condition are effective at detecting change over time (Watson, 1997). There is no certainty that trend due to management can be separated from the changes wrought by environmental fluctuations.

An alternative view is that measuring trend by comparing condition ratings over time is unnecessary. Instead, analysis and interpretation of change in attributes such as shrub populations (Watson, 1997) or landscape function (Tongway and Ludwig, 1997) is sufficient, and does not preclude judging whether the change is desirable or not for grazing or any other use. Whatever the approach, a reasonably accurate determination of measured trend or change over time should be the goal of any monitoring programme.

Estimates at a single point in time of 'apparent trend' have depended on current measures of plant composition, plant age, distribution, vigour, litter accumulation and soil surface condition (Wagner, 1989). There is no evidence that these can be related to 'measured trend' and their use may lead managers to incorrect conclusions about the effects of grazing or other management actions. Many of the indicators used probably reflect the effect of current or recent climatic conditions as much or more than the grazing history of the area.

Scale

As previously mentioned, the notions of 'condition', 'health' and 'trend' are intimately associated with spatial and temporal scale. Unless a location is absolutely uniform, and an assessment covers it entirely, any ground-based measure will sample a subset of the whole and will have a specific spatial context. For instance, an area classified as 'at risk' due to erosion might be a component of a mosaic of areas that release and trap erosion products, so that the system overall might be 'healthy' (Friedel and Laycock, 1996). A great deal of ground-based assessment has been developed without regard for larger-scale environmental processes.

Monitoring changes in condition is also dependent on the time frame of assessment. The longer the time interval between assessments, the greater the change might be; on the other hand, the longer the interval, the harder it will be to detect when the change occurred and what caused it (Watson, 1997). Monitoring at intervals that are too short may not detect actual changes because of sampling and other errors.

Satellite data offer a perspective up to a regional scale, without the resolution of ground-based information but with much more comprehensive coverage (Fig. 10.2). Fine-scale processes are not detectable and the ability to make short-term predictions from the data is low. On the other hand, measurements can be repeated at regular time intervals and, where archived satellite data are available, retrospective measurements can also be made. Predictions are possible but on an extended time scale. Ground-based and remote sensing methods are not substitutes for one another. They occupy different parts of the space–time continuum and the respective data will thus provide different insights into the condition and trend of landscapes.

In general, this chapter deals with biophysical and ecological monitoring from management unit up to regional scale. Appropriate measures will be different at each level (e.g. tussock size, patchiness of cover, regional rainfall response) and should integrate properties at finer scales. As a result, conclusions drawn from the data will also differ at each level. We do not attempt to deal with economic or social indicators of sustainability but these also have to be addressed particularly at regional to national scale, for policy development or resource allocation (Pickup and Stafford Smith, 1993; West, 1999).

Principles of Range Monitoring

This section provides a broad framework for range monitoring. Some issues relating to particular methodologies are simply summarized here and are addressed in detail in the next main section.

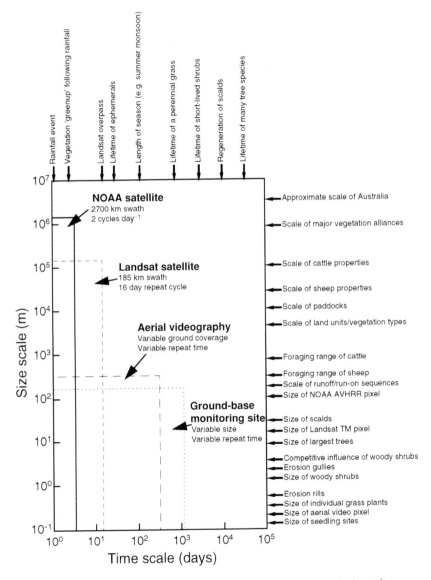

Fig. 10.2. Temporal and spatial scales appropriate to monitoring in Australian rangelands (adapted from Graetz and Pech, 1987).

Getting started: range inventory

Rangeland monitoring has to be preceded by inventory. Inventory and monitoring have different purposes, even if methodologies might be quite similar. The general purpose of an inventory is usually to estimate the kind, amount, quality, condition, location or other attributes of the rangeland resource at a given time (Laycock, 1990). Sometimes, a great deal of resource information is collected during inventory, covering landforms, vegetation attributes, land surface characteristics and details of soil profiles and substrates (McDonald *et al.*, 1990), which is inappropriate for monitoring, but necessary to assess the capability of land to support particular uses.

The purpose of monitoring is to document change in the rangeland resource over time. This change is estimated by repeated assessments using either ground-based methods or remotely sensed data. The different objectives of inventory and monitoring often result in different approaches to collection and interpretation of data. Whereas inventories provide the basis for developing a management plan, monitoring provides information to evaluate management objectives in that plan.

Setting objectives

Management objectives should deal with aspects of the vegetation or soil that the manager wishes to change. Monitoring objectives then deal with the specific attributes of the vegetation or soil that must be monitored to determine if the management objectives have been met. A management objective might be to change the composition of vegetation from 30% cover of shrubs to 10–15%. If that is the only vegetation parameter defined in the management objectives, a monitoring objective may be simply to monitor the shrub cover over time with the appropriate methodology then defined.

Management objectives are affected by the scale of the management unit and the time frame of the management decisions (Table 10.2). It follows that monitoring objectives must be set to match. For example, a management objective to distribute grazing more evenly in a paddock might be linked to a monitoring objective to determine paddock-wide change in herbage cover over time, rather than to determine change in herbage composition, which is a community-scale attribute.

Monitoring objectives must specify what type of information is important to evaluate the success of management. This will depend on who wants the information and what it is to be used for (Table 10.3) (Holm, 1993).

Specific monitoring objectives need to be set for the management unit as a whole. Too often, monitoring is started with the idea of 'let's measure everything and then we will know if anything changes in the future'. This

Table 10.2. Management objectives for grazed rangelands are pitched at various spatial and temporal scales (from Brown and Smith, 1993), and monitoring objectives should be scaled accordingly.

Factor	Scale			
	Organism	Community	Catena	Landscape
Process	Effects on individuals	Grazing by individuals	Grazing by groups	Grazing by herds
Emergent property	Growth/ reproduction	Plant succession	Soil/vegetation changes	Geomorphic changes
Temporal scale	Days–seasons	Seasons–years	Years–decades	Decades–centuries
Spatial scale	cm^2–m^2	m^2–ha	ha–km^2	km^2
Management unit		Vegetation community	Paddock/ pasture	Pastoral property/ranch
Management decisions		Range improvements	Season of use, stocking rate, livestock distribution	Enterprise mix, grazing regimes, kind/class of livestock

approach invariably leads to failure, because the monitoring effort has no real purpose.

Developing a sampling strategy

Devising a strategy for monitoring requires a very clear understanding of how the system of interest operates. Underlying ecological processes will control the kinds of responses to grazing or other uses that are possible. When does rainfall or snowmelt occur? When and how long is the growing season? Is it regular or stochastic? Which strategies do the plants use to cope with the prevailing climatic conditions? Is perenniality to be expected, or are plant cover and composition naturally highly variable? Are soils naturally eroding and, if they are, where are the products of wind and water erosion deposited? Are they retained within the system or are they deposited outside? How do erosion and deposition affect productivity? How are elements of the landscape (e.g. fertile patches, vegetation communities) distributed? Of all the processes at work, which are the most critical? Answers to these questions will help to resolve what methods are likely to be most useful, whether they are plant-based, soil-based, some integration of both, a landscape functional analysis to include hydrological behaviour, or remotely sensed indices.

Knowledge of the way grazing occurs is also essential. Does it occur within a single vegetation community or across several? Is it continuous

Table 10.3. The purposes of monitoring have consequences for the precision, accuracy and frequency of measurement (adapted from Brown *et al.*, 1998).

Level	Purpose	Characteristic needs	Methodologies
Enterprise	Improved short- and long-term productivity through adaptive management	Frequent low precision feedback; must satisfy the producer; needs to be at the scale of the appropriate management unit (e.g. paddock, property)	Producer-developed benchmark performance indicators; photos; requires only representative points
Government	Ensuring that the public interest is met, both in terms of sustainable land use (property scale) and industry success (sub-regional scale)	Intermittent assessment with precision that can detect trend on individual properties and across regions; may need to be legally defensible, though strong credibility may lessen this requirement	Hierarchical system linking precision at ground points with broad-scale assessment, possibly remotely sensed (e.g. Bastin *et al.*, 1993)

or seasonal? If the scale of grazing is within or exceeds the scale of a community, what are the appropriate indicators and how should they be evaluated (Fig. 10.2)? What are the temporal and spatial scales of management decision making? The temporal scale of repeated measurements has to be related to likely time scales of environmental change and management response. Timing should be related to 'decision points' (Brown *et al.*, 1998), when a manager can take the appropriate adaptive action.

Scale is also an important consideration when regional-level monitoring is the goal. Can lower-level measurements simply be scaled up? They probably cannot, due to increasing complexities of spatial pattern. And can system outputs provide useful indications of internal processes? They almost certainly cannot on their own. For example, if quantity and quality of water yield of a grazed catchment are used to integrate management impacts, deleterious change to vegetation may go undetected until water yield is affected (Brown and Howard, 1996).

Since monitoring will be constrained by administrative resources, efforts should perhaps be focused on areas at greatest risk.

Applying methods

There are some further general considerations before monitoring gets under way. Decisions regarding which techniques to use are also driven by financial and time costs, the availability of the technology and its ease of use. For a given ground-based method, how many measurements are enough? Trade-offs between error and the number of samples are almost inevitable, given limitations of time and money. So how different must measurement locations be, or how much change will occur over time, before the differences can be detected? Both the statistical error of a method and the observer error affect precision. The risk of not detecting change (trend) is greater than the risk of falsely identifying a change, due to inherent environmental variability and relatively few replicate samples.

Another issue, related to precision, is accuracy or the spatial and temporal resolution of measurements for the purpose of monitoring. There is no point in accurately measuring the amount of individual forage species if the key process is the shifting balance between the forage and tree/shrub layer. Nor is there need to make weekly measurements if change due to grazing is occurring over intervals of years and managers can only realistically make stocking adjustments, for example, yearly. Too frequent sampling may merely detect short-term rainfall responses. On the other hand, if measurement resolution is too coarse, critical events may be missed.

During monitoring, recording the causes of change needs to be an integral part of activities. Weather events, changing stocking practices or livestock distribution, fire, flood or insect plagues are just a few influences that can shape outcomes. This will be particularly critical if monitoring includes benchmark locations that might experience different conditions.

Using the outcomes

Management objectives have already been discussed. How the outcomes will be used must be an important consideration in initial planning. If the intent is advisory, involving the landholder should be part of the process (Table 10.3). Burnside and Chamala (1994) suggested two roles for the landholder: one as a learner and one as a knowledge giver. In the first, participating in gathering ground-based data builds management knowledge and skills, while in the second the landholder contributes to a larger body of knowledge by helping to interpret trend. If learning by doing is to succeed, feedback at enterprise level (Table 10.3) has to be frequent and preferably paddock by paddock (Brown *et al.*, 1998), in order to maintain interest. This means a two-tiered system: a frequent, low precision one for landholders, probably incorporating photos, and a less frequent, higher precision one for monitoring agencies.

Methods of Range Monitoring

Choosing methods is strongly affected by what the management objectives are and who wants the information. In some cases, repeated ground-level photographs at a fixed location are all that is needed to illustrate overall change, and engage the interest of landholders. Photographs are a quick and inexpensive means of recording the appearance of the vegetation and can be a useful supplement to other measurement techniques in all monitoring endeavours (Smith, 1990). However, by themselves, they are rarely an effective means of quantifying change.

Whenever change has to be quantified, the decision is then whether to use ground-based or remotely sensed measurements, or a combination of both.

Ground-based monitoring: what, how, where and when?

Once monitoring objectives are set, what methods are appropriate? Management objectives are often stated in terms of outputs (improving livestock or wildlife carrying capacity, water yield, reduction of erosion, etc.). Those outputs can be measured directly but often do not satisfy the intent of monitoring. For the most part, the vegetation and soil determine the level of those outputs and thus are the focus of most rangeland monitoring efforts (Smith, 1990).

What and how to measure

The number of methods available for monitoring vegetation is endless and it is beyond the scope of this chapter to outline all those available. Chapters 4, 5, 7 and 9 deal with methods in detail and Elzinga and Evenden (1997) provided an annotated bibliography of more than 1400 publications dealing with vegetation monitoring, mostly from the US. Publications such as Bureau of Land Management (1996) contain detailed descriptions of a wide variety of vegetation sampling methodologies but they do not always provide much information to assist the user on how to pick appropriate methods. The reader is also referred to the *African Journal of Range and Forage Science* and the *Rangeland Journal* for additional African and Australian references.

In vegetation monitoring, there are several attributes that can be used to characterize vegetation. In a grassland, one can choose amongst a number of measures, from dry matter yield, through aerial and basal cover, to frequency and presence/absence. Each has advantages and disadvantages, and the choice depends on the management and monitoring objectives. Dry matter yield gives a good indication of total productivity. If it is combined with botanical composition, it also gives a good indication of edible forage, provided it is known which species are eaten and which are not. However, it can vary markedly in the short term (weeks to months) as a result of rainfall and utilization. It can also vary significantly over short distances, including metre scale, and this being the case it should be assessed with quadrats that are large enough to encompass at least some of the finer variation. The quadrats should also be distributed so as to sample larger-scale variation fully. Equipment such as disc pasture meters is inappropriate in sparse and patchy vegetation, because of the inordinately large numbers of readings necessary to achieve acceptable precision (Chapter 7).

Aerial cover may be a useful surrogate for dry matter yield, if the ground layer is of uniform structure, though cover, like dry matter yield, will vary in the short term. The limitation where structure is non-uniform is that broad flat plants will score high values, whereas dense upright plants such as bunch grasses may not. Basal cover is much less subject to rapid fluctuation, but it is so low in some rangelands that it is difficult to measure with any precision, because of the time required. It is most likely to be practical for assessing abundant perennials. Both aerial and basal cover can be assessed with quadrat- and point-based techniques, but point-based techniques are of limited value in sparse, patchy vegetation. Point-based measures of aerial cover, however, are useful in circumstances where remotely sensed estimates of cover and cover classes need verification (described below), or where estimates of percentage of bare ground are required.

If botanical composition is to be assessed, the issue of area-based versus point-based measures becomes very important. Abundant species are likely to be readily recorded by either type of technique but, if species are uncommon, the chances of encountering them with point samples can be very low indeed unless operators use very large numbers of points, which can be both time consuming and tiring. The choice then depends on how important rare species are to the assessment.

Point-based assessments have been modified to record nearest plant data (Everson *et al.*, 1990) to reduce the sample size needed for a particular level of precision, but the measure is then no longer of cover. Instead it provides an index of relative abundance. In vegetation where perennials are sparse, and short-lived species come and go, this technique will indicate a declining proportion of perennials at times when short-lived species are common, though perennials may be stable in absolute terms. Another point-based method provides absence frequency (Neuteboom *et al.*, 1992), or distance to the nearest plant base, as a way of characterizing bare patch size frequencies. It would be of most value in moister perennial grasslands in a research context where fine scale patterns are of interest.

Use of the Levy bridge apparatus, which provides clusters of point data, is more problematic than the wheelpoint apparatus (Fig. 10.3), because observations are not independent (Everson *et al.*, 1990) and the data are strongly affected by localized distribution patterns of species even in relatively dense grasslands.

Species frequency, assessed in quadrats, also gives a measure of relative abundance, but one that is quite independent of plant size and/or weight. It is fast, and can be assessed in classes such as size or phenological state, but values give little indication of ecological or production significance. It can also be affected by spatial patterning, depending on how quadrats are distributed and how many are assessed. Scoring species for presence or

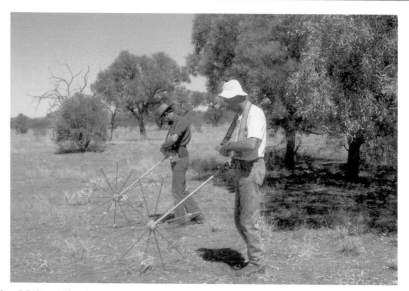

Fig. 10.3. Wheelpoint apparatus, for estimating aerial or basal cover of the understorey, as a one-person operation. The apparatus can be strapped to a belt, leaving the operator with hands free to record data on a small data logger slung from the neck in a comfortable position.

absence only is also fast but it is less likely to be useful for monitoring. Rather, it is more appropriate for detecting differences amongst vegetation types, unless a site is being radically altered by use.

Where yield and species composition and frequency of the ground layer are all of interest, the three can be assessed in a single quadrat-based procedure. One well-established procedure is BOTANAL (Chapter 4), which is practical for a diversity of vegetation types, from tropical to arid, and which allows other optional attributes of the quadrats or surrounds to be recorded as well. The calibration procedure of BOTANAL may be impractical under some circumstances for monitoring, because of the time needed for selecting reference standards and for calibration at every monitoring location. Distance between locations may preclude revisiting existing reference standards. However, the procedure can be streamlined with the use of easily transportable photographic standards for yield. A folio of photographs can be accumulated for different seasonal conditions, but estimates should be checked against calibration quadrats from time to time. Computer-based data recording systems are recommended.

In all situations where observers are conscious of spatial variation, such as patterns of tree groves or patch grazing, they may stratify their sampling to characterize the patches adequately or they may simply obtain a mean assessment, if that is considered sufficient for the purpose. If the latter, then we recommend annotating individual measurements just the same, in case additional interpretation is needed later. Ground-based measures can only provide summary values for patch data. Distribution patterns are best assessed with remotely sensed information.

Demographic techniques are generally unlikely to be useful for monitoring ground-layer species for management purposes, though they have value for research. However, they may be very valuable for shrubs and trees. Several approaches to monitoring shrubs and trees are possible, depending on the importance of changes in their populations to the overall management objectives. If, for instance, shrubs are a critical source of forage for stock, then survivorship curves and birth and death rates are important indicators. Individual cohorts have to be recorded on fixed transects or plots (Chapter 6). Shrub counts and density estimates are inadequate for detecting demographic change, since they do not discriminate adequately between existing plants and recruitment. Determining sample size in order to detect changes in rates has been discussed in detail by Watson (1997) for shrublands.

On the other hand, if changes in vegetation structure are important only, for example, for the impact of the overstorey on the ground layer, then counting and density estimates may be sufficient. If a management objective is to maintain a certain cover of trees, it may be sufficient to know if a new cohort of tree seedlings is establishing or whether the mature cover is increasing to the extent that a management burn may be necessary. In the former case, rapid visual estimates of seedling density in broad classes whilst walking representative transects may be adequate.

For mature trees, measurement of densities using distance-based estimates are likely to be imprecise since trees are not always randomly distributed, as the underlying model assumes. Cover estimates using line-intercept and point-based techniques, like distance-based estimates, can be very time consuming and difficult to use in wooded areas, and they also sample only a small subset of likely spatial variation. A useful alternative which can assess extensive areas relatively quickly and easily is the variable plot technique, using a Bitterlich gauge (Fig. 10.4). Gauge angles and the number of observation points can be adjusted for different tree/shrub densities, to achieve broad spatial coverage. The technique gives total crown coverage of individuals, whereas the line- and point-based methods usually disregard areas of overlap and give net crown cover (Friedel and Chewings, 1988).

The focus thus far has been on *composition* and *structure* of vegetation, but soils also provide important indicators of change. As discussed above in the section about defining range condition, soil monitoring has depended largely on assessing features of water and wind erosion and, since it has been assumed that vegetation will change before soil, vegetation has demanded greater attention. But soil change is not restricted to erosion and it may precede vegetation change. Hence, there is a third major attribute of rangeland systems to be considered, that of *function* (Noss, 1990).

Standard scoring schemes for erosion (e.g. Anonymous, 1995) are qualitative and may be insufficiently sensitive to detect significant change in

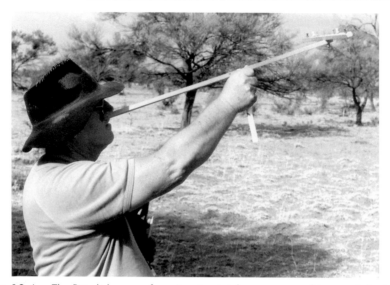

Fig. 10.4. The Bitterlich gauge for estimating total crown cover of trees and shrubs. Various pin spacings on the cross-bar provide gauge angles appropriate to different densities of trees and shrubs.

function at the stage of initiation. Tongway (1994) and Tongway and Hindley (1995) have devised soil condition assessments that integrate larger landscape processes, capacity for storage of moisture and nutrients, suitability as plant habitat, and stability, to provide predictions of trend. They provide a simple array of observations and tests, which can be selected to suit local conditions. The areal extent of sampling depends on the scale of landscape pattern. This approach assumes a developing understanding of processes and may be time consuming, but the quality of information is potentially high.

Herrick and Whitford (1999) recommended one of these tests, soil stability in water, as a core indicator of active soil organic matter, an integrator of a diversity of finer-scale processes. They proposed a flexible approach to monitoring, incorporating information at multiple scales, and including optional measures such as penetrometer resistance (for soil compaction) and infiltration capacity, depending on site characteristics and monitoring needs.

Monitoring systems that have been developed in Australia for large regional vegetation alliances are described in various manuals (e.g. Anonymous, 1995; Sullivan and Egan, 1996), covering diverse aspects of vegetation and soil, site selection and, in some cases, data management. For reviews of some approaches to monitoring vegetation, see Gardiner and Norton (1983) and Friedel (1990).

Selection of monitoring locations

Sampling to document long-term changes in vegetation or soil attributes is typically done at two levels: the primary monitoring locations and the subsamples (transects, quadrats, points) taken to characterize each location. Because most rangelands to be monitored are so large and encompass so much spatial variability in soils, vegetation and other characteristics, it is seldom efficient to select monitoring locations at random (Smith, 1990).

Sampling at each monitoring location should be done in an area as uniform as possible with respect to vegetation type, soil, slope, aspect and topographic position. The areas sampled should be large enough to represent the local variation in plants and soil characteristics, as well as any patterns induced by patch grazing. Locations should be carefully identified, perhaps using global positioning system coordinates, to ensure that the same area is sampled subsequently, and any atypical areas to be excluded should be carefully defined.

Issues to consider include the following:

- If an individual management unit (either a paddock or a series of paddocks) encloses several types of vegetation, and they are of different preference for livestock, then they must be stratified. Whether one or all are subsequently monitored depends on the importance of each for production or other values, and the cost of obtaining the information.

- If vegetation types are not absolutely distinct, and some means of separating unique types is required, then the attributes used to identify vegetation types must be independent of those used to assess their condition (Foran *et al.*, 1986, compared with Martens *et al.*, 1990). So, if condition is to be assessed by the vegetation composition of the ground layer, then vegetation types should be determined by, for example, underlying topography, soils and overstorey species.

- If livestock do not graze uniformly across a paddock or vegetation community, then where should sampling be located along the gradient of grazing? Selecting fixed distances from watering points can be risky, due to the possibility of local environmental variation or an unknown history of use, for example, of fire. Differences that are unrelated to livestock grazing may be detected as a consequence. Fortunately, multivariate analysis (Chapter 2) applied to numerous samples from the same vegetation type can help to cluster similar locations and minimize subjectivity.

Other means of deciding where to locate ground-based monitoring also involve elements of subjectivity. Anomalies in remotely sensed data can pinpoint places of likely interest – for instance, where response to rainfall is above or below expectation. There may be one-off reasons for following the fate of a particular spot too – for example, because of a new placement of supplements which alters livestock distributions.

Time and frequency of measurement
The season of measurement of vegetation is important because standing crop, botanical composition, cover, height and density of plant species change through the year, depending on soil and weather conditions, life history and phenology of the species involved. Because there is no one best time to measure all species, monitoring is often done at about the same time of the year, near the time of peak above-ground standing crop.

It may be desirable to measure vegetation more than once a year but this must be determined by the management and monitoring objectives and the available time and manpower. The frequency of measurement should relate to the rate of change in the key indicators, so that intervals of two or more years may be sufficient in relatively stable situations. It is possible for measurement to be strategic rather than regular if change is irregular and driven by episodic events such as irregular rainfall or fire.

Short-term monitoring to detect levels of utilization is sometimes used as an inexpensive substitute for long-term monitoring, but utilization of individual tussocks cannot be scaled up to infer long-term community-level impacts of grazing (Frost *et al.*, 1994; McKinney, 1997).

Data analysis
Due to the spatial and temporal diversity of rangelands and the purposes of monitoring, it is to be expected that non-parametric statistics and multivariate analysis will often be appropriate tools. Methods of multivariate analysis are addressed in detail in Chapter 2.

Monitoring programmes should never be established without a clear view of how data will be analysed and the time frame for the task. If analyses are deferred, it will be difficult to check anomalies, to ascertain if adequate information has been obtained to support interpretations and to use the data for education and training and timely feedback to land managers.

Remotely sensed methods

Using remote sensing for rangeland monitoring means that the data are digital and can potentially be analysed in a semi-automated and repeatable way. Where these data are derived from satellite-borne sensors, wide-area coverage is available on a regular basis and contemporary data can often be complemented with access to an archive allowing a historical perspective of landscape change to be obtained (Chapter 9). The various spectral bands of remotely sensed data are commonly processed to an index of vegetation cover or phenology. Vegetation cover may be estimated directly from the raw data (e.g. visible red band of MSS; Graetz *et al.*, 1988), while ratioing the red and infrared bands produces an index of vegetation greenness and cover (the commonly used normalized difference vegetation index; e.g. Tucker *et al.*, 1986). More commonly, various bands of the multispectral data are transformed to a perpendicular vegetation index dataspace (Tueller, 1989) which shows a gradation between bare soil and maximum cover (e.g. the PD54 index of Pickup *et al.*, 1993). Other ratios have been developed for specific purposes – for example, Karnieli's (1997) spectral crust index, which uses the visible blue and red bands to distinguish cyanobacterial soil crusts. Alternatively, mixture modelling techniques can be used to map, say, the amount of tree and shrub cover within pixels (McCloy and Hall, 1991). However, even with unmixing techniques, the pixel resolution of high-resolution satellite data generally does not allow discrete information to be extracted about vegetation composition or small-scale erosion features (rills and small gullies). Instead, each pixel must be regarded as a mixture of soil, vegetation, litter, shadow and other components. Despite this limitation, vegetation cover generally provides a useful surrogate of landscape stability (i.e. degree of soil surface protection against erosion) and the amount of vegetation available for grazing in the rangelands.

There are many examples in the remote sensing and rangelands literature of where satellite data have been successfully used to assess and monitor rangeland vegetation throughout the world (e.g. Tappan *et al.*, 1992). Maximum value is perhaps obtained when the spectral, spatial and temporal dimensions of remotely sensed data are combined. One such approach, the grazing gradient method (Pickup *et al.*, 1994) (Fig. 10.5), has been used to assess the condition of 38,000 km^2 of rangeland in central Australia (Bastin *et al.*, 1993). Such an assessment procedure could conceivably be extended through the analysis of archived data and ongoing monitoring to detect trend (Pickup *et al.*, 1998).

Remote sensing using either satellite or airborne data can serve as a stand-alone technique for range assessment and monitoring, or it can be used with ground-based monitoring data to extrapolate the spatial extent of ground data. A key component with the latter approach is that the two data sources are compatible, i.e. both contribute complementary information about vegetation and soil attributes at a relevant scale. For example, it should be possible to relate ground-based cover measurements of vegetation components that are spectrally distinct in the visible and near-infrared bands to an index of vegetation cover derived from remotely sensed data if the ground data are collected across multipixel-sized areas (Chapter 9). It would not be possible, however, to relate the composition of herbage biomass measured within subpixel areas to remotely sensed data because the information conveyed by both data types does not converge. The scale of comparison is inappropriate, herbage components at the level of individual species are generally not spectrally distinct and biomass is difficult to estimate from remotely sensed data (particularly satellite data) because of its height dimension (see also Chapter 7).

There are several issues to be considered where remotely sensed data are to be used for rangeland monitoring. Here some of these issues

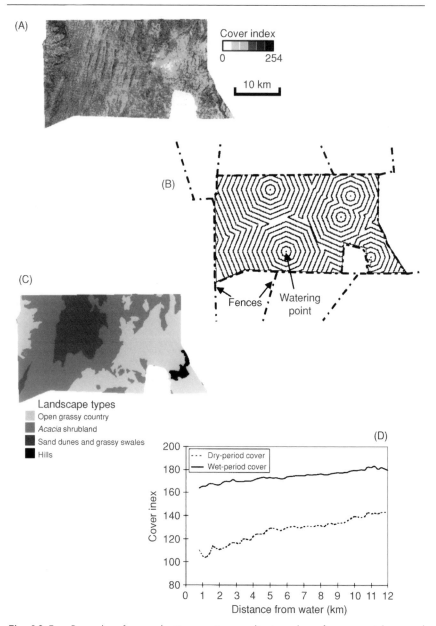

Fig. 10.5. Procedure for conducting grazing gradient analyses from remotely sensed satellite data. (A) Calculate index of vegetation cover from radiometrically standardized and geometrically rectified satellite image. (B) Digitize locations of fences and watering points, and calculate distance from nearest source of water. (C) Stratify landscape types according to grazing preference. (D) Calculate average cover levels at increasing distance from water. In this example, there is a pronounced grazing gradient to 5 km from water in the dry-period satellite data for the *Acacia* shrubland landscape type. This gradient is much less apparent in the wet-period data, indicating that the vegetation substantially recovers from grazing.

are briefly discussed; further detail can be found in Tueller (1989) and in Chapter 9.

Which remotely sensed data?

The choice will be influenced by the size of the area to be monitored, the minimum spatial and spectral resolution required to discriminate features of interest, and the temporal frequency of monitoring. For example, Advanced Very High Resolution Radiometer (AVHRR) data are suitable for continental-scale monitoring of vegetation growth (e.g. Tappan *et al.*, 1992) or mapping of extensive wildfires (Matson *et al.*, 1987) whereas Landsat Multi-Spectral Scanner (MSS) or Thematic Mapper (TM) data are more suitable for monitoring grazing-induced land degradation when such degradation occurs at a scale of one to many hectares (Bastin *et al.*, 1995). Airborne scanners or aerial videography may supply suitable data for the detailed study of small areas but these instruments may be logistically less attractive than high-resolution sensors on satellites if frequent wide-area coverage is required. Air photography at a variety of scales is another widely used form of remotely sensed imagery. Air photos can assist in locating ground-based monitoring sites and extrapolating the outcomes from monitoring to other similar locations. They can also provide valuable information about landscape pattern to assist in interpreting satellite imagery. In addition, photos can be scanned and analysed digitally.

What preprocessing is required?

Change detection as part of monitoring will require that multi-temporal images are co-registered (and perhaps rectified to a map base) and radio-metrically calibrated (Chapter 9).

What analysis procedure?

Combining the spectral, spatial and temporal dimensions of remotely sensed data should increase their power for rangeland monitoring. The value of the data is also enhanced when explicit models exist to determine grazing impact. For example, in large paddocks where grazing intensity decreases with increasing distance from stock watering points, calculating average cover levels (or cover variance) from satellite data can identify gradients of cover change attributable to grazing (Pickup *et al.*, 1994). Repeating these analyses after major rainfall events will show the degree to which vegetation recovers from grazing (Bastin *et al.*, 1993). Further insight into vegetation resilience within and between paddocks can be obtained by mapping the magnitude of scaled vegetation response to rainfall (Pickup *et al.*, 1994). Comparing the response of vegetation cover to rainfall in areas close to water with that at more distant locations after a series of major rain-falls should provide a useful measure of trend (Pickup *et al.*, 1998). Testing of this last approach within a number of large paddocks in central Australia has shown that an improving response ratio through time equates with an upward trend, while declining values are indicative of a deteriorating trend.

In some rangelands, not all grazing is due to domestic livestock. In Australia, large numbers of kangaroos, feral goats and rabbits can significantly contribute to total grazing pressure. The larger herbivores are dependent on surface water and are not constrained by conventional fences. In this situation, interpreting remotely sensed data using underlying models of animal distribution based on watering points is problematic without complementary ground-based surveys (e.g. Landsberg et al., 1994) to determine the abundance of different herbivores. Rabbits are not dependent on free water and although they reduce cover levels in the vicinity of warrens, they do not contribute to grazing gradients with increasing distance from watering points.

In rangeland environments where grazing gradients do not develop, other forms of spatial analysis of remotely sensed data may provide insights into grazing impact. Fenceline contrasts apparent in satellite data have been used to develop local range condition assessment methodologies (Mackay and Zietsman, 1996; Ringrose et al., 1997), while differences in behaviour over time of perennial, ephemeral and woody species have provided information on the plant species mix of various areas in the semiarid and subhumid rangelands of Western Australia (Wallace et al., 1994). Degradation in the tropical tallgrass rangelands of northern Australia occurs through loss of perennial grasses, increased runoff and formation of bare eroded areas and is often poorly related to distance from water (Ash et al., 1997). Although not yet established, analyses of change in the size, shape and arrangement of bare patches derived from high-resolution remotely sensed data (e.g. aerial videography) could provide useful information to complement ground-based monitoring of this form of degradation (see 'What and how to measure', above).

Verification of results

Analyses of remotely sensed data may be verified with varying rigour: from cursory ground inspection through to detailed on-ground data collection and statistical analysis (e.g. Foran, 1987). Often, the effort and cost of acquiring ground-truth data detracts from the feasibility of remotely sensed data. In some situations, aerial videography can replace ground-based methods as a source of useful information about vegetation cover components and can usefully verify high resolution satellite data (Pickup et al., 2000). Airphotos can be used as a visual aid to interpret landscape pattern and possible cover change being analysed with satellite data. Alternatively, they can be scanned and processed digitally to verify satellite data. In this case, it is important that if multiple photos are scanned, the data are radiometrically standardized to remove any compounding effects of bidirectional reflectance.

Interpretation and Use of Assessments

While it is beyond the scope of this chapter to explore interpretation and use of assessments in detail, we emphasize that, when planning a monitoring system, consideration should be given to the way that land managers will act on the outcomes. A clear link from management to monitoring objectives has already been advocated, but are the data useful afterwards? There is no value in collecting detail if the capacity to manage at a fine level is not there. History shows there is always a danger of data collection for its own sake.

Conclusions

Some authors suggest that there should be a single, coherent model to explain the dynamics of rangeland ecosystems (Committee on Rangeland Classification, 1994), and some would like a universal set of indicators of range health (Busby *et al.*, 1996) or a common methodology (Heard *et al.*, 1986). While these goals might seem desirable in a very broad sense, we have argued that rangeland dynamics vary with the forces that drive them, and methods must be tailored to fit not only particular environmental characteristics, but also management objectives and the customers for the information.

In addition, the requirement for simple and objective methods (e.g. Heard *et al.*, 1986) is unrealistic. Rangeland environments are not simple and so it is unlikely that simple procedures will provide the necessary information for good management. Nor is it likely that truly objective methods can ever be devised. As we have shown, subjective knowledge and judgement are important elements at all stages of monitoring, from the selection of methods to the interpretation of the outcomes. Objective methods applied blindly are bound to fail because we shall not recognize when they are inappropriate. We should be trying to marry the best aspects of our subjective insights with new knowledge gained as objectively as possible.

Monitoring should be part of a larger plan of management and implementation. Table 10.4 highlights some of the complementary activities that would be needed to make monitoring effective in a particular context. These include not just issues of scientific models and methods, but cultural, economic and political factors as well. We need to recognize the holistic nature of monitoring if is to be useful ultimately.

Finally, we emphasize that monitoring is about detecting change. Most effort to date has gone into assessing condition or health at a single point in time. Reliable measurement of change, combined with understanding of its causes, are the key to effective management action.

Table 10.4. Example of actions that should be taken by various groups to achieve effective monitoring for management decision making on pastoral properties (from Brown *et al.*, 1998).

Factor	Resource managers	Researchers	Government
Planning	• Commit to ongoing monitoring as integral part of property management	• Process-oriented research (not small-scale replicated plots) • Take account of landscape-scale processes and real-world variability	• Adopt ethos of stable resource condition on pastoral leases • Improve quality and focus of land management research that – involves producers – results in improved property management
Implementation	• Gain experience with suitable monitoring methods • Critically evaluate relevance of results	• Use goal-oriented research teams • Involve resource managers in experimental design • Conduct on-property research for adaptive management (not as site demonstrations)	• Establish performance criteria required for resource condition • Commit to funding larger integrated research projects • Adopt more sophisticated property planning approaches
Outcomes	• Adopt greater flexibility in management planning • Incorporate results into adjusted property management	• Make research outputs tangible – e.g. indicators that can be easily measured • Use adult education programmes to involve resource managers in results	• Be unambiguous in response to resource management problems • Given budget limits, clearly communicate how and why research funding decisions are made

References

Anonymous (1995) *The Western Australian Rangeland Monitoring System. Arid Shrublands Manual. Field Operations.* Department of Agriculture, Perth, Australia, 34 pp.

Ash, A.J., McIvor, J.G., Mott, J.J. and Andrew, M.H. (1997) Building grass castles: integrating ecology and management of Australia's tropical tallgrass rangelands. *Rangeland Journal* 19, 123–144.

Bastin, G.N., Pickup, G., Chewings, V.H. and Pearce, G. (1993) Land degradation assessment in central Australia using a grazing gradient method. *Rangeland Journal* 15, 190–216.

Bastin, G.N., Pickup, G. and Pearce, G. (1995) Utility of AVHRR data for land degradation assessment: a case study. *International Journal of Remote Sensing* 16, 651–672.

Behnke, R.H. and Scoones, I. (1993) Rethinking range ecology: implications for rangeland management in Africa. In: Behnke, R.H., Scoones, I. and Kerven, C. (eds) *Range Ecology at Disequilibrium.* Overseas Development Institute, London, pp. 1–30.

Bonvissutto, G. and Somlo, R. (1995) Guias de condición para los principales tipos de campo de dos áreas ecológicas de Patagonia – Argentina. In: Somlo, R. and Becker, G. (eds) *Seminario Taller sobre Producción, Nutrición y Utilización de Pastizales.* Grupo Regional Patagónico de Ecosistemas de Pastoreo, FAO–UNESCO/MAB–INTA, Bariloche, Argentina, pp. 95–96.

Bosch, O.J.H. and Kellner, K. (1991) The use of a degradation gradient for the ecological interpretation of condition assessment in the western grassland biome of southern Africa. *Journal of Arid Environments* 21, 21–29.

Brown, J.R. and Howard, B.M.F. (1996) Bridging the gap between monitoring and its application for management at regional and landscape scales. In: West, N.E. (ed.) *Rangelands in a Sustainable Biosphere. Proceedings of the Fifth International Rangeland Congress, Volume II.* Society for Range Management, Denver, Colorado, pp. 107–109.

Brown, J.R. and Smith, D.W. (1993) Using soil survey information for site description: a landscape approach. In: Kimble, J.M. (ed.) *Utilization of Soil Survey Information for Sustainable Land Use. Proceedings of 8th International Soil Management Workshop July 1992.* USDA Soil Conservation Service, National Soil Survey Centre, Lincoln, Nebraska, pp. 77–82.

Brown, J.R., Stafford Smith, M. and Bastin, G. (1998) Monitoring for resource management. In: Tothill, J. and Partridge, I. (eds) *Tropical Grassland Society of Australia Occasional Paper No. 9.* Tropical Grassland Society of Australia, St Lucia, Queensland, pp. 57–66.

Bureau of Land Management (1996) *Sampling Vegetation Attributes.* Interagency Technical Reference, National Applied Resource Science Center, Denver, Colorado, 163 pp.

Burnside, D.G. and Chamala, S. (1994) Ground-based monitoring: a process of learning by doing. *Rangeland Journal* 16, 221–237.

Busby, F.E., Ruyle, G.B. and Joyce, L.A. (1996) Minimum ecosystem function: a strategy to integrate methods to classify, inventory, and monitor rangelands. In: West, N.E. (ed.) *Proceedings of the Fifth International Rangeland Congress, Vol. II.* Society for Range Management, Denver, Colorado, pp. 101–104.

Clements, F.E. (1916) *Plant succession.* Publication No. 242. Carnegie Institute, Washington DC, 512 pp.

Committee on Rangeland Classification (1994) *Rangeland Health: New Methods to Classify, Inventory, and Monitor Rangelands.* Board on Agriculture, National Research Council, Washington DC, 180 pp.

Dankwerts, J.E. and Adams, K.M. (1991) Dynamics of rangeland ecosystems. *Proceedings of the Fourth International Rangeland Congress, Volume 3.* Association Française de Pastoralisme, Montpellier, France, pp. 1066–1069.

Dyksterhuis, E.J. (1949) Condition and management of range land based on quantitative ecology. *Journal of Range Management* 2, 104–115.

Ellis, J.E. and Swift, D.M. (1988) Stability of African pastoral ecosystems: alternate paradigms and implications for development. *Journal of Range Management* 41, 450–459.

Elzinga, C.L. and Evenden, A.G. (1997) *Vegetation Monitoring: an Annotated Bibliography.* General Technical Report INT-GTR-352, Forest Service, US Department of Agriculture, Intermountain Research Station, Ogden, Utah, 184 pp.

Everson, T.M., Clarke, G.P.Y. and Everson, C.S. (1990) Precision in monitoring plant species composition in montane grasslands. *Vegetatio* 88, 135–141.

Foran, B.D. (1987) Detection of yearly cover change with Landsat MSS on pastoral landscapes in central Australia. *Remote Sensing of Environment* 23, 333–350.

Foran, B.D., Bastin, G.N. and Shaw, K. (1986) Range assessment and monitoring in arid lands: the use of classification and ordination in range survey. *Journal of Environmental Management* 22, 67–84.

Friedel, M.H. (1990) Some key concepts for monitoring Australia's arid and semi-arid rangelands. *Australian Rangeland Journal* 12, 21–24.

Friedel, M.H. (1991) Range condition assessment and the concept of thresholds: a viewpoint. *Journal of Range Management* 44, 422–426.

Friedel, M.H. and Chewings, V.H. (1988) Comparison of crown cover estimates for woody vegetation in arid rangelands. *Australian Journal of Ecology* 13, 463–468.

Friedel, M.H. and Laycock, W.A. (1996) Rangeland inventory and monitoring: theory and conceptual foundations: Chairpersons' summary and comments. In: West, N.E. (ed.) *Proceedings of the Fifth International Rangeland Congress, Volume II.* Society for Range Management, Denver, Colorado, pp. 110–112.

Frost, W.E., Smith, E.L. and Ogden, P.R. (1994) Utilization guidelines. *Rangelands* 16, 256–259.

Gardiner, G. and Norton, B.E. (1983) Do traditional methods provide a reliable measure of trend? In: Bell, J.F. and Atterbury, T. (eds) *Proceedings International Conference on Renewable Resource Inventories for Monitoring Changes and Trends.* Oregon State University, Corvallis, Oregon, pp. 618–622.

Graetz, R.D. and Pech, R.P. (1987) Detecting and monitoring impacts of ecological importance in remote arid lands: a case study in the southern Simpson Desert of South Australia. *Journal of Arid Environments* 12, 269–284.

Graetz, R.D., Pech, R.P. and Davis, A.W. (1988) The assessment and monitoring of sparsely vegetated rangelands using calibrated Landsat data. *International Journal of Remote Sensing* 9, 1201–1222.

Harrington, G.N., Wilson, A.D. and Young, M.D. (1984) Management of rangeland ecosystems. In: Harrington, G.N., Wilson, A.D. and Young, M.D. (eds) *Management of Australia's Rangelands.* CSIRO Australia, East Melbourne, pp. 3–13.

Heady, H.F. and Child, R.D. (1994) *Rangeland Ecology and Management.* Westview, Boulder, Colorado, 519 pp.

Heard, C.A.H., Tainton, N.M., Clayton, J. and Hardy, M.B. (1986) A comparison of five methods for assessing veld condition in the Natal midlands. *Journal of the Grassland Society of Southern Africa* 3, 70–76.

Herrick, J.E. and Whitford, W.G. (1999) Integrating soil processes into management: from microaggregates to macrocatchments. In: Eldridge, D. and Freudenburger, D. (eds) *Proceedings of the Sixth International Rangeland Congress,*

Vol. I. VI International Rangeland Congress, Inc., Aitkenvale, Queensland, pp. 91–95.

Holling, C.S. (1973) Resilience and stability of ecological systems. *Annual Review of Ecology and Systematics* 4, 1–23.

Holm, A.McR. (1993) *The Western Australian Rangeland Monitoring Program – an Overview.* Miscellaneous Publication 27/93, Department of Agriculture Western Australia, Perth, pp. 13–20.

Humphrey, R.R. (1949) Field comments on the range condition method of forage survey. *Journal of Range Management* 2, 1–10.

Karnieli, A. (1997) Development and implementation of spectral crust index over dune sands. *International Journal of Remote Sensing* 18, 1207–1220.

Kinloch, J.E. and Friedel, M.H. (1996) Seed banks and soil loss in grazed arid grasslands – some preliminary results. In: *Conference Papers Australian Rangeland Society 9th Biennial Conference, September 1996, Port Augusta.* Australian Rangeland Society, Adelaide, pp. 243–244.

Landsberg, J., Stol, J. and Muller, W. (1994) Telling the sheep (dung) from the goats'. *Rangeland Journal* 16, 122–134.

Landsberg, J., James, C.D., Morton, S.R., Hobbs, T.J., Stol, J., Drew, A. and Tongway, H. (1997) The effects of artificial sources of water on rangeland biodiversity. *Final Report to the Biodiversity Group, Environment Australia.* Environment Australia and CSIRO, Canberra, 208 pp.

Laycock, W.A. (1990) Inventory concepts for rangelands. In: Lund, H.G. and Preto, G. (eds) *Global Natural Resource Monitoring Assessments: Preparing for the 21st Century.* American Society of Photogrammetry and Remote Sensing, Bethesda, Maryland, pp. 200–209.

Laycock, W.A. (1991) Stable states and thresholds of range condition on North American rangelands: a viewpoint. *Journal of Range Management* 44, 427–433.

Laycock, W.A. (1994) Implications of grazing vs. no grazing on today's rangelands. In: Vavara, M., Laycock, W.A. and Pieper, R.D. (eds) *Ecological Implications of Livestock Herbivory in the West.* Society for Range Management, Denver, Colorado, pp. 250–280.

Lendon, C. and Lamacraft, R.R. (1976) Standards for testing and assessing range condition in central Australia. *Australian Rangeland Journal* 1, 40–48.

Ludwig, J.A. and Tongway, D.J. (1995) Spatial organisation of landscapes and its function in semi-arid woodlands. *Landscape Ecology* 10, 51–63.

Mackay, C.H. and Zietsman, H.L. (1996) Assessing and monitoring rangeland condition in extensive pastoral regions using satellite remote sensing and GIS techniques: application in the Ceres Karoo region of South Africa. *African Journal of Range and Forage Science* 13, 100–112.

Martens, J.C., Dankwerts, J.E., Stuart-Hill, G.C. and Aucamp, A.J. (1990) Use of multivariate techniques to identify vegetation units and monitor change on a livestock production system in a semi-arid savanna of the eastern Cape. *Journal of the Grassland Society of Southern Africa* 7, 184–189.

Matson, M., Stephens, G. and Robinson, J. (1987) Fire detection using data from the NOAA-N satellites. *International Journal of Remote Sensing* 8, 961–970.

McCloy, K.R. and Hall, K.A. (1991) Mapping the density of woody vegetative cover using Landsat MSS digital data. *International Journal of Remote Sensing* 12, 1877–1885.

McDonald, R.C., Isbell, R.F., Speight, J.G., Walker, J. and Hopkins, M.S. (1990) *Australian Soil and Land Use Survey: Field Handbook*, 2nd edn. Inkata Press, Melbourne, 198 pp.

McKinney, E. (1997) It may be utilization, but is it management? *Rangelands* 19(3), 4–7.

Milton, S.J. and Hoffman, M.T. (1994) The application of state-and-transition models to rangeland research and management in arid succulent and semi-arid grassy Karoo, South Africa. *African Journal of Range and Forage Science* 11, 18–26.

Moir, W.H. (1989) History of development of site and condition criteria in the Bureau of Land Management. In: Lauenroth, W.K. and Laycock, W.A. (eds) *Secondary Succession and the Evaluation of Rangeland Condition*. Westview, Boulder, Colorado, pp. 49–76.

National Rangeland Management Working Group (Australia) (1994) *Rangeland Issues Paper*. ANZECC/ARMCANZ, Canberra, 28 pp.

Nelson, T., Holechek, J.L., Valdez, R. and Cardenas, M. (1997) Wildlife numbers on late and mid seral Chihuahuan Desert rangelands. *Journal of Range Management* 50, 593–599.

Neuteboom, J.H., Lantinga, E.A. and Loo, E.N. van (1992) The use of frequency estimates in studying sward structure. *Grass and Forage Science* 47, 358–365.

Noss, R.F. (1990) Indicators for monitoring biodiversity: a hierarchical approach. *Conservation Biology* 4, 355–364.

Paruelo, J., Bertiller, M., Schlichter, T. and Coronato, F. (eds) (1993) Secuencias de deterioro en distintos ambientes patagónicos. Su caracterización mediante el modelo de Estados y Transiciones. *Documento del Proyecto Lucha contra la Desertificación de la Patagonia*. INTA-GTZ, Bariloche, Argentina, 110 pp.

Petraitis, P.S., Latham, R.E. and Niesenbaum, R.A. (1989) The maintenance of species diversity by disturbance. *Quarterly Reviews in Biology* 64, 393–418.

Pickup, G. and Stafford Smith, D.M. (1993) Problems, prospects and procedures for assessing the sustainability of pastoral land management in arid Australia. *Journal of Biogeography* 20, 471–487.

Pickup, G., Chewings, V.H. and Nelson, D.J. (1993) Estimating changes in vegetation cover over time in arid rangelands using Landsat MSS data. *Remote Sensing of Environment* 43, 243–263.

Pickup, G., Bastin, G.N. and Chewings, V.H. (1994) Remote sensing-based condition assessment for non-equilibrium rangelands under large-scale commercial grazing. *Ecological Applications* 4, 497–517.

Pickup, G., Bastin, G.N. and Chewings, V.H. (1998) Identifying trends of land degradation in non-equilibrium rangelands. *Journal of Applied Ecology* 35, 365–377.

Pickup, G., Bastin, G.N. and Chewings, V.H. (2000) Measuring rangeland vegetation with high resolution airborne videography in the blue-near infrared spectral region. *International Journal of Remote Sensing* 21, 339–351.

Pieper, R.D. and Beck, R.F. (1990) Range condition from an ecological perspective: modifications to recognise multiple use objectives. *Journal of Range Management* 43, 550–552.

Ringrose, S., Vanderpost, C. and Matheson, W. (1997) Use of image processing and GIS techniques to determine the extent and possible causes of land management/fenceline induced degradation problems in the Okavango area, northern Botswana. *International Journal of Remote Sensing* 18, 2337–2364.

Sampson, A.W. (1919) *Plant Succession in Relation to Range Management.* Bulletin 791, US Department of Agriculture, Washington DC, 76 pp.

Smith, E.L. (1989) Range condition and secondary succession: a critique. In: Lauenroth, W.K. and Laycock, W.A. (eds) *Secondary Succession and the Evaluation of Rangeland Condition.* Westview, Boulder, Colorado, pp. 103–141.

Smith, E.L. (1990) Monitoring concepts for rangelands. In: Lund, H.G. and Preto, G. (eds) *Global Natural Resource Monitoring and Assessments: Preparing for the 21st Century.* American Society of Photogrammetry and Remote Sensing, Bethesda, Maryland, pp. 210–220.

Society for Range Management (1989) *A Glossary of Terms used in Range Management.* Society for Range Management, Denver, Colorado, 20 pp.

Stoddart, L.A., Smith, A.D. and Box, T.W. (1975) *Range Management*, 3rd edn. McGraw-Hill, New York, 532 pp.

Sullivan, S.A. and Egan, J.L. (1996) *Data Collection Methods for Land Resource Monitoring, Northern Territory.* Technical Report 96/1, Northern Territory Department of Lands, Planning and Environment, Darwin, 78 pp.

Tainton, N.M. (1981) The ecology of the main grazing lands of South Africa. In: Tainton, N.M. (ed.) *Veld and Pasture Management in South Africa.* Shuter & Shuter and University of Natal, Pietermaritzburg, South Africa, pp. 25–56.

Tappan, G.G., Tyler, D.J., Wehde, M.E. and Moore, D.G. (1992) Monitoring rangeland dynamics in Senegal with Advanced Very High Resolution Radiometer data. *Geocarta International* 7, 87–98.

Tolba, M.K. (1992) Preface. In: Middleton, N.J. and Thomas, D.S.G. (eds) *World Atlas of Desertification.* UNEP, Edward Arnold, London, pp. iv–v.

Tongway, D. (1994) *Rangeland Soil Condition Assessment Manual.* CSIRO Division of Wildlife and Ecology, Canberra, 69 pp.

Tongway, D. (1995) Monitoring soil productive potential. *Environmental Monitoring and Assessment* 37, 303–318.

Tongway, D. and Hindley, N. (1995) *Manual for Soil Condition Assessment of Tropical Grasslands.* CSIRO Division of Wildlife and Ecology, Canberra, 60 pp.

Tongway, D.J. and Ludwig, J.A. (1997) The nature of landscape dysfunction in rangelands. In: Ludwig, J., Tongway, D., Freudenberger, D., Noble, J. and Hodgkinson, K. (eds) *Landscape Ecology, Function and Management: Principles from Australia's Rangelands.* CSIRO Australia, Collingwood, Australia, pp. 49–61.

Tucker, C.J., Justice, C.O. and Prince, S.D. (1986) Monitoring the grasslands of the Sahel 1983–1985. *International Journal of Remote Sensing* 7, 1571–1582.

Tueller, P.T. (1989) Remote sensing technology for rangeland management. *Journal of Range Management* 42, 442–453.

Unity in Concepts and Terminology Task Group (1995) New concepts for assessment of range condition. *Journal of Range Management* 48, 271–282.

Wagner, R.E. (1989) History and development of site and condition criteria in the Bureau of Land Management. In: Lauenroth, W.K. and Laycock, W.A. (eds) *Secondary Succession and the Evaluation of Rangeland Condition.* Westview, Boulder, Colorado, pp. 35–48.

Wallace, J.F., Holm, A.McR., Novelly, P.E. and Campbell, N.A. (1994) Assessment and monitoring of rangeland vegetation composition using multitemporal Landsat data. *Proceedings 7th Australasian Remote Sensing Conference*, Melbourne, pp. 1102–1109.

Watson, I.W. (1997) Continuous and episodic demography of arid zone shrubs in Western Australia, 1983–1993. PhD thesis, Macquarie University, Sydney, 394 pp.

West, N.E. (1999) Accounting for rangeland resources over entire landscapes. In: Eldridge, D. and Freudenburger, D. (eds) *Proceedings of the Sixth International Rangeland Congress, Vol. II.* VI International Rangeland Congress, Inc., Aitkenvale, Queensland, pp. 726–736.

West, N.E., McDaniel, K., Smith, E.L., Tueller, P.T. and Leonard, S. (1994) *Monitoring and Interpreting Ecological Integrity of Arid and Semi-Arid Lands of the Western United States.* Range Improvement Task Force, New Mexico State University, Las Cruces, New Mexico, 21 pp.

Westoby, M., Walker, B. and Noy-Meir, I. (1989) Opportunistic management for rangelands not at equilibrium. *Journal of Range Management* 42, 266–274.

Williams, R.E., Allred, B.W., Denio, R.M. and Paulsen, H.A. (1968) Conservation, development, and use of the world's rangelands. *Journal of Range Management* 21, 355–360.

Wilson, A.D. (1989) The development of systems of assessing the condition of rangeland in Australia. In: Lauenroth, W.K. and Laycock, W.A. (eds) *Secondary Succession and the Evaluation of Rangeland Condition.* Westview, Boulder, Colorado, pp. 77–102.

Wilson, A.D., Tongway, D.J., Graetz, R.D. and Young, M.D. (1984) Range inventory and monitoring. In: Harrington, G.N., Wilson, A.D. and Young, M.D. (eds) *Management of Australia's Rangelands.* CSIRO Australia, East Melbourne, pp. 113–127.

World Resources Institute (1986) *World Resources 1986: An Assessment of the Resource Base that Supports the Global Economy.* Basic Books, New York, 353 pp.

Measuring Chemical Composition and Nutritive Value in Forages

A.T. Adesogan[1], D.I. Givens[2] and E. Owen[3]

[1]Welsh Institute of Rural Studies, Llanbadarn Campus, University of Wales, Aberystwyth, UK; [2]ADAS Nutritional Sciences Research Unit, Drayton Manor Drive, Stratford-upon-Avon, Warwickshire, UK; [3]Department of Agriculture, University of Reading, Reading, UK

Introduction

Since feed accounts for one of the greatest costs of livestock production, it is important that diets are formulated to optimize animal productivity. For grazing animals, this can be achieved by knowledge of how species, grazing management and fertilization can optimize dietary quality. In pen- or stall-fed animals, accurate ration formulation is largely dependent on knowledge of the nutritive value and chemical composition of the feed ingredients used. Forages are often the dietary component with the most variability in nutritive value; forage quality analysis is, therefore, integral for proper accurate rationing. This chapter aims to appraise critically some of the existing forage evaluation methods.

Sampling

Unlike concentrates, the chemical composition of forages varies with physiological age, time of grazing or harvest, variety, species, degree of contamination and botanical fraction. Furthermore, valid results can only be obtained when the sample analysed truly represents the forage under study. Improper sampling is one of the largest but most overlooked sources of variation in forage analyses (Linn and Martin, 1991). Proper sampling can be ensured by subsampling and mixing samples taken randomly from different parts of the forage being evaluated. However, this process is labour intensive and can be subject to bias.

The sample taken must be appropriate for the objectives of the investigation. Consequently, Johnson (1982) recommended that plant parts of equivalent physiological age should be used when monitoring changes in element concentrations over time, whole plants should be analysed for mineral uptake trials and samples that are similar in form and composition to what is eaten by animals should be used in feed evaluation experiments. This is particularly difficult in grazed pastures, yet it is integral, especially in tropical pastures, which can contain large amounts of low-quality stem that animals often avoid.

Alexander (1960) showed that silage corers could provide representative samples of clamped forages, provided two full cores are taken at midway points of the two halves of the same diagonal of the silo. Corers that leave the silo undisturbed are preferable to those that express moisture and give higher apparent dry matter (DM) contents (Rees et al., 1983). It is important to realize that, while clamps are now up to 4 m high, corers have not changed in size since they were used for 2 m silage clamps in the 1960s (Crawshaw, 1993). Thus, additional care is required to obtain representative samples in clamps, and with baled silages over-representation of the central part of the bale should be avoided.

Sample Preparation

Most samples undergo some form of processing before analysis to ensure uniformity and homogeneity. This is normally achieved by oven-drying and subsequently grinding the sample. Oven-drying at temperatures above 80°C can cause thermochemical degradation, while slow drying at temperatures below 50°C causes DM loss by respiration and enzymatic conversions (Smith, 1973). Prolonged exposure to temperatures in excess of 100°C can also lead to the formation of Maillard products in forages that are digestible in vitro but not in vivo. Oven-drying at 60°C for about 48 h in a well-ventilated oven followed by grinding is therefore preferable, particularly for fresh forages. However, oven-drying is not recommended for silages, because it causes underestimation of DM due to losses of volatile constituents such as ethanol, volatile nitrogen (N) and volatile fatty acids (VFAs). Ideally, undried samples should be used for silage analysis. Alternatively, to reduce losses of volatile substances, samples should be immersed in liquid N and chopped with a commercial food processor, or freeze-dried and milled.

Where cost or other reasons preclude the use of the methods outlined above, oven-drying of silage samples can be practised provided the volatile materials lost are accounted for with appropriate correction equations (Dulphy and Demarquilly, 1981; Porter et al., 1984). If not, chemical constituents and energy values expressed on an oven DM basis could be overestimated, while digestibility values could be underestimated. The existing correction equations are largely species specific, and most require separate quantification of VFAs that are erroneously assumed to have constant volatility (Givens *et al.*, 2000). A simpler correction procedure postulated by Givens (1986) entails adding a correction factor of 19 g DM kg^{-1} to the oven DM value, but this approach may not be sufficiently accurate for some purposes.

Chemical Analysis

In vivo measurements like those described in Chapter 15 provide the most accurate estimations of forage quality. They are not appropriate for analysing large numbers of samples, as they are usually expensive, labour intensive, protracted and disliked by the public in certain countries. Consequently several 'less animal-based' techniques are used to estimate the nutritive value. Ideally, such techniques should be cheap, routinely practicable, accurate and simple, preferably involving one stage; they should allow between- and within-species comparisons and should cope with large data sets (Clancy and Wilson, 1966; Weiss, 1993). As can be seen in the ensuing sections, many of the existing analytical techniques do not meet all these criteria.

Protein analysis

The protein concentration of forages can be determined from N estimates. The Kjeldahl technique is quite sensitive to N concentration and gives accurate results. It can be used for fresh or oven-dried samples and there are now modern Kjeldahl systems that automate and speed up the traditional procedure. Such systems are not as fast and convenient for analysing large numbers of samples as the automatic N analysers based on the Dumas combustion method. An example of the latter are the LECO N determinators, which may give slightly less accurate results but involve fewer analytical steps, use small sample sizes and allow the analysis of several samples in a day. Combustion methods often give higher values than Kjeldahl measurements, because they measure some additional N-containing compounds (e.g. nitrates).

The protein result obtained by Kjeldahl and LECO methods are based on a conversion factor that reflects the quantity of N in the protein. Although the commonly quoted factor of 6.25 suffices for general analysis, when precision is required the factor used should accurately reflect the N concentration of the protein in the forage. The protein determined by these methods is 'crude' and not 'true' protein, because the analytical result includes non-protein nitrogen (NPN). True protein can be measured by using high-pressure liquid chromatography to determine the individual amino acids in a sample. However, this method is expensive and it underestimates protein concentration when the 6.25 conversion factor is used to convert N results to protein (Salawu, 1997). Alternatives include using the ninhydrin assay or colorimetric techniques. Amino acid quantification by the ninhydrin assay is quite sensitive but the reagent is difficult to prepare and use and hence colorimetric techniques are often preferred. A rapid and more economical adaptation of the ninhydrin assay for analysing crude silage extracts was recently developed by Winters *et al.* (1999).

Colorimetric methods such as the Bradford, Biuret and Lowry assays can also be used to determine true protein concentration. These techniques largely measure soluble N; therefore it is important to pre-digest or adequately macerate samples before they are analysed. The Biuret/microbiuret method is not absolute, since the colour obtained depends on the protein in the sample being analysed (Cole, 1969). It therefore requires standardization against the Kjeldahl or another method. It is also important to remember that the Biuret method measures only peptide N and neglects the non-protein N fraction (Cole, 1969). The Lowry method (a more sensitive version of the Biuret test, due to the presence of Folin phenol reagent) and the dye-binding Bradford method also quantify peptides, but the dye-binding capacity is related to sample particle size (Cole, 1969) and the size of the peptides present. Since some of the dyes used also bind to starch (Cole, 1969), dye-binding methods may be unsuitable for analysis of starch-containing forages. Colorimetric methods may give inaccurate protein estimates in tannin-containing forages (Kilkowski and Gross, 1999).

Cell wall analysis

Most predictions of forage nutritive value are based on estimates of cell wall fractions, because the greatest determinant of the extent of digestion is the degree of lignification and cell wall content.

Cell wall contents in forages were traditionally estimated by measuring the crude fibre (CF) content. Various methods are available for such determinations but, though relatively easy, they give an inaccurate measure of fibre content and produce predictions of digestibility that vary with cutting date, species and maturity (Kivimae, 1960). Predictions of digestibility from lignin content are often more accurate than those from CF. However, the equations often vary with forage species and analytical method (Weiss, 1993). Lignin analysis is also expensive and complicated and the results obtained are affected by the degree of contamination with other substances (Kivimae, 1960).

The Van Soest (1967) scheme gives more insight into fibre digestibility by separating the total fibre fraction (neutral detergent fibre, NDF) from the less digestible fibre fraction (acid detergent fibre, ADF). Some authors have associated relatively high errors with the prediction of digestibility and energy value from NDF or ADF contents (Abrams *et al.*, 1988). For starch-containing forages such as maize silage and whole-crop wheat, the inclusion of an amylase digestion step gives more accurate results.

Bioassays

In vitro digestion with rumen fluid

Of the currently available *in vitro* digestibility techniques, the rumen-fluid pepsin method of Tilley and Terry (1963) is one of the most useful for predicting digestibility *in vivo* (Fig. 11.1). It produces values that are numerically similar to *in vivo* values for many forages (Clancy and Wilson, 1966). However, the method requires fistulated animals to obtain rumen fluid and long incubation periods (Wilkins, 1974). It is also thought to have poor reproducibility (Wainman *et al.*, 1981), partly due to variability in rumen fluid composition and activity (Clancy and Wilson, 1966). To avoid the latter, similar herbages should be compared in the same experiment if possible and standards should be included in the run to enable subsequent adjustment of digestibility results to values for the fixed standard (Tilley and Terry, 1963).

The technique is based on the premise that the final residue is similar to the faeces voided by animals eating the forages. This assumption is not strictly true, because metabolic faecal N, which is present in *in vivo* but not

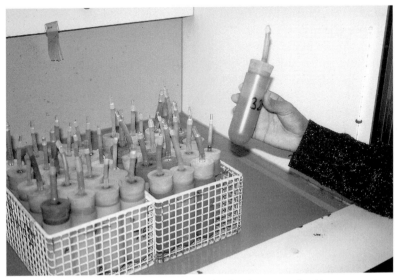

Fig. 11.1.   Digestion tubes containing samples for the rumen fluid/pepsin *in vitro* digestibility technique (Tilley and Terry, 1963).

in vitro residues, can cause lower protein digestibility *in vivo* (Ibbotson *et al.*, 1982). Also, the *in vitro* indigestible residue may contain bacterial residues and other substances, which would have been digested in the distal parts of the digestive tract *in vivo*. To overcome these problems, Van Soest *et al.* (1966) introduced a technique that measures true digestibility *in vitro* by replacing the acid-pepsin step of the Tilley and Terry (1963) technique with a neutral detergent digestion step. The result was a shorter, yet accurate procedure for true digestibility estimations, but it still requires using rumen fluid and has the attendant problems.

Faeces have been successfully used instead of rumen fluid as a source of inoculum for *in vitro* digestibility estimates (Akhter *et al.*, 1999). Although the digestibility value obtained is generally lower than that with rumen fluid, good relationships were found between both techniques.

Several workers have found that, though accurate for fresh forages, the rumen-fluid pepsin technique gives less accurate predictions of digestibility in other forages (Givens *et al.*, 1989, 1995; Adesogan *et al.*, 1998). This is attributable to *in vivo* and *in vitro* differences in sample form, particle outflow, N supply to the microbes and the production of Maillard products.

In vitro digestion with enzymes

To avoid using rumen fluid, several cellulase-based techniques have been used to estimate forage digestibility. These are usually comparable or superior to cell wall measurements as predictors of nutritive value. In general, cellulase-based methods are simple and highly reproducible (Wainman *et al.*, 1981). However, they can be expensive and require a constant supply of cellulase of constant activity. Differences in cellulase activity can account for up to 15 digestibility units (g kg^{-1} DM) and hinder between-laboratory interpretation of results (De Boever *et al.*, 1988). This problem can be avoided by using standards or regressing cellulose digestibility on mass of cellulase used (De Boever *et al.*, 1988).

The majority of enzymatic techniques for estimating *in vitro* digestibility in the literature can be classified into three groups, involving: (i) one-stage cellulase solubilization; (ii) neutral detergent pre-treatment preceding cellulase solubilization (ND); and (iii) pepsin pre-treatment preceding cellulase solubilization (PC). Jones and Hayward (1975) noted that although PC gave a better prediction, the single-stage cellulase technique was significantly correlated with digestibility and was adequate for initial screening of samples. While some results indicate that the PC procedure is more accurate, others favour the ND procedure. The PC method is easier to manipulate, is prone to fewer errors (McLeod and Minson, 1982) and requires fewer hours to complete than the ND technique (Dowman and Collins, 1982). When starch-rich forages such as maize silage or whole-crop wheat are analysed, it is important to include a starch hydrolysis step in both procedures (Dowman and Collins, 1982). Nevertheless, several workers have shown that none of the techniques based on cellulase (or on rumen fluid) provides consistently accurate predictions of the *in vivo* digestibility or energy value of starch-rich forages (Dowman and Collins, 1982; Adesogan *et al.*, 1998).

In situ rumen degradability

The *in situ* rumen degradability technique is theoretically superior to *in vitro* digestibility techniques because it provides information on the dynamics of forage digestion. Unlike many other feed evaluation techniques, it does not require a constant electricity supply and can therefore be used conveniently in less developed countries. Huntington and Givens (1995) reviewed the methodology of the technique and identified the following as important sources of variation in results obtained from such trials: sample preparation, washing and drying procedure, animal effects, bag type (Fig. 11.2), pore size and modelling. They also suggested methods of standardizing the technique and highlighted areas requiring further research. Additional problems with the rumen degradability technique include correction for particulate losses, particularly from starch-rich forages, and choosing the appropriate outflow rate. Particulate losses through the pores of *in situ* rumen degradability bags exaggerate the immediately soluble fraction and thereby disproportionately influence the curve fitting process (Dhanoa *et al.*, 1995) and overestimate effective degradability. The magnitude of the losses depends on the washing method and bag characteristics. Compared

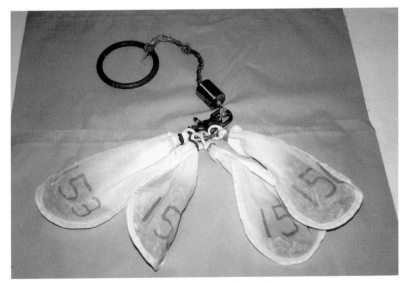

Fig. 11.2.   Polyester bags for rumen degradability trials.

with hand washing, machine washing is more thorough and consistent and it produces more reproducible results although increasing particulate losses (Cockburn *et al.*, 1993). Such particulate losses should be accounted for using true solubility values determined in cold water with filter paper.

The models of Lopez *et al.* (1994) and Weisbjerg *et al.* (1990) can also be used to account for particulate losses in forages. However, both models assume that the rate of degradation of the fine particles lost is similar to that of the material remaining in the bag. This does not hold true for all forages.

The widely used exponential model of Ørskov and McDonald (1979) seems to be unsuitable for describing the degradation of forages that contain appreciable starch and cell wall contents, as these degrade at different rates (Givens *et al.*, 1993). The model also appears to be inappropriate for describing N degradability in forages containing high soluble N values, because the fitted line often resembles a straight line. Also, conventional methods of calculating effective degradability may be unsuitable for such forages because of possible differences in the rates of passage of the cell wall and starch fractions (Hill and Leaver, 1993).

In vitro fermentation with rumen fluid

The gas production technique of Menke *et al.* (1979) was developed to predict *in vivo* digestibility by simulating the *in vivo* fermentation of feedstuffs (Fig. 11.3). The Menke technique and its variants (Pell and Schofield, 1993; Theodorou and France, 1993) are superior to digestibility and

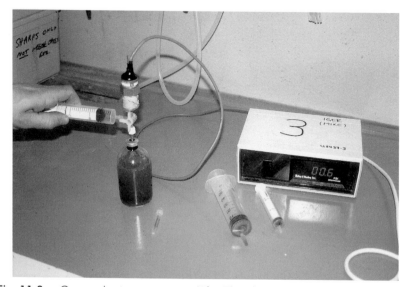

Fig. 11.3. Gas production equipment. (After Theodorou and France, 1993.)

degradability techniques because they account for contributions from soluble and insoluble feed fractions while providing information on the dynamics of forage fermentation. Additionally, when nutrient content is not limiting, gas production measures microbial growth (Pell and Schofield, 1993). However, the use of the gas production technique as an index of the nutritive value is hampered by the dependence of total gas production on sample size (Menke *et al.*, 1979), sample form and the composition of the end products of fermentation. A marked shift in the proportions of VFA produced can occur when feeds with different composition are fermented and the ratio of fermented to degraded carbohydrate and yield of gaseous products per mole of hexose fermented are not constant (Beever, 1993). The production of gas by the reaction of fermentation end products with the buffer also complicates interpretion of gas production profiles, especially as such indirect gas production is rarely accounted for. Caution is therefore required when interpreting gas production profiles and the validity of any interpretations should be ensured by accounting for the end products of the fermentation.

An additional problem in using gas production measurements to estimate ruminal fermentation is that the profile must be described with an 'appropriate' model to enable the estimation of the parameters of the curve. Traditionally, exponential models such as that of Ørskov and McDonald (1979) were used but several better-fitting models have been recently proposed (France *et al.*, 1993; Williams *et al.*, 1994).

Near-infrared Reflectance Spectroscopy

The NIRS technique is based on the relationship between the spectrum produced when light is passed through a sample and chemical constituents within the sample that are associated with certain wavelength regions of light absorbance. Regression relationships developed between NIRS spectral data and laboratory or *in vivo* measurements can be used to predict the nutritive value of future samples. The technique requires no chemical reagents, produces no pollutants and offers cheap, non-destructive, fast, accurate, quantitative and qualitative feedstuff evaluation (De Boever *et al.*, 1995). Although empirical in nature and involving complex statistical procedures, NIRS is increasingly being used for forage evaluation because it accurately estimates various forage quality parameters. Several authors have also demonstrated the superiority of NIRS over chemical, rumen fluid and enzymatic methods at predicting digestibility and energy value (Adesogan *et al.*, 1998). The major disadvantages of NIRS are the cost of purchasing the equipment and the requirement for extensive calibration, using large frequently updated data sets (> 100 samples). Attendant problems include the transfer of wet chemistry errors to prediction errors (Barber *et al.*, 1989) and the need to validate the calibrations with independent data sets.

Internal cross-validation (De Boever *et al.*, 1995) and spectral dissimilarity selection techniques (Baker and Barnes, 1990) enable the use of relatively small data sets for validation.

NIRS scanning of fresh forages is preferable to prevent the volatilization that accompanies drying, especially in silages. Where dry scanning is practised, the use of a repeatability file and the standard normal variate detrending (SNV-D) process (Baker and Barnes, 1990) is recommended, to reduce variability due to moisture content and particle size differences, respectively. Relevant derivative transformations are also advocated since they reduce the effect of variable path length and resolve overlapped bands, thereby decreasing the standard error of prediction (Abrams *et al.*, 1988; Baker and Barnes, 1990).

The right choice of the regression technique and mathematical treatment are essential for developing accurate NIRS prediction equations. Multiple stepwise regression (MSR) was widely used traditionally but gives only limited spectral information. Multiple partial least squares (MPLS) (Shenk and Westerhaus, 1991) and principal components analysis (PCA) (Cowe and McNichol, 1985) use more spectral data and are superior to MSR (Shenk and Westerhaus, 1991; Baker *et al.*, 1994). However, they require analysis of several samples and are thus less appropriate for small populations.

A good understanding of the wavelength regions associated with the various chemical constituents is integral for proper interpretation of NIR spectra. Barton and Burdik (1981) claimed that the choice or method of wavelength selection is the single element that limits the use of spectrometers in predicting nutritive parameters. Further, they stressed that wavelengths employed in the prediction of bioassay measurements should reflect constituents that are part of the chemical parameter of interest whilst minimizing the number of wavelengths used.

Tannins

Tannins are of interest in that small amounts can prevent bloat, reduce protein degradation in the rumen and reduce losses of gaseous N. However, high concentrations can depress digestibility of organic matter and protein (Kumar and D'Mello, 1995). Tannins fall into two major groups: hydrolysable tannins, which are potentially toxic to ruminants; and condensed tannins (proanthocyanidins), which tend to have beneficial effects on protein digestion, and are more common in forage legumes (Reed, 1994).

Several authors have reviewed the analytical methods for measuring tannins (Desphande *et al.*, 1986; Reed, 1994). The methods available can be classified into those involving colorimetry, protein precipitation and gravimetry (Salawu, 1997). The results of such tests do not necessarily reflect the ability of condensed tannins to alter the site of protein digestion (Reed, 1994).

Colorimetric methods

The vanillin–HCl method (Broadhurst and Jones, 1978) is preferable to other methods such as the Prussian blue and Folin–Dennis method (Folin and Ciocalteu, 1927) because of its specificity, simplicity and sensitivity (Desphande *et al.*, 1986). It is specific for flavan-3-ols and proantho-cyanidins and is more suitable for samples containing low amounts of the latter (Scalbert *et al.*, 1989). Although the traditional vanillin–HCl method is technically more difficult than other methods, due to its dependence on timing, solvent type and temperature (Price *et al.*, 1978, cited by Salawu, 1997), simpler field-based spot tests have been developed (LeFeuvre and Jones, 1997). The butanol–HCl method (Bate-Smith, 1975), which is specific for proanthocyanidins and flavan-3,4-diols (Reed, 1994), is more popular (Salawu, 1997). The Folin–Dennis method is less specific as it determines total free phenolic hydroxyl groups.

Generally, colorimetric methods suffer from differences between the extinction coefficients of the standards employed and those of the compounds in the sample being analysed, leading to inaccurate estimations of polyphenol content (Reed, 1994). This was considered as the largest cause for the deviation of tannin concentrations in the literature.

Protein precipitation methods

Although protein precipitation techniques may be less useful for tannin quantification, they are often more useful for estimating their protein-binding ability (Reed, 1994). The radial diffusion assay (Hagerman, 1987), which involves tannin–bovine serum–albumin complexes, is particularly simple, involves no interference with other proteins and is therefore suit-able for routine analysis of samples. Haemoglobin precipitation techniques that require a supply of fresh blood can suffer from interference with absorbance measurements due to soluble complex induced turbidity in the supernatant (Salawu, 1997). Protein precipitation techniques also require the use of standards and the attendant inaccuracies.

Gravimetric methods

No standards are required for the techniques involving precipitation with polyvinylpyrolidone (Makkar *et al.*, 1993) or trivalent ytterbium (Reed *et al.*, 1985). The ytterbium method allows direct comparisons between the tannin content and nutritional effects, such as protein precipitation and enzyme inhibition. The method does not precipitate all polyphenols and the repeatability of the original procedure is poor in plants with low levels of polyphenols (Reed, 1994).

Minerals and Trace Elements

Several minerals are important in animal nutrition, particularly P, Ca and Na, though many minor elements such as Co have also been shown to limit animal production. The methods used for analysis of minerals and trace elements in forages and other feeds were reviewed by AFRC (1988). In general, forages are prepared for mineral and trace element analysis by dry ashing at 550°C or wet-acid digestion (e.g. AOAC, 1990). Prepared solutions are then usually analysed by atomic absorption spectrophotometry for individual elements or by inductively coupled plasma emission spectrophotometry for multiple elements. As proposed by Cherney (2000), there are no simple techniques that can be routinely used for vitamin analysis in forages.

Conclusion

This chapter has appraised several major methods of forage analysis. Although none of the methods is flawless, they provide valuable insight about forage quality, without which accurate rationing would be virtually impossible. The method chosen in a particular situation should depend on the level of accuracy required, affordability and availability of reagents and equipment and technical expertise.

References

Abrams, S.M., Shenk, J.S. and Harpster, H.W. (1988) Potential of near infrared reflectance spectroscopy for analysis of silage composition. *Journal of Dairy Science* 71, 1955–1959.

Adesogan, A.T., Givens, D.I. and Owen, E. (1998) Prediction of the *in vivo* digestibility of whole crop wheat from *in vitro* digestibility, chemical composition, *in situ* rumen degradability, *in vitro* gas production and near infrared reflectance spectroscopy. *Animal Feed Science and Technology* 74, 59–272.

AFRC (1988) AFRC Technical Committee on Responses to Nutrients, Report No. 3. Characterisation of Feedstuffs: Other Nutrients. *Nutrition Abstracts and Reviews (Series B)* 58, 549–571.

Akhter, S., Owen, E., Theodorou, M.K., Butler, E.A. and Minson, D.J. (1999) Bovine faeces as a source of microorganisms for the *in vitro* digestibility assay of forages. *Grass and Forage Science* 54, 219–226.

Alexander, R.H. (1960) The sampling of silage pits by coring. *Journal of Agricultural Engineering Research* 5, 118–122.

AOAC (1990) Minerals in animal feed. Atomic absorption spectrophotometric method. In: *Official Methods of Analysis of the Association of Official Analytical Chemists*, 15th edn. AOAC, Arlington, Virginia, 84 pp.

Baker, C.W. and Barnes, R. (1990) The application of near infrared spectroscopy to forage evaluation in ADAS. In: Wiseman, J. and Cole, D.J.A. (eds) *Feedstuff Evaluation*. Butterworths, London, pp. 337–351.

Baker, C.W., Givens, D.I. and Deaville, E.R. (1994) Prediction of organic matter digestibility *in vivo* of grass silage by near infrared reflectance spectroscopy: effect of calibration method, residual moisture and particle size. *Animal Feed Science and Technology* 50, 17–26.

Barber, G.D., Offer, N.W. and Givens, D.I. (1989) Predicting the nutritive value of silage. In: Haresign, W. and Cole, D.J.A. (eds) *Recent Advances in Animal Nutrition*. Butterworths, London, pp. 141–158.

Barton, F.E. II and Burdick, D. (1981) Prediction of forage quality with near infrared reflectance spectroscopy. In: *Proceedings of the XIV International Grassland Congress*. Lexington, pp. 532–534.

Bate-Smith, E.C. (1975) Phytochemistry of proanthocyanidins. *Phytochemistry* 16, 1421.

Beever, D.E. (1993) Rumen function. In: Forbes, J.M. and France, J. (eds) *Quantitative Aspects of Ruminant Digestion and Metabolism*. CAB International, Wallingford, UK, pp. 187–215.

Broadhurst, R.B. and Jones, W.T. (1978) Analysis of condensed tannins using acidified vanillin. *Journal of the Science of Food and Agriculture* 29, 788.

Cherney, D.J.R. (2000) Characterisation of forages by chemical analysis. In: Givens, D.I., Owen, E., Omed, H. and Axford, R.E. (eds) *Forage Evaluation in Ruminant Nutrition*. CAB International, Wallingford, UK, pp. 281–300.

Clancy, M.J. and Wilson, R.K. (1966) Development and application of a new chemical method for predicting the digestibility and intake of herbage samples. In: *Proceedings of the Xth International Grassland Congress*. Helsinki, pp. 445–453.

Cockburn, J.E., Dhanoa, M.S., France, J. and Lopez, S. (1993) Overestimation of solubility when using dacron bag methodology. *Proceedings of the 1993 Winter Meeting of the British Society of Animal Science, Scarborough*, Paper 188.

Cole, E.R. (1969) Alternative methods to the Kjeldahl estimation of protein nitrogen. *Review of Pure and Applied Chemistry* 19, 109–130.

Cowe, I.A. and McNichol, J.W. (1985) The use of principal components in the analysis of near infrared spectra. *Applied Spectroscopy* 39, 257–266.

Crawshaw, R. (1993) Evaluation of grass silage. In: *Proceedings of the British Grassland Society Winter Meeting, Great Malvern, Worcestershire, 16–17 November 1992*, pp. 97–108.

De Boever, J.L., Cottyn, B.G., Vanacker, J.M. and Boucque, C.V. (1995) The use of NIRS to predict the chemical composition and the energy value of compound feeds for cattle. *Animal Feed Science and Technology* 51, 243–253.

De Boever, J.L., Cottyn, B.G., Andries, J.I., Buysse, F.X. and Vanacker, J.M. (1988) The use of a cellulase technique to predict digestibility, metabolizable and net energy of forages. *Animal Feed Science and Technology* 19, 247–260.

Desphande, S.S., Cheryan, M. and Salunkhe, D. (1986) Tannin analysis of food products. *CRC Critical Reviews in Food Science and Nutrition* 24, 401–449.

Dhanoa, M.S., France, J., Siddons, R.C., Lopez, S. and Buchanan-Smith, J.G. (1995) A non-linear compartmental model to describe forage degradation kinetics during incubation in polyester bags in the rumen. *British Journal of Nutrition* 73, 3–15.

Dowman, M.G. and Collins, F.C. (1982) The use of enzymes to predict the digestibility of animal feeds. *Journal of the Science of Food and Agriculture* 33, 689–696.

Dulphy, J.P. and Demarquilly, C. (1981) Problèmes particuliers aux ensilages. In: Dermaquilly, C. (ed.) *Prévision de la Valeur Nutritive des Ruminants.* INRA, Versailles, France, pp. 81–104.

Folin, O. and Ciocalteu, V. (1927) On tyrosine and tryptophane determination in proteins. *Journal of Biology and Chemistry* 73, 627.

France, J., Dhanoa, M.S., Theodorou, M.K., Lister, S.J., Davies, D.R. and Isac, D. (1993) A model to interpret gas accumulation profiles associated with *in vitro* degradation of ruminant feeds. *Journal of Theoretical Biology* 163, 99–111.

Givens, D.I. (1986) New methods for predicting the nutritive value of silage. In: Stark, B. and Wilkinson, M. (eds) *Developments in Silage – 1986.* Chalcombe, Marlow, UK, pp. 66–75.

Givens, D.I., Everington, J.M. and Adamson, A.H. (1989) Chemical composition, digestibility *in vitro*, and digestibility and energy value *in vivo* of untreated cereal straws produced on farms throughout England. *Animal Feed Science and Technology* 26, 323–335.

Givens, D.I., Moss, A.R. and Adamson, A.H. (1993) The digestion and energy value of whole crop wheat treated with urea. *Animal Feed Science and Technology* 43, 51–64.

Givens, D.I., Cottyn, B.G., Dewey, P.J.S. and Steg, A. (1995) A comparison of the neutral detergent–cellulase method with other laboratory methods for predicting the digestibility *in vivo* of maize silages from three European countries. *Animal Feed Science and Technology* 54, 55–64.

Givens, D.I., Owen, E. and Adesogan, A.T. (2000) Current procedures, future requirements and the need for standardization. In: Givens, D.I., Owen, E., Omed, H. and Axford, R.E. (eds) *Forage Evaluation and Ruminant Nutrition.* CAB International, Wallingford, UK., pp. 449–474.

Hagerman, A.E. (1987) Radial diffusion method for determining tannins in plant extracts. *Journal of Chemical Ecology* 13, 437–449.

Hill, J. and Leaver, J.D. (1993) The intake digestibility and rate of passage of whole crop wheat by growing heifers. *Proceedings of the 1993 Winter Meeting of the British Society of Animal Production, Scarborough,* Paper 98.

Huntington, J.A. and Givens, D.I. (1995) The *in situ* technique for studying the rumen degradation of feeds: a review of the procedure. *Nutrition Abstracts and Reviews (Series B)* 65, 65–93.

Ibbotson, C.F., Phillips, M.C., Turner, P.J. and Delaney, M. (1982) The alkali treatment of whole crop cereals. II. Farm scale feasibility trial with barley. *Experimental Husbandry* 38, 154–162.

Johnson, A.D. (1982) Sample preparation and chemical analyses of vegetation. In: Mannetje, L. 't (ed.) *Measurement of Grassland Vegetation and Animal Production.* Commonwealth Agricultural Bureaux (CAB), Farnham Royal, UK, 260 pp.

Jones, I.H. and Hayward, M.V. (1975) The effect of pepsin pretreatment of herbage on the prediction of dry matter digestibility from solubility in fungal cellulase solutions. *Journal of the Science of Food and Agriculture* 26, 711–718.

Kilkowski, W.J. and Gross, G.G. (1999) Color reaction of hydrolysable tannins with Bradford reagent, coumasie brilliant blue. *Phytochemistry* 51, 363–366.

Kivimae, A. (1960) Estimation of the digestibility of grassland crops from their chemical composition. *Proceedings of the VIIIth International Grassland Congress.* Reading, pp. 466–470.

Kumar, R. and D'Mello, J.F.P. (1995) Antinutritional factors in forage legumes. In: D'Mello, J.F.P. and Davendra, C. (eds) *Tropical Legumes in Animal Nutrition.* CAB International, Wallingford, UK, pp. 95–133.

LeFeuvre, R.P. and Jones, R.J. (1997) Spot test for presence of condensed tannins. *Leucaena News,* July Issue Number 4, p. 3.

Linn, J.G. and Martin, N.P. (1991) Forage quality analyses and interpretation. *Veterinary Clinics of North America – Food Animal Practice* 7(2) 509–523.

Lopez, S., France, J. and Dhanoa, M.S. (1994) A correction for particulate matter loss when applying the polyester-bag method. *British Journal of Nutrition* 71, 135–137.

Makkar, H.P.S., Blummel, M., Morowy, N.K. and Becker, K. (1993) Formation of complexes between polyvinyl pyrrolidones or polyethylene glycol and tannins, and their implication in gas production and true digestibility in *in vitro* techniques. *British Journal of Nutrition* 73, 897–913.

McLeod, M.N. and Minson, D.J. (1982) Accuracy of predicting digestibility by the cellulase technique: the effect of pre-treatment of forage samples with neutral detergent or acid pepsin. *Animal Feed Science and Technology* 7, 83–92.

Menke, K.H., Raab, L., Salewski, A., Steingass, H., Fritz, D. and Schneider, W. (1979) The estimation of the digestibility and metabolizable energy content of ruminant feedingstuffs from gas production when they are incubated with rumen liquor *in vitro. Journal of Agricultural Science, Cambridge* 93, 217–222.

Ørskov, E.R. and McDonald, I. (1979) The estimation of protein degradability in the rumen from incubation measurements weighted according to rate of passage. *Journal of Agricultural Science* 92, 499–503.

Pell, A.N. and Schofield, P. (1993) Computerized monitoring of gas production to measure forage digestion *in vitro. Journal of Dairy Science* 76, 1063–1073.

Porter, M.G., Patterson, D.G., Steen, R.W.J. and Gordon, F.J. (1984) Determination of dry matter and gross energy of grass silage. In: *Proceedings of the Seventh Silage Conference.* Queens University, Belfast, pp. 89–90.

Price, M.L., Van Scoyoc, S. and Butler, L.G. (1978) A critical review of the vanillin–HCl reaction as an assay for proanthocyanidins (condensed tannins): modification of solvent for estimation of the degree of polymerisation. *Journal of Agriculture and Food Chemistry* 26, 1214–1218.

Reed, J.D. (1994) Nutritional toxicology of tannins and related polyphenols in forage legumes. In: *Proceedings of the Toxic Legumes Symposium held at the 86th Annual Meeting of the American Society of Animal Science.* Minneapolis, pp. 1516–1527.

Reed, J.D., Horvarth, P.J., Allen, M.S. and Soest, V. (1985) Gravimetric determination of soluble phenolics including tannins from leaves by precipitation with trivalent ytterbium. *Journal of the Science of Food and Agriculture* 36, 255–261.

Rees, D.V.H., Audsley, E. and Neale, M.A. (1983) Apparatus for obtaining an undisturbed core of silage and for measuring the porosity and gas diffusion in the sample. *Journal of Agricultural Engineering Research* 28, 107–114.

Salawu, M.B. (1997) The nutritive value of the leguminous browse *Calliandra calothyrsus* and the role of tannins in ruminant feeds. PhD thesis, University of Aberdeen, UK.

Scalbert, A., Monties, B. and Janin, G. (1989) Tannins in wood: Comparison of different estimation methods. *Journal of Agricultural and Food Chemistry* 37, 1324–1329.

Shenk, J.S. and Westerhaus, M.O. (1991) Population definition, sample selection and calibration procedures for near infrared reflectance spectroscopy. *Crop Science* 31, 469–474.

Smith, D. (1973) Influence of drying and storage conditions on non-structural carbohydrate analysis of herbage tissues – a review. *Journal of the British Grassland Society* 28, 129–134.

Theodorou, M.K. and France, J. (1993) Rumen microorganisms and their interactions. In: Forbes, J.M. and France, J. (eds) *Quantitative Aspects of Ruminant Digestion and Metabolism.* CAB International, Wallingford, UK, pp. 145–163.

Tilley, J.M.A. and Terry, R.A. (1963) A two stage technique for the *in vitro* digestion of forage crops. *Journal of the British Grassland Society* 18, 104–111.

Van Soest, P.J. (1967) Development of a comprehensive system of feed analysis and its application to forages. *Journal of Animal Science* 26, 119–128.

Van Soest, P.J., Wine, R.H. and Moore, L.A. (1966) Estimation of the true digestibility of forages by the *in vitro* digestion of cell walls. In: *Proceedings of the Xth International Grassland Congress.* Helsinki, pp. 438–441.

Wainman, F.W., Dewey, P.J.S. and Boyne, A.W. (1981) *Compound Feedingstuffs for Ruminants.* Third Report, Feedingstuffs Evaluation Unit, Rowett Research Institute, Aberdeen, UK, 49 pp.

Weisbjerg, M.R., Bhargava, P.K., Hvelplund, T. and Madsen, J. (1990) *Use of Degradation Curves in Feed Evaluation.* Report No. 679, National Institute of Animal Production, Beretning fra Statens Husdyrbrugsforsog, Denmark, 33 pp.

Weiss, W.P. (1993) Predicting energy values of feeds. *Journal of Dairy Science* 76, 1801–1811.

Wilkins, R.J. (1974) *The nutritive value of silages.* Proceedings of the Eighth Nutrition Conference for Feed Manufacturers, Butterworths, Nottingham, pp. 167–189.

Williams, B.A., Boer, H., Diekema, B. and Tamminga, S. (1994) A progressive carbon balance for the *in vitro* fermentation of wheat straw using the cumulative gas production technique. *Proceedings of the Society of Nutritional Physiology* 3, 184.

Winters, A., Lloyd, J., Lowes, K., Jones, R. and Merry, R. (1999) A rapid and economical technique for predicting free amino acid content in legume silage. In: *Proceedings of the XII International Silage Conference.* Upsalla, Sweden, p. 168.

Measuring Physical, Chemical and Biological Soil Parameters in Grasslands

12

J. Bouma[1], J.P. Curry[2] and V.J.G. Houba[3]

[1]Department of Environmental Sciences, Laboratory for Soil Science and Geology, Wageningen University, Wageningen, The Netherlands; [2]Department of Environmental Resource Management, Faculty of Agriculture, University College, Belfield, Dublin, Ireland; [3]Department of Environmental Sciences, Wageningen University, Wageningen, The Netherlands

Introduction

Numerous methods are used for measuring physical, chemical and biological soil properties. Not many are specifically focused on grassland soils but when methods are applied to grassland soils they can produce data sets that are distinct from data obtained for other forms of land use. The objective of this chapter is to discuss the main physical, chemical and biological processes in grassland soils with reference to published methodologies:

- Relationships between physical, chemical and biological processes. Increasingly a holistic, systems approach is being taken as the three basic processes are strongly interrelated.
- The importance of choosing any particular method. All too often researchers jump into a project using familiar methods without considering if they are appropriate.
- The importance of sampling techniques and intensity. The number of samples and their location in the field are subject to specific conditions when dealing with grasslands.
- The need for quality control. Producing data is never a problem; producing good and reliable data is the big challenge. All potential sources of error have to be considered: sampling procedures, pre-treatment of samples, and the measurement procedures and final calculations themselves, including additional errors that can arise if further calculations are required to arrive at the final data set.

The section on soil biology illustrates the significance of soil physical and chemical conditions for biological processes. When describing physical conditions, emphasis is given to so-called land qualities, which characterize dynamic physical conditions during the growing season, rather than measurement of single parameters. In the soil chemical section, special attention is paid to the importance of proper pre-treatment of samples and to the wide range of results that can be found when using different analysis procedures.

Measurement of Physical Parameters to Characterize Land Qualities

Physical parameters, such as porosity, bulk density, particle density, shear resistance, infiltration rate, moisture retention and permeability, do not have much significance by themselves, but derive their meaning in the broader context of dynamic physical processes occurring in grasslands throughout the year. Soil moisture regimes govern fluxes of water and solutes and hence physical conditions in terms of water and oxygen content and temperature at any given time. Rather than focusing on the single parameters mentioned above, attention is increasingly focused on more comprehensive 'land qualities', which are 'attributes of land that have a significant impact on functioning of the land' (FAO, 1983). Land qualities can only be assessed using expert knowledge or models and measured soil characteristics (e.g. soil texture, organic matter content and the physical parameters mentioned above).

Relevant examples of physical land qualities for grassland in The Netherlands are moisture supply capacity (MSC), trafficability (T) and drainage status (e.g. Bouma, 1981, 1984). Grasslands in different agroecological zones will have to be characterized by different land qualities. Socio-economic settings are also critical when deciding which land qualities are important. For instance, trafficability is often important with intensive, mechanized grassland management, but is of negligible consequence in extensive grazing systems. The drainage status expresses the duration of the period in which the soil is very wet and is, therefore, only important in soils with high groundwater tables or with perched water tables. On the other hand, moisture supply capacity will be relevant everywhere. Measurement of physical characteristics is discussed in the context of important land qualities. This provides a logical link between physical characteristics, their measurement and their practical application and relevance.

In this chapter, MSC and T will be used as examples, but the basic principles also apply to other land qualities. MSC is defined as the capacity of a soil to supply water to a growing crop or pasture. It is governed by weather patterns over the years, groundwater levels, soil structure, basic physical properties of the root zone, rooting patterns and the specific demands of a given species. Trafficability, defined and measured in number of days, is the capacity of a soil to allow traffic without causing adverse effects on soil structure. It is governed by climate, soil characteristics and typical threshold soil moisture contents for compactibility. The following sections discuss how MSC and T can be derived at different knowledge levels and which physical data are needed, including the corresponding measurement techniques.

Knowledge levels

Most methodology books and manuals have a strong technological and disciplinary focus. However, studies on grassland systems require an interdisciplinary systems-oriented approach. Selection of methodologies and approaches should reflect not only technical but also interdisciplinary aspects, while questions raised by stakeholders should play a central role. Bouma and Hoosbeek (1996) have proposed consideration of different knowledge levels when defining input of professional expertise. They use two scales, one ranging from qualitative to quantitative and the other from deterministic to empirical (Fig. 12.1). Using the diagram, it is possible to distinguish user expertise (K1), expert knowledge (K2), use of simple empirical methods or models (K3) and use of ever more complex models and methods (K4 and K5). The diagram in Fig. 12.1 has to be interpreted differently at different spatial scales. This chapter will focus on the field level, because this is where the interest of farmers and research workers lies. At the regional scale, questions are asked by planners and politicians and may relate to optimal land use patterns.

Deriving data for moisture supply capacity

At K1 level, farmers have only a broad understanding of MSC as they observe wilting or death of grass, which may differ at different spots in the field and under different weather conditions. However, they may find it difficult to define exactly why wilting occurs. There can be many reasons, including low rainfall, high evaporative demand, low water-holding capacities in the root zone and shallow rooting. This knowledge level will involve little or no measurement.

At K2 level, reasons can often be better explained because of available expertise. At this level, standard data tables are often used (e.g. Landon, 1991). In such tables, available water is defined as a function of soil texture and rooting depth, which can easily be estimated in the field. Assessments at K2 level are highly generalized but are based on measurements made elsewhere. Many questions can be answered using K2-level knowledge, without requiring sophisticated data-intensive methodology (Bouma, 1983a).

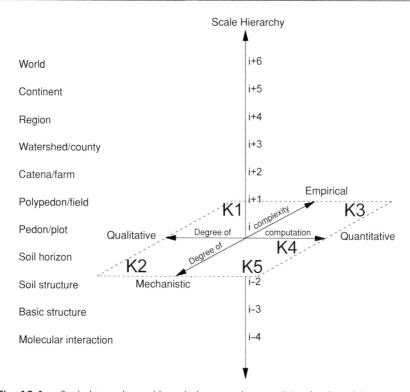

Fig. 12.1. Scale hierarchy and knowledge type diagram (Hoosbeek and Bryant, 1992; Bouma and Hoosbeek, 1996). Classification of models and data based on hierarchical scale level, degree of computation and degree of complexity. Knowledge types: K1 = qualitative–empirical (User); K2 = qualitative–mechanistic (Expert); K3 = quantitative–empirical (Specialist: simple comprehensive models); K4 = quantitative–mechanistic/empirical (Specialist: complex comprehensive models); K5 = quantitative–mechanistic (Specialist: complex models of aspects).

At K3 level, capacity-type models (such as the DSSAT models; e.g. Ritchie, 1995) are used in which the rooting zone is considered as a black box containing water between 'field capacity' (traditionally corresponding to 0.3 kPa) and 'wilting point' (15 kPa) (e.g. Landon, 1991). Excess water is assumed to drain to the subsoil, while rain falling on soil having a moisture deficit is supposed to be absorbed in the root zone. In sloping soils a runoff component is also included. Again, tables are available to estimate moisture retention curves as a function of texture but measurements of water contents at different pressure heads, defining the limits of water availability, can also be made (Cassel and Klute, 1986). Bouma (1983b) discussed ten methods for measuring moisture retention properties, emphasizing operational aspects such as representative elementary volumes of samples, reliability and accuracy, ease of operation, level of expertise required and cost.

K4 models, such as the WAVE model (Vanclooster *et al.*, 1994), are more deterministic and also consider dynamic flow processes. Hydraulic conductivity (*K*) has to be known for both saturated and unsaturated soil. Many methods for measuring *K* have been proposed (Amoozegar and Warrick, 1986; Klute and Dirksen, 1986) and have been discussed by Bouma (1983a) in terms of operational aspects. Infiltration rates are often measured separately. This can be done by using infiltrometers placed at the soil surface after cutting the grass (Bouwer, 1986) or by sprinkling, where the infiltration rate is defined as soon as an increasing sprinkling rate leads to surface ponding of water (Peterson and Bubenzer, 1986).

K5 models consider detailed processes, such as the occurrence of bypass flow and internal catchment, which describes rapid downward flow of water along continuous macropores through an unsaturated soil matrix and accumulation of free water in dead-end pores (e.g. Bouma, 1991). Also, irregular wetting patterns due to poor soil wettability can be described with complex simulation models (e.g. Dekker and Ritsema, 1995). Recently, the concept of water accessibility was introduced by Droogers *et al.* (1997), describing the effects of large dense clods, which cannot be penetrated by roots, on water availability. Even though the water inside the clod may be 'available' (because it may have a pressure head between −30 and −1500 kPa), it may not be accessible when the root cannot 'pull' the water from the inside to the outside of the clod. This can be a problem in grassland on clayey soils where soil traffic under wet conditions, by either machinery or cattle, may result in compaction and formation of large clods in surface soil.

Deriving data for trafficability

At Kl level, farmers are perfectly able to estimate trafficability in terms of ability to travel on the land or to allow grazing, but this cannot be quantified.

At K2 level, experts can apply their knowledge, based on relationships between soil water content and soil stability (e.g. Bouma, 1983b; Droogers *et al.*, 1996). Van Wijk (1988) asked farmers to indicate when they considered soil to be trafficable. They then measured the corresponding soil pressure heads and found that farmers' experience corresponded with characteristic pressure heads in different grassland soils in the range of −5 kPa to −12 kPa. These values were used later to derive the number of trafficable days from simulations (K4 level) of soil moisture regimes for a series of years. Thus, the effect of different weather conditions on soil moisture contents and the associated mechanical stability can be derived.

The K3 and higher levels allow simulations of soil moisture regimes in varying degrees of detail, as was discussed above for MSC. These simulations estimate moisture contents of the soil, which, in turn, determine mechanical stability. The lower plastic limit has been used to indicate the onset of soil plasticity (e.g. Droogers et al., 1996).

Selection of the most appropriate methods

Different methods can be used to characterize soil and physical land qualities that are important for grassland management. K2 methods are usually rather simple and low-cost, but costs increase as methods become more sophisticated. However, running a complicated K4 or K5 model with inadequate data is unwise and is bound to lead to pseudo-accuracy. It may be preferable to run a simpler K3 model with a lower data demand. Running a complicated model is justified only when the additional expense of deriving data for such a model is necessary to satisfy the objectives of the study. As stated above, a K2 approach may be quite satisfactory in many cases, certainly in areas of the world where few data are available.

Moisture regimes as drivers of soil processes

The previous examples illustrate the importance of the soil moisture regime for physical land qualities. Chemical and biological processes are also strongly affected by such regimes as they govern fluxes of solutes, air and heat and, thereby, growing conditions for plants and soil flora and fauna. Recent research suggests the following guidelines for characterizing soil moisture regimes:

- Descriptive drainage classes are defined in soil surveys (USDA, 1953). Based on profile morphology, broad differences in soil wetness are indicated at a K2 level in terms of well, imperfectly, poorly and very poorly drained.
- Many methods are available to measure soil moisture contents (Gardner, 1986). Measurements can now routinely be made everywhere as user-friendly equipment has been automated. On-site monitoring using transducer tensiometers and TDR (time domain reflectometry) is attractive and possible also in developing countries (Topp et al., 1980). Also, remote sensing can measure plant stress, which is often an indicator of moisture deficiency.
- Since monitoring is quite costly and limited to actual conditions, simulation modelling is commonly used to predict moisture regimes for different weather conditions covering many years. Many models are now available. Simple K3 models are usually satisfactory for general

application (e.g. Ritchie, 1995). K4/K5 models need moisture retention data and, sometimes, also hydraulic conductivity data.

- *In situ* instantaneous profile methods using tensiometry and TDR are the best, but they are very time consuming and costly (e.g. Klute, 1986). Samples can also be taken for laboratory analysis, using the multiple-outflow method (Van Dam *et al.*, 1994). Also data are needed to express heterogeneity aspects (e.g. Booltink, 1994).
- Samples taken in the field for measuring bulk density, moisture retention and *K* should be representative. Small standard cylinders (100 cm^3) are often not suitable because some soils need large samples to be representative, while others need small ones (e.g. Bouma, 1989, 1997). Various techniques have been defined for bulk density, including methods where some soil is excavated and weighed while the excavated volume is determined by filling the cavity with sand or with water contained inside a plastic liner (Blake and Hartge, 1986).
- We advocate use of K3 simulation techniques for well-defined soil types and agroecological zones. It is not possible to extend this type of simple characterization to all soils but regression analysis can relate complex soil characteristics, needed for the simulations, to simple ones that can be measured directly. Such relations are referred to as pedotransfer functions (e.g. Vereecken *et al.*, 1986; Bouma, 1989, 1997; Tietje and Tapkenhinrichs, 1993). Pedotransfer functions for hydraulic characteristics have been developed for major soils in The Netherlands (Wosten *et al.*, 1994). They require data on bulk density, organic matter content and texture, which can be obtained rather easily.
- Properties of any given soil type vary greatly following different management practices. A 'genoform' of a given soil type describes the natural soil profile but various 'phenoforms' can result from different types of management (Droogers and Bouma, 1997). We advocate definition of grassland phenoforms for major soil units by field measurements and use of simulation techniques to express their dynamic behaviour in terms of yields in different years and the associated water and nutrient regimes.

Soil Chemical Attributes

Soil chemical attributes are related to soil fertility, which in turn is a function of the parent material and the age of soils. Soil fertility is not a single parameter and is related not only to chemical but also to biological and physical characteristics. The importance of chemical data for grassland soils depends on the intensity of the production system. For intensive systems, soil chemical data, together with fertilizer experiments, are necessary to amend nutrient deficiencies. However, this is not an option for more extensive systems and certainly not for native grasslands or rangelands.

Sampling and pre-treatment

Soil analytical data are obtained by sampling a field or a soil profile. Samples are usually dried, ground and sieved. From this, a suitable subsample is taken for analyses.

Variation in the analytical results of samples from the same field are caused by horizontal and vertical field heterogeneity, changes caused by pre-treatment of the sample, and analytical errors, including subsampling.

Field heterogeneity

Most variation in analytical data is caused by variation in the field. In the horizontal direction there are often pronounced differences in chemical and physical properties, even in fields without obviously different soil types. This can occur at very short distances, as demonstrated by Schuffelen et al. (1945), who measured extractable K values for 59 samples of 10×10 cm taken from within 1 m². The highest value obtained was twice and the lowest value was half the mean value. The same or greater heterogeneity can occur at larger scales. Thus an adequate number of samples must be collected and analysed, both to estimate the mean accurately and to describe the variability within the field (Table 12.1).

Vertical variation in soil chemical composition can be expected. Cationic nutrients are usually located mainly in the surface layer, where the cation exchange capacity (CEC) is usually higher. For anions such as nitrate, sulphate and chloride the situation is usually different, since these anions are rather mobile and can be moved downwards by rain or, in dry conditions, can be concentrated in the upper soil layers due to upward movement of water. Sampling from 0 to 5 cm can give very different values compared with 0–10 or 0–15 cm.

These examples demonstrate the difficulty of taking a sample that is representative for an area or profile. There is no standard procedure

Table 12.1. Data for standard and detailed sampling of two different fields in Illinois (USA) (Peck and Melsted, 1967).

Soil test	Units	Data	Mansfield field Standard sampling	Mansfield field Detailed sampling	Urbana field Standard sampling	Urbana field Detailed sampling
pH	–	Mean	6.59	6.55	6.37	6.21
		CV (%)	2.8	0.44	1.35	0.43
P	mg kg⁻¹	Mean	14.35	14.72	10.96	13.73
		CV (%)	13.6	4.75	12.1	3.10
K	mg kg⁻¹	Mean	130.3	133.5	123.2	125.2
		CV (%)	2.59	0.60	3.86	1.08

applicable to all soils and conditions. Points to keep in mind when sampling are as follows:

- A series of cores should be taken according to some systematic random pattern.
- Separate soil cores or replicate sets of composite samples should be analysed to determine statistical and agronomic significance of results of the field composite sample.
- The number of soil cores to be bulked depends on the heterogeneity of the soil, the degree of accuracy desired, and the element to be determined. For example, from a study of four apparently uniform fields, Leo (1963) calculated that from two to over 500 cores were necessary for a representative composite sample with a coefficient of variation (CV) of 10% of the mean. The optimum number of cores varied depending on the element (Mg, 2–89; N, 11–569; P, 6–321; K, 28–193) and on the method of fertilization. More cores were needed where fertilizers had been heavily banded for several years.
- There is a possible need for taking separate composite samples to represent different horizons of soil profiles or root zones, or else different parts of the sampling area with different soil types (stratified sampling).
- Contamination of soil samples by crop residues, manure and newly applied fertilizer must be avoided and also atypical areas near fertilizer loading points, borders, gates, watering troughs, etc.

In The Netherlands a minimum of 50–60 cores are taken for grassland on a maximum area of 2 ha. However, sampling at this intensity may be impossible under extensive conditions. The cores must be evenly distributed, avoiding irregularities in the field. If fewer cores are taken the standard deviation (SD) will increase considerably, whereas taking more cores than 50–60 has much less effect on the SD. For example, when one field was sampled, the CV declined as the number of cores increased from 5 to 150, as follows: 5 (CV 40%), 10 (28%), 20 (23%), 30 (20%), 40 (16%), 50 (15%) and 150 cores (8%). The standard sampling depth in The Netherlands is 0–5 cm (though this will be increased to 10 cm in the near future) for grassland and 0–30 cm for arable land.

Sample pre-treatment
The sample taken in the field should be dried at 40°C as quickly as possible to stop microbiological processes; it should then be ground or crushed (to a fraction < 2 mm), sieved (to remove roots and gravel), mixed and stored until analysis (ISO 11464)[1]. A higher drying temperature may lead to

---

[1] ISO numbers refer to publications listed in the References section and obtainable from the Sales Department, International Standards Organization, Central Secretariat 1, Rue de Varembé, PO Box 56, CH 1211 Genève, Switzerland.

chemical conversions. Even at a drying temperature of 30–40°C, changes in inorganic N and exchangeable Mn concentrations will occur (Houba *et al.*, 1994). Ovens should preferably have forced air ventilation and soil should be spread out in a layer not thicker than 2–3 cm. Soil structure is destroyed with grinding and sieving and this could have consequences for extractable nutrients (Houba *et al.*, 1993). Dried samples are preferred for chemical analysis, because subsampling is easier and samples can be stored more conveniently. However, even storage of dry soil samples under laboratory conditions can influence some chemical soil properties, especially when weak unbuffered extractions are used (Houba and Novozamsky, 1998). Special precautions should be taken in preparing soil samples for trace element analysis to avoid contamination of the sample. For the determination of carbonates and organic matter, or where a small subsample is being used for analysis, a second grinding down to 250 µm is needed to obtain a representative subsample (ISO 11464).

Since soils very often contain fractions > 2 mm (gravel, stones, etc.) the proportion of this fraction in the whole sample should be measured. It is then possible to express subsequent analyses on the basis of the fraction < 2 mm or on the basis of the original complete soil sample.

Subsampling and analytical errors
Additional sources of errors introduced in the laboratory are small compared with those caused by subsampling and, in particular, field sampling. For proper subsampling the complete dry sample should be spread out on a paper and mixed carefully, avoiding dust formation. Then the sample is quartered and two quarters are mixed again. The process is repeated with these two quarters until the desired subsample size is achieved. It is often possible to reduce the analytical error to 2–3%, while the error due to subsampling may be about 5% and that due to field sampling about 15%. To keep the analytical error as low as possible, every laboratory should introduce measures to check the analytical results by introduction of control reference samples and by participation in national and international inter-laboratory comparisons (Houba *et al.*, 1996a). The between-laboratory error is nearly always higher than the within-laboratory error (Table 12.2).

Chemical Methods

Soil chemical data can be a very useful tool in many types of grassland research. When an experiment is being planned all aspects of any proposed analyses (sampling, pre-treatment, choice of methods, etc.) should be discussed with a person with general knowledge of chemical soil and plant analysis and who knows the capabilities of the laboratory concerned. Too often, too many analyses for the wrong elements are routinely requested.

Table 12.2. Between- and within-laboratory variation for some chemical parameters estimated in soil samples.

Parameter/ element	Units	Between-laboratory variation			Within-laboratory variation		
		Median	MAD[a]	n[b]	Median	MAD[a]	n[b]
Total N	g kg^{-1}	2.78	0.11	188	2.57	0.05	4
Total C	g kg^{-1}	32.4	2.69	157	33.8	1.05	4
Total P	mg kg^{-1}	1300	44	189	1220	55	4
pH-H$_2$O	–	7.50	0.10	249	7.49	0.06	4
CaCO$_3$	%	9.61	0.79	133	8.30	0.05	4
fraction < 2 μm	%	26.0	1.90	80	26.6	0.60	4
CEC (1 M ammonium acetate)	cmol + kg^{-1}	19.7	1.90	101	21.7	0.89	4

[a]Median of Absolute Deviations
[b]Number of independent determinations

Soil characteristics

The Soil Science Society of America Handbook (Sparks, 1996) is recommended as a guide to standard analytical procedures. Also in recent years a number of useful international standardized soil procedures (sampling, chemical, physical and biological methods) have been developed by the International Organization for Standardization (ISO) in Switzerland. Soil characteristics, such as granular composition or particle size analysis (ISO 11277), organic matter (ISO 14235) and the potential CEC (CEC estimated at a buffered pH of 7 or 8) (ISO 13536) are parameters that are more or less stable in time and do not change easily. However, it is important to realize that some determinations are just 'agreed upon' and not necessarily 'correct'. An example is the particle size analysis by hydrometers or pipetting methods, which have been standardized to enable comparisons of different data sets. For the determination of particle size composition, organic matter is usually oxidized using a mild oxidant, e.g. H$_2$O$_2$, which is assumed not to have any influence on mineral particles. Dissolving of cementing agents and carbonates is not always done, since the acids used for this purpose could influence certain mineral particles present in certain types of soils. In particular, the presence of carbonates will have a large influence on the quantity of mineral fractions of certain sizes. Although the granular composition is performed on a subsample < 2 mm, earlier milling or crushing could influence the final data.

For the determination of organic matter, two basic methods are used: (i) directly, via ignition of the soil at elevated temperatures and determination of the loss-on-ignition; and (ii) indirectly, via the determination of the C content of the soil and recalculation of C into organic matter by multiplication by an empirical factor (often 2) (ISO 14235).

The direct method has the advantage of being quick but the disadvantage is the contribution to the loss in weight by other components than organic matter (water bound to clay minerals and oxides, carbonates at higher ignition temperatures, salts, etc.). In principle, this method is very applicable to soils not containing high quantities of clay minerals, oxides and carbonates. In all other cases correction factors have to be estimated empirically.

For the measurement of soil pH-water, 1 M KCl or 0.01 M $CaCl_2$ is used as equilibrium solution. The preferred solution for most soils is 0.01 M $CaCl_2$ since the salt concentrations are best compared with the mean salt concentration in soil solution. Moreover, Ca^{2+} is the main cation in most agricultural soils. Since pH is an intensity parameter, even a volume-to-volume extraction could be used, since the extraction ratio has almost no effect on the estimated value.

Nutritional parameters

For estimation of chemical soil fertility status, there is an overwhelming number of extraction procedures used all over the world. In principle, every extracting solution is relevant for estimation of the nutritional status of soils when the relationship between the crop yield or quality parameter versus the concentration in the soils for the element under study is known. Field fertilizer experiments should be the basis of the established relationships. Fertilizer recommendation systems, developed and tested in certain areas having specific soil types, crops and climatological conditions, cannot be used for other areas, soil types and crops without testing under field conditions.

Almost every country in the world has developed its own methods for determination of nutritional parameters. The extracting agents used include strong acidic or alkaline solutions, complexing agents, concentrated buffered and unbuffered salt solutions, weak unbuffered salt solutions and even water. Each method is relevant for fertilizer recommendation purposes when tested, preferably in field experiments. The weak unbuffered extractants have the advantage that the amount of nutrients estimated is a better measure of the available nutrient that can be taken up by a crop directly and easily. The more concentrated extractants always dissolve part of the less directly available buffer of nutrients and elements present in organic matter, minerals and salts.

Recently, the use of 0.01 M $CaCl_2$ as a standard soil extractant was proposed. This solution estimates the availability of elements at the pH existing in the soil. From a laboratory point of view this extractant has many advantages: soil chemical basis, costs of chemicals, simple single procedure, simultaneous detection of several nutrients and elements, etc. (Houba *et al.*, 1996b; Van Erp *et al.*, 1998).

The Soil Biota

The composition of the soil biota is extremely variable, with typical biomass ranges for the major components in temperate grassland being $10–90 \times 10^3$ g m^{-2} for plant roots, 200–500 g m^{-2} for fungi, 100–200 g m^{-2} for bacteria, 0–200 g m^{-2} for actinomycetes, and 50–250 g m^{-2} for invertebrates in soils where lumbricid earthworms are abundant. The soil microbial biomass largely controls the rates of turnover and mineralization of organic substrates in terrestrial ecosystems, while the fauna significantly influence these processes by ingesting and turning over microbial biomass and organic matter and by physically altering the soil environment.

Soil bacteria are mostly adsorbed on to soil particles and tend to occur in small soil pores (< 10 µm). As is the case for all soil microorganisms, their distribution and abundance are very patchy, reflecting the distribution of roots and other organic resources. Soil bacteria play a major part in the decomposition of organic residues, non-symbiotic N_2 fixation (*Azotobacter*, *Bacillus* and *Clostridium*) and symbiotic N_2 fixation (*Rhizobium*, *Bradyrhizobium*). Others are plant pathogens (*Agrobacterium*, *Pseudomonas*, *Erwinia*, *Acrinomycetes*), sulphur oxidizers (*Thiobacillus*), nitrifiers (*Nitrosomonas* and *Nitrobacter*) or denitrifiers (*Pseudomonas* and *Alcaligenes*).

Fungi generally dominate the soil microbial biomass, especially in acidic soils, their most important role being the decomposition of organic matter. Some (e.g. *Rhizoctonia*, *Verticillium* and *Fusarium*) can be important plant parasites, while those that form symbiotic mycorrhizal associations with plant roots (vesicular arbuscular mycorrhizae, VAM) have a very important role in regulating nutrient uptake, disease resistance, water relations and plant growth.

Most actinomycetes are free-living saprophytes involved in the degradation of very recalcitrant polymers such as chitin, cellulose and hemicellulose; some are plant pathogenic. Algae, being photoautotrophic, are largely restricted to the soil surface and have a key role in the primary colonization of bare soil. Some are capable of symbiotic and non-symbiotic N_2 fixation.

The soil fauna is abundant and diverse, with a wide range of feeding habits. Detritivores feeding on dung, decaying organic matter and associated microflora usually comprise 60–90% of the invertebrate biomass in grassland; herbivores normally constitute less than 30% and predators/parasites less than 20%. Soil invertebrates range from less than 10 µm for the smallest protozoa to several metres in length for giant Australian earthworms. They can be assigned to three broad categories based on size:

microfauna (mainly protozoa and nematodes), mesofauna (enchytraeid worms and smaller arthropods) and macrofauna (earthworms, molluscs and larger arthropods), which correlate roughly with the degree to which they interact with their habitat. Microfauna inhabit water films; mesofauna inhabit air-filled pore spaces and are largely restricted to existing pores; while macrofauna can create their own spaces by burrowing and thus influence soil structure.

The distribution of soil animals is highly variable in time and space. Peak densities tend to occur in spring and autumn in temperate grasslands and during the wet season in tropical grasslands. The majority of soil arthropods occupy the top 5–10 cm layer of undisturbed temperate soils, with surface concentration tending to be marked in podzolic soils and less so in mull soils, where the organic matter is more evenly distributed in the profile. Nematodes tend to have a greater depth distribution, reflecting root depth. The majority of earthworms occur in the top 10–20 cm of undisturbed soils but deep-burrowing species can be found to depths of several metres. Seasonal changes occur in the vertical distribution patterns of most soil invertebrate groups, with pronounced downward shifts to escape drought or cold.

Measuring soil microbial biomass

Microbial population density and biomass may be assessed directly or indirectly. A representative number of soil samples is taken and these are combined, mixed and sieved to obtain a homogeneous sample for study. Up to 20 core samples c. 3 cm in diameter and 20 cm deep per site or treatment plot are normally required. Comparisons between sites or experimental treatments are often based on one or two annual samplings (usually in spring and autumn in temperate sites), but much more frequent sampling (several times per month) is required for detailed study of population dynamics.

Direct counting and culturing methods

Bacterial cells in small volumes of soil suspension spread thinly on a glass slide and stained with acridine orange can be counted directly by fluorescent microscopy (Schinner et al., 1996), while fungal hyphae can be rapidly counted by the membrane filtration techniques (Parkinson, 1982). Direct counting methods do not discriminate between viable and non-viable bacterial cells, while total fungal hyphal length can significantly overestimate live fungal biomass unless an appropriate correction factor is applied. The extent of VAM colonization can be assessed by light-microscopic examination of root segments cleared with KOH and stained with trypan blue (Phillips and Hayman, 1970).

Plate count techniques involve incubating dilute soil suspensions mixed with nutrient agar in Petri dishes, and estimating the number of viable bacteria on the basis of subsequent colony development. These techniques are very selective as only a fraction of the soil community can be readily cultured.

Most probable number (MPN) dilution methods are often used for estimating numbers of physiologically similar organisms with particular growth characteristics, such as algae, protozoa, rhizobia and bacteria associated with the N cycle, based on the detection of specific qualitative attributes of the microorganisms of interest (Woomer, 1994).

While the above techniques are valuable tools, they are usually time consuming and technically demanding, and the biomass estimates derived from them are difficult to relate to microbial activity in the field.

Indirect methods

A variety of biochemical techniques is available for estimating microbial biomass indirectly, the most commonly used being chloroform fumigation and incubation (CFI) and chloroform fumigation and extraction (CFE). CFI involves killing living soil biomass by fumigation with chloroform (Jenkinson, 1988). The dead biomass becomes a substrate for organisms that survive fumigation or are added in a soil inoculum, and the increase in CO_2 evolution that occurs when the fumigated sample is incubated can be related to the size of the microbial biomass. The ratio of biomass C values derived from direct count estimates of biovolume to those derived from CFI range from 0.86 to 1.25 for temperate arable and grassland soils in the UK (Powlson, 1994).

The CFE method is considered to be more robust than CFI, and more reliable over a greater range of soil pH (Sparling and West, 1988). Fumigated and non-fumigated control samples are extracted with 0.5 M K_2SO_4, and the organic C contents of extracts are determined. Microbial biomass C is determined by difference, and the method also allows microbial biomass values for N, P and S to be determined.

Other indirect methods include measurement of substrate-induced respiration (SIR) and ergosterol content. SIR is determined by incubating soil samples amended with glucose and measuring the maximum initial respiratory response, which is proportional to the amount of microbial C present in the sample (Anderson and Domsch, 1978). A conversion factor derived from calibration with CFI allows values to be converted to mg biomass C. Ergosterol is the predominant sterol of most fungi, and the ergosterol content of soil provides an indirect measure of fungal biomass (Parkinson and Coleman, 1991).

Bioassay methods such as CFI, CFE and SIR do not differentiate between dormant and active microbial biomass, nor between bacterial and fungal biomass. They can give misleading results when the organic matter content of the sample is high, when soil is waterlogged and when pH is very low (Powlson, 1994). However, they are suitable for comparative purposes and for modelling labile C and nutrient turnover (Jenkinson and Parry, 1989).

Novel methods

Recent approaches to characterizing soil microbial communities include metabolic profiling and BIOLOG plating (Garland and Mills, 1991), fatty acid profiling (Cavigelli *et al.*, 1995), immunological methods (Schloter *et al.*, 1995) and molecular techniques involving specific DNA and RNA probes or more broad-scale analysis of community DNA (Tiedje *et al.*, 1999). Molecular techniques are particularly promising in relation to the study of microbial biodiversity and community response to environmental stress.

Estimating soil invertebrate populations

There is no single procedure that will give reliable estimates for the populations of all groups of soil fauna. The following account considers the most widely used sampling and extraction methods; further information may be found in Southwood (1978), Edwards (1991) and Dunger and Fiedler (1997).

Sampling

The numbers of samples, their distribution and size vary with the group being studied. For microfauna, small core samples (2.5 cm diameter) are preferred, and for mesofauna 5 cm diameter samples are often used. Samples for macrofauna generally range from 10 cm diameter cores for smaller insect larvae up to 25×25 cm quadrats for the larger lumbricid earthworms. Samples are normally taken at random or in a stratified random manner from within the study area. A less formal method of ensuring representative sampling is to take samples at intervals following a W-shaped pattern. This approach is often taken for nematodes, which tend to be very patchy in distribution. A sampling depth of 5–10 cm is usually adequate for arthropods in temperate soils; but for earthworms, nematodes in arid soils and other deep-dwelling forms, sampling to depths of 25–50 cm may be necessary.

The number of samples per site is frequently a compromise between what is desirable and what can be handled. For microfauna, large numbers of samples are usually taken, pooled and subsampled for extraction; for mesofauna and macrofauna, samples are usually treated separately. A useful guideline is that the number of samples should be such that the standard error does not exceed 5–10% of the mean population estimate, depending on the level of precision required. Simple core samplers made from metal tubing sharpened at one end may be adequate in light organic soils, but usually more elaborate corers designed to minimize sample disturbance and compaction are required.

Soil protozoa are counted by microscopic observation using dried soil smears, soil agar films, water–soil suspensions, staining and fixation, membrane filtration, or MPN estimation (Ingham, 1994). Larger invertebrates such as earthworms, larger insect larvae and myriapods may be sampled by hand-sorting blocks of soil, which are excavated with a spade or purpose-made metal sampler. Mesofauna and smaller macrofauna are not efficiently sampled by hand-sorting and must be extracted using appropriate techniques.

Spatial heterogeneity often complicates the application of standard methods of data analysis to soil biological parameters. However, recently developed techniques such as geostatistics allow heterogeneity and the underlying reasons for it to be systematically explored (Stein *et al.*, 1992).

Extraction

Mechanical methods such as sieving, flotation, sedimentation, differential wetting and centrifugation may be used singly or in combination to separate animals from soil. Mechanical methods may be the only option for heavy clay and arid soils; however, they tend to be laborious and time consuming, animals may be damaged during extraction, and it can be difficult to distinguish between animals that were alive or dead at the time of sampling.

With behavioural or dynamic methods, animals are induced to leave the substrate under the influence of stimuli such as heat, desiccation, flooding or repellent chemicals. Dynamic methods are easier to use than mechanical and animals are recovered in good condition; however, only active stages are extracted, and the efficiency of extraction varies with group, soil conditions and season. Dry extraction involves heating the soil sample from above and collecting the animals that leave the sample as it dries out. Variants of this approach are widely used for soil arthropod extraction and are most efficient when steep temperature and humidity gradients are maintained between the top and bottom of the sample. Wet extraction involves immersion of the sample in water with or without heating, and works well for animals such as nematodes, enchytraeid worms and dipterous larvae, which are susceptible to desiccation so cannot be recovered by dry extraction. Dilute solutions of formalin applied to the soil surface can effectively expel larger earthworm species with well-defined burrows from the soil, but are less efficient for sampling smaller endogenic species. Large numbers of earthworms can also be expelled from soil by applying an electrical current through an electrode powered by a portable generator. The problem of delimiting the area sampled has been addressed in the design of the octet machine (Thielemann, 1986), which can give results comparable to the formalin method under favourable conditions.

The surface fauna

The above-ground invertebrate biomass is normally small compared with that in the soil and litter (Curry, 1994), but may be relevant to improved understanding of the soil community. Pitfall trapping is a useful way of collecting a wide range of surface-active invertebrates where estimates of activity rather than absolute abundance are adequate. Refuge traps of the 'defined area' type placed on the soil surface provide a reliable and non-destructive means of estimating slug population density (Ferguson et al., 1989). Quantitative surveys of the fauna on the surface and in low vegetation are generally conducted by means of portable suction samplers (Dietrick, 1961). The efficiency of sampling can be increased by enclosing the area to be sampled within a tent and then removing the animals by suction (e.g. the 'quick trap' method; Turnbull and Nicholls, 1966).

When studying soil insects it may be necessary to know the numbers of adults emerging from a given area within a particular period of time. Positively phototactic animals (mainly *Diptera* and *Hymenoptera*) can be sampled by means of conical or pyramid-shaped emergence traps covered with dark cloth and fitted with transparent collecting containers at the apex.

Assessing the Role of Organisms in Soil Processes

Chapter 13 gives details of methods for quantifying microbially mediated N transformations.

Organic matter decomposition

Soil respiration, measured as CO_2 output or O_2 uptake, is a useful indicator of microbial activity associated with degradation of organic matter. Soil respiration can be measured in the field, where results tend to be very variable and do not distinguish between microbial and plant respiration, or in the laboratory using sieved soil. Litter breakdown rates are also good indicators of soil biological activity and can give valuable information on system response to disturbance. Nylon mesh bags containing known mass of leaf litter are placed on the soil surface or buried in the soil; bags are recovered at intervals, the remaining litter mass is determined and the rate of decomposition is assessed on the basis of ash-free dry mass loss over time. Mesh size of *c.* 1 mm is usually used, but this will exclude most macrofauna and decomposition rates may be underestimated in habitats where macrofauna are abundant. If larger meshes are used there is a risk of litter fragments being lost, thus leading to overestimation of decomposition rates.

Decomposition rates are strongly influenced by the nature of the litter and by climate (Swift et al., 1979) and these influences need to be taken into account when planning litterbag experiments.

Food webs and nutrient cycling

Conceptual models of detrital food webs provide a useful tool for evaluating the contribution of different groups of soil organisms to nutrient cycling (Hunt *et al.*, 1987). The main taxa are assigned to trophic groups based on their feeding habits, and C and nutrient utilization by the main groups together with rates of transfer between groups are calculated (Hutchinson and King, 1980; Curry, 1994). There are many sources of error associated with the construction of whole ecosystem nutrient budgets based on sometimes questionable assumptions about feeding relationships and food chain transfer efficiencies.

Stable isotope techniques offer potential for more directly and precisely estimating nutrient cycling among key groups of organisms. Studies involving ^{15}N-enriched litter have provided valuable information on the contribution of earthworms to N turnover (Blair *et al.*, 1995b), while differences in the natural abundance of ^{15}N between legumes and non-legumes (Schmidt *et al.*, 1997) and of ^{13}C between C_3 and C_4 plants (Martin *et al.*, 1992) offer novel methods for identifying the sources of C and N assimilated by earthworms and other organisms and for the quantification of C and N fluxes in the soil.

Microcosm and mesocosm studies

Food web studies do not take account of non-feeding interactions between soil biota and their habitat; much additional information can be gained from manipulative experiments carried out under controlled conditions. Microcosm experiments are often conducted in the laboratory using small containers and highly simplified ecosystems. An example of a relatively complex microcosm study is that of the interactive effects of bacteria, fungi, and bacterial- and fungal-feeding nematodes on N cycling and plant growth in blue grama grass (Ingham *et al.*, 1985).

Experiments carried out under field conditions in enclosed 'mesocosms', which are partially permeable to their surroundings while retaining the complexity of undisturbed soil, may give information that is more directly applicable to natural ecosystems (Odum, 1984). The impact of different groups of biota, for example, can be studied in intact soil monoliths, which are defaunated by deep freezing and replaced in the field wrapped in nets of various mesh size to allow free gas and water exchange with the surrounding environment. By varying the mesh size, access of fauna can be restricted to certain size classes or prevented entirely.

Other forms of manipulation could include use of biocides to selectively eliminate or suppress different elements of the biota. However, the biocides available are not entirely selective and none have effects that are strictly limited to their target group (Ingham, 1985). Blair *et al.* (1995a) reduced earthworm numbers in some field enclosures by electro-shocking and increased the density in others by adding worms as a means of evaluating their impact.

Impact on soil properties

Methods for studying interrelationships between soil biota and soil structure were extensively reviewed in Brussaard and Kooistra (1993). Valuable techniques for studying effects at the microsite level include microscopic examination of thin resin-impregnated soil sections (Fitzpatrick, 1993), which can be combined with fluorescent staining to study the distribution of organisms associated with particular features (Altemuller and Van Vliet-Lanoe, 1990). Techniques for studying the role of organisms in stabilization of soil structure at the level of smaller aggregates and biospore linings include optical and fluorescent microscopy, scanning electron microscopy including EDAX, transmission electron microscopy and computer-aided tomography (Oades, 1993).

Rhizotrons facilitate non-destructive study of root-related processes by means of glass-walled observation galleries (Lussenhop and Fogel, 1993). Data collection and analysis are labour intensive, but video recording and image analysis techniques can greatly improve the quantity and value of the information obtained. Rhizotrons are expensive to install and mini-rhizotrons offer greater flexibility but less opportunity for direct observation. However, this could improve with the availability of mini-rhizotron video cameras (Lussenhop and Fogel, 1993).

Important research issues relating to macro-invertebrates include their impact on macroporosity, transport processes, aggregate formation and stability, and their role in soil and organic matter mixing and in soil C and nutrient storage and depletion (Blair *et al.*, 1995b; Tomlin *et al.*, 1995). Techniques for studying preferential flows of air, water and solutes in macroporous soils were reviewed by Edwards *et al.* (1993) and Tomlin *et al.* (1995). The structure of earthworm burrows may be investigated by careful (and tedious) excavation (Ligthart *et al.*, 1993; McKenzie and Dexter, 1993), and by non-destructive but very expensive techniques such as X-ray computed tomography (Joschko *et al.*, 1993) and magnetic resonance imaging (Ligthart *et al.*, 1993).

Negative impacts on sward productivity

Significant damage to grassland swards may be caused by a wide range of soil-dwelling invertebrates (Curry, 1994). Examples include: root-feeding nematodes in prairie grasslands; slugs, which can affect ley establishment and clover persistence in temperate soils; chafer larvae such as grass grub, which causes widespread damage to New Zealand pasture; and seed-harvesting ants, which can significantly reduce the legume content of semiarid grasslands. Improved temperate pastures are also susceptible to diseases caused by soil-borne pathogens, notably foliar diseases in ryegrass, root rot in grasses and legumes caused by *Fusarium* spp. and clover rot caused by *Sclerotinia trifoliorum* (Priestley *et al.*, 1988).

A common method of assessing the impact of pests or disease is to eliminate the organisms of interest by means of pesticides in glasshouse or field plot experiments and to assess the effects on herbage yield and quality by comparing treated with untreated controls. However, the effects of pesticides are not confined to the target organisms and it is possible that at least part of the response to pesticides may be due to other factors, such as a temporary increase in the supply of mineral N resulting from the killing of organisms such as earthworms (Davidson *et al.*, 1979).

Conclusion

This chapter has discussed several methods of soil analysis and particular considerations on their use. As has been stressed, there are many methods and often certain ones are preferred by different laboratories in different countries. A similar approach can be found in a special issue of the *Australian Journal of Experimental Agriculture* edited by Sparrow *et al.* (1998).

References

Altemuller, H.J. and Van Vliet-Lanoe, B. (1990) Soil thin section fluorescence microscopy. In: Douglas, L.A. (ed.) *Soil Micromorphology*. Elsevier, Amsterdam, pp. 565–579.

Amoozegar, A. and Warrick, A.W. (1986) Hydraulic conductivity of saturated soils: field methods. In: Klute, A. (ed.) *Methods of Soil Analysis. Part I. Agronomy 9.* American Society of Agronomy, Madison, Wisconsin, pp. 735–770.

Anderson, J.P.E. and Domsch, K.H. (1978) A physiological method for the quantitative measurement of microbial biomass in soils. *Soil Biology and Biochemistry* 10, 215–221.

Blair, J.M., Bohlen, P.J., Edwards, C.A., Stiner, B.R., McCartney, D.A. and Allen, M.F. (1995a) Manipulation of earthworm populations in field experiments in agroecosystems. *Acta Zoologica Fennica* 196, 48–51.

Blair, J.M., Parmelee, R.W. and Lavelle, P. (1995b) Influences of earthworms on biogeochemistry. In: Hendrix, P.F. (ed.) *Ecology and Biogeography of Earthworms in North America*. Lewis Publishers, Boca Raton, Florida, pp. 127–158.

Blake, G.R. and Hartge, K.H. (1986) Bulk density. In: Klute, A. (ed.) *Methods of Soil Analysis. Part I. Agronomy 9.* American Society of Agronomy, Madison, Wisconsin, pp. 363–375.

Booltink, H.W.G. (1994) Field-scale distributed modelling of bypass flow in a heavily textured soil. *Journal of Hydrology* 163, 65–84.

Bouma, J. (1981) Soil survey interpretation: estimating use-potentials of clay soil under various moisture regimes. *Geoderma* 26, 165–177.

Bouma, J. (1983a) Use of soil survey data to select measurement techniques for hydraulic conductivity. *Agricultural Water Management* 6, 177–190.

Bouma, J. (1983b) Soil behavior under field conditions: differences in perception and their effects on research. *Geoderma* 60, 1–15.

Bouma, J. (1984) Estimating moisture related land qualities for land evaluation. In: *Land Use Planning Techniques and Policies*. Special Publication no. 12, Soil Science Society of America, American Society of Agronomy, Madison, Wisconsin, pp. 61–76.

Bouma, J. (1989) Using soil survey data for quantitative land evaluation. In: Stewart, B.A. (ed.) *Advances in Soil Science 9*. Springer Verlag, New York, pp. 177–213.

Bouma, J. (1991) Influence of soil macroporosity on environmental quality. *Advances in Agronomy* 46, 1–37.

Bouma, J. (1997) Long-term characterization: monitoring and modeling. In: Lal, R., Blum, W.H., Valentin, C. and Stewart, B.A. (eds) *Methods for Assessment of Soil Degradation. Advances in Soil Science*, 18, JCRC Press, Boca Raton, Florida, pp. 337–358.

Bouma, J. and Hoosbeek, M.R. (1996) The contribution and importance of soil scientists in interdisciplinary studies dealing with land. In: Wagenet, R.J. and Bouma, J. (eds) *The Role of Soil Science in Interdisciplinary Research*. Special Publication number 45, Soil Science Society of America, Madison, Wisconsin, pp. 1–15.

Bouwer, H. (1986) Intake rate: cylinder infiltrometer. In: Klute, A. (ed.) *Methods of Soil Analysis. Part I. Agronomy 9*. American Society of Agronomy, Madison, Wisconsin, pp. 825–843.

Brussaard, L. and Kooistra, M.J. (eds) (1993) *Soil Structure and Soil Biota Interrelationships. Geoderma* 56; 57 (1,2) (special issue).

Cassel, D.K. and Klute, A. (1986) Water potential: tensiometry. In: Klute, A. (ed.) *Methods of Soil Analysis. Part I. Agronomy 9*. American Society of Agronomy, Madison, Wisconsin, pp. 563–594.

Cavigelli, M.A., Robertson, G.P. and Klug, M.J. (1995) Fatty acid methyl ester profiles as measures of soil microbial community structure. *Plant and Soil* 170, 99–113.

Curry, J.P. (1994) *Grassland Invertebrates: Ecology, Influence on Soil Fertility and Effects on Plant Growth*. Chapman & Hall, London, 437 pp.

Davidson, R.L., Shackley, A., Wolfe, V.J. and Donelan, M.J. (1979) Anomalous increases in pasture yield after use of insecticides on soil. In: Crosby, T.K. and Pottinger, R.P. (eds.) *Proceedings of the 2nd Australasian Conference on Grassland Invertebrate Ecology*. Government Printer, Wellington, New Zealand, pp. 30–32.

Dekker, L.W. and Ritsema, C.J. (1995) Fingerlike wetting patterns in two water-repellant loam soils. *Journal of Environmental Quality* 24, 324–333.

Dietrick, E.J. (1961) An improved backpack motor fan for suction sampling of insect populations. *Journal of Economic Entomology* 54, 394–395.

Droogers, P. and Bouma, J. (1997) Soil survey input in exploratory modelling of sustainable soil management practices. *Soil Science Society American Journal* 61, 1704–1710.

Droogers, P., Fermont, A. and Bouma, J. (1996) Effects of ecological soil management on workability and trafficability of a loamy soil in the Netherlands. *Geoderma* 73, 131–145.

Droogers, P., Van der Meer, F.B.W. and Bouma, J. (1997) Water accessibility to plant roots in different soil structure occuring in the same soil type. *Plant and Soil* 188, 83–91.

Dunger, W. and Fiedler, H.J. (1997) *Methoden der Bodenbiologie*, 2nd edn. Fischer, Jena, Germany, 539 pp.

Edwards, C.A. (1991) Methods for assessing populations of soil-inhabiting invertebrates. *Agriculture, Ecosystems and Environment* 34, 145–176.

Edwards, W.M., Shipitalo, M.J. and Owens, L.B. (1993) Gas, water and solute transport in soils containing macropores: a review of methodology. *Geoderma* 57, 31–49.

FAO (1983) *Guidelines: Land evaluation for rainfed agriculture*. Soils Bulletin 52. Food and Agriculture Organization, Rome.

Ferguson, C.M., Barratt, B.P. and Jones, P.H. (1989) A new technique for estimating the density of the grey field slug, *Deroceras reticulatum*. In: Henderson, I.F. (ed.) *Slugs and Snails in World Agriculture*. British Crop Protection Council, Farnham, Monograph No. 41, pp. 331–336.

Fitzpatrick, E.A. (1993) *Soil Microscopy and Microbiology*. Wiley, Chichester, UK, 304 pp.

Gardner, W.H. (1986) Water content. In: Klute, A. (ed.) *Methods of Soil Analysis. Part I. Physical and Mineralogical Methods. 2nd edn. Monograph 9*. American Society of Agronomy/Soil Science Society of America, Madison, Wisconsin, pp. 493–545.

Garland, J.L. and Mills, A.L. (1991) Classification and characterisation of heterogeneous microbial communities on the basis of patterns of community-level sole-carbon source utilisation. *Applied Environmental Microbiology* 57, 2351–2359.

Houba, V.J.G. and Novozamsky, I. (1998) Influence of storage time and temperature of air-dried soils on pH and extractable nutrients using 0.01 mol/L $CaCl_2$. *Fresenius Journal of Analytical Chemistry* 360, 362–365.

Houba, V.J.G., Chardon, W.J. and Roelse, K. (1993) Influence of grinding of soil on apparent chemical composition. *Communications in Soil Science and Plant Analysis* 24, 1591–1602.

Houba, V.J.G., Novozamsky, I. and Van der Lee, J.J. (1994) Aspects of pre-treatment of soils for inorganic chemical analysis. *Química Analítica* 13, S94–S99.

Houba, V.J.G., Uittenbogaard, J. and Pellen, P. (1996a) Wageningen Evaluating Programmes for Analytical Laboratories (WEPAL), organization and purpose. *Communications in Soil Science and Plant Analysis* 27, 421–431.

Houba, V.J.G., Lexmond, Th.M., Novozamsky, I. and Van der Lee, J.J. (1996b) State of the art and future developments of soil analysis for bioavailability assessment. *Science of the Total Environment* 178, 21–28.

Hunt, H.W., Coleman, D.C., Ingham, E.R., Ingham, R.E., Elliott, E.T., Moore, J.C., Rose, S.L., Reid, C.P.P. and Morley, C.R. (1987) The detrital food web in a short-grass prairie. *Biology and Fertility of Soils* 3, 57–68.

Hutchinson, K.J. and King, K.L. (1980) The effects of sheep stocking level on invertebrate abundance, biomass and energy utilization in a temperate, sown grassland. *Journal of Applied Ecology* 17, 369–387.

Ingham, E.R. (1994) Protozoa. In: Weaver, P.W. *et al.* (eds) *Methods of Soil Analysis, Part 2. Microbiological and Biochemical Properties.* Soil Science Society of America, Madison, Wisconsin, pp. 491–515.

Ingham, R.E. (1985) Review of the effects of 12 selected biocides on target and non-target soil organisms. *Crop Protection* 4, 3–32.

Ingham, R.E., Trofymow, J.A., Ingham, E.R. and Coleman, D.C. (1985) Interactions of bacteria, fungi and their nematode grazers: effects on nutrient cycling and plant growth. *Ecological Monographs* 55, 119–140.

ISO 11277 *Soil quality – Determination of particle size distribution of mineral soils.* International Standards Organization, Geneva, Switzerland.

ISO 11464 *Soil quality – Pretreatment of samples for physico-chemical analyses.* International Standards Organization, Geneva, Switzerland.

ISO 13536 *Soil quality – Determination of the potential cation exchange capacity and exchangeable cations using barium chloride solution buffered at pH = 8.* International Standards Organization, Geneva, Switzerland.

ISO 14235 *Soil quality – Determination of organic carbon in soil by sulfochromic determination.* International Standards Organization, Geneva, Switzerland.

Jenkinson, D.S. (1988) Determination of microbial biomass carbon and nitrogen in soil. In: Wilson, J.R. (ed.) *Advances in Nitrogen Cycling in Agricultural Ecosystems.* CAB International, Wallingford, UK, pp. 368–386.

Jenkinson, D.S. and Parry, L.C. (1989) The nitrogen cycle in the Broadbalk wheat experiment: a model for the turnover of nitrogen through the soil microbial biomass. *Soil Biology and Biochemistry* 21, 535–541.

Joschko, M., Müller, P.C., Kotzke, K., Döhring, W. and Larink, O. (1993) Earthworm burrow system development assessed by means of X-ray computed tomography. *Geoderma* 56, 209–221.

Klute, A. (1986) *Methods of Soil Analysis. Part I. Physical and mineralogical methods,* 2nd edn. Monograph 9, American Society of Agronomy/Soil Science Society of America, Madison, Wisconsin, 485 pp.

Klute, A. and Dirksen, C. (1986) Hydraulic conductivity and diffusivity: laboratory methods. In: Klute, A. (ed.) *Methods of Soil Analysis. Agronomy 9.* American Society of Agronomy, Madison, Wisconsin, pp. 687–732.

Landon, J.R. (1991) *Booker Tropical Soil Manual.* Longman Scientific and Technical, New York, 520 pp.

Leo, M.W.M. (1963) Heterogeneity of soil sampling. *Journal of Agriculture and Food Chemistry* 11, 432–434.

Ligthart, T., Peek, G.J.W. and Taber, E.T. (1993) A method for the three-dimensional mapping of earthworm burrow systems. *Geoderma* 57, 129–141.

Lussenhop, J. and Fogel, R. (1993) Observing soil biota *in situ. Geoderma* 56, 25–36.

Martin, A., Balesdent, J. and Mariotti, A. (1992) Earthworm diet related to soil organic matter dynamics through ^{13}C measurements. *Oecologia* 91, 23–29.

McKenzie, B.M. and Dexter, A.R. (1993) Size and orientation of burrows made by the earthworms *Aporrectodea rosea* and *A. caliginosa. Geoderma* 56, 233–241.

Oades, J.M. (1993) The role of biology in the formation, stabilization and degradation of soil structure. *Geoderma* 56, 377–400.

Odum, E.P. (1984) The mesocosm. *BioScience* 34, 558–562.

Parkinson, D. (1982) Filamentous fungi. In: Page, A.L., Miller, R.H. and Keeney, D.R. (eds) *Methods of Soil Analysis,* part 2. American Society of Agronomy/Soil Science Society of America, Madison, Wisconsin, pp. 949–968.

Parkinson, D. and Coleman, D.C. (1991) Microbial populations, activity and bio-
mass. *Agriculture, Ecosystems and Environment* 34, 3–33.
Peck, T.R. and Melsted, S.W. (1967) Field sampling for soil testing. In: Stelley, M.
(ed.) *Soil Testing and Plant Analysis. 1. Soil testing.* Special Publication Series
No. 2, Soil Science Society of America, Madison, Wisconsin, pp. 25–35.
Peterson, A.E. and Bubenzer, G.D. (1986) Intake rate: sprinkler infiltrometer.
In: Klute, A. (ed.) *Methods of Soil Analysis. Agronomy 9.* American Society of
Agronomy, Madison, Wisconsin, pp. 845–867.
Phillips, J.M. and Hayman, J.D. (1970) Improved procedures for clearing roots
and staining parasitic and vesicular–arbuscular mycorrhizal fungi for rapid
assessment of infection. *Transactions of the British Mycological Society* 55,
158–161.
Powlson, D.S. (1994) The soil microbial biomass: before, beyond and back. In:
Ritz, K., Digton, J. and Giller, K.E. (eds) *Beyond the Biomass.* Wiley, Chichester,
UK, pp. 3–20.
Priestley, R.H., Thomas, J.E. and Sweet, J.B. (1988) *Diseases of Grasses and Herbage
Legumes.* National Institute of Agricultural Botany, Cambridge, 37 pp.
Ritchie, J.T. (1995) International consortium for agricultural systems applications
(ICASA): establishment and purpose. *Agricultural Systems* 49, 329–335.
Schinner, F., Öhlinger, R., Kandler, E. and Margesin, R. (eds) (1996) *Methods in Soil
Biology.* Springer-Verlag, Berlin, 426 pp.
Schloter, M., Assmus, B. and Hartmann, A. (1995) The use of immunological
methods to detect and identify bacteria in the environment. *Biotechnology
Advances* 13, 75–90.
Schmidt, O., Scrimgeour, C.M. and Hanley, L.L. (1997) Natural abundance of ^{15}N
and ^{13}C in earthworms from a wheat and a wheat–clover field. *Soil Biology and
Biochemistry* 29, 1301–1308.
Schuffelen, A.C., Hudig, J. and Uittenwaal, B.W.G. (1945) Scheikundige verschillen
in de bouwvoor in horizontale richting en op korten afstand. *Landbouwkundig
Tijdschrift* 56–57, 457–465.
Southwood, T.R.E. (1978) *Ecological Methods,* 2nd edn. Chapman & Hall, London,
542 pp.
Sparks, D.L. (ed.) (1996) *Methods of Soil Analysis. Part 3: Chemical Methods.* Book
series 5, Soil Science Society of America, Madison, Wisconsin, 1390 pp.
Sparling, G.P. and West, A.W. (1988) A direct extraction method to estimate soil
microbial C: calibration *in situ* using microbial respiration and ^{14}C labelled
cells. *Soil Biology and Biochemistry* 20, 337–343.
Sparrow, L.A., Anderson, C.A. and Muir, L.L. (eds) (1998) *Moving Towards Precision
with Soil and Plant Analysis.* CSIRO Publishing, Melbourne.
Stein, A., Bekker, R.M., Bloom, J.H.C. and Rogaar, H. (1992) Spatial variability of
earthworm populations in a permanent polder grassland. *Biology and Fertility of
Soils* 14, 260–266.
Swift, M.J., Heal, O.W. and Anderson, J.M. (1979) *Decomposition in Terrestrial Eco-
systems.* Blackwell, Oxford, 372 pp.
Thielemann, U. (1986) Elektrischer regenwurmfans mitt der Oktett-methode.
Pedobiologia 29, 295–302.
Tiedje, J.M., Brempong-Asuming, S., Nuesslein, K., Marsh, T.L. and Flynn, S.J.
(1999) Opening the black box of soil microbial diversity. *Applied Soil Ecology* 13,
109–122.

Tietje, O. and Tapkenhinrichs, M. (1993) Evaluation of pedotransfer functions. *Soil Science Society American Journal* 56, 1371–1379.

Tomlin, A.D., Shipitalo, M.J., Edwards, W.M. and Protz, K. (1995) Earthworms and their influence on soil structure and infiltration. In: Hendrix, P.F. (ed.) *Earthworm Ecology and Biogeography in North America.* Lewis, Boca Raton, Florida, pp. 159–183.

Topp, G.C., Davis, J.L. and Annan, A.P. (1980) Electromagnetic determination of soil water content measurements in coaxial transmission lines. *Water Resources Research* 16, 574–582.

Turnbull, A.L. and Nicholls, C.F. (1966) A 'quick trap' for area sampling of arthropods in grassland communities. *Journal of Economic Entomology* 59, 1100–1104.

USDA (1953) *Soil Survey Manual.* US Department of Agriculture Handbook 18. USDA, Washington DC.

Van Dam, J.C., Stricker, J.N.M. and Droogers, P. (1994) Inverse method to determine soil hydraulic functions from multistep outflow experiments. *Soil Science Society American Journal* 58, 647–652.

Van Erp, P., Houba, V.J.G. and Van Beusichem, R. (1998) One hundredth molar calcium chloride extraction procedure. Part I: A review of soil chemical, analytical, and plant nutritional aspects. *Communications in Soil Science and Plant Analysis* 29, 1603–1623.

Van Wijk, A.L.M. (1988) *Drainage, Bearing Capacity and Yield (Losses) on Low Moor Peat Pasture Soils in the Netherlands.* Report No. 20. Institute of Land and Water Management Research, Wageningen, The Netherlands, 15 pp.

Vanclooster, M., Viane, P., Diels, J. and Christiaens, K. (1994) *WAVE, a mathematical model for simulating water and agrochemicals in the soil and vadose environment.* Reference and User Manual. Institute of Land and Water Management, University-Leuven, Belgium, 154 pp.

Vereecken, H., Diels, J., Van Orshoven, J., Feyen, J. and Bouma, J. (1986) A procedure to identify different groups of hydraulic conductivity and moisture retention curves for soil horizons. *Soil Science Society American Journal* 56, 1371–1379.

Woomer, P.L. (1994) Most probable number counts. In: Weaver, R.W. *et al.* (eds) *Methods of Soil Analysis, Part 2. Microbiological and Biochemical Properties.* Soil Science Society of America, Madison, Wisconsin, pp. 59–79.

Wosten, J.H.M., Veerman, G.J. and Stolte, J. (1994) *Water Retention and Hydraulic Conductivity Characteristics of Top- and Subsoils in the Netherlands.* The Staring Series, Technical Document 18. Winand Staring Centre, Wageningen, The Netherlands.

Measuring and Monitoring Nitrogen and Phosphorus Flows and Losses in Grassland Systems

13

S.C. Jarvis[1] and O. Oenema[2]

[1]Institute of Grassland and Environmental Research, North Wyke Research Station, North Wyke, Okehampton, Devon, UK; [2]Wageningen University and Research Centre, Alterra, Wageningen, The Netherlands

Introduction

Previously, the need for information on nitrogen (N) and phosphorus (P) flows in grassland systems was driven by agronomic and economic considerations. Although these remain important, emphasis has, in many circumstances, changed to the environmental consequences of losses of N and P. Thus, particularly in western Europe, there are legislative and public pressures to reduce losses and improve soil, air and water quality. In addition, increasing pressures for greater efficiency in resource utilization in agriculture have prompted renewed interest in N and P, and development of methods to improve understanding.

Grasslands have complex nutrient cycles and transfers, particularly for N, and we describe the requirements for measuring and assessing the key components of both elements.

N and P Budgeting

Nutrient budgets are powerful tools for nutrient management planning at both farm and governmental levels (e.g. Jarvis *et al.*, 1996a; Romsted *et al.*, 1997) and involve estimation of pools and flows within a system to facilitate better understanding of inputs and outputs/losses.

Budget studies may differ in approach, scale and data acquisition strategy (Smaling and Fresco, 1993; Smaling and Oenema, 1997). Three approaches are commonly used for grassland farms. The first, a *farm gate balance*, is a 'black-box' approach requiring records of N and P inputs and outputs entering and leaving the system. Differences between input and output are measures of depletion or enrichment. Uncontrollable inputs, e.g. by atmospheric deposition or biological N_2 fixation, and losses are not included. Farm gate balances are now widely used in policy analysis (e.g. Brouwer and Hellegers, 1997).

A *surface balance* determines fluxes across the soil surface. Differences between inputs and outputs in crop uptake are again measures of net loading or depletion of the soil. Because surface balances also include uncontrollable inputs, they provide more accurate estimates of enrichment or depletion than farm gate balances. However, this is also a black-box approach, providing no information about the fate of surplus N and P or causes of change.

A *system balance* provides information about inputs, outputs, losses and internal cycling. The system is generally divided into different compartments, e.g. soil, crop, livestock and animal manures. Each compartment may be further subdivided into different pools, e.g. soil inorganic and organic pools. Determining changes in flows between various compartments and pools provides detailed information about nutrient use efficiency and the controlling factors. System balances are commonly used in research and are also appropriate for nutrient management planning.

This chapter gives details of methods and approaches used to construct different balances or provide detailed knowledge of N or P in grasslands.

Inputs and Outputs

External inputs

Pastures receive external inputs of N and P from the atmosphere. This may be by wet (N and P) or dry (N) deposition and can be quantified by using conventional rainfall and filter collection devices or assessment of interception by vegetation (Rowland and Grimshaw, 1989). Atmospheric inputs range between 0 and 1 kg P ha^{-1}, but may reach > 50 kg N ha^{-1} year^{-1}. The other major N input is biological fixation of atmospheric N_2. Other additional 'external' inputs of P come from weathering of minerals in the (sub)soil.

The main inputs to intensive systems are from fertilizers, biological fixation of N_2 and purchase of manures, feeds and concentrates. These can be quantified accurately from certified contents of purchased inputs and farm or experimental records.

Measurement of biological nitrogen fixation

Many pastures rely on biological fixation of atmospheric N_2. The current interest in organic farming has increased requirements to quantify fixation. Controls over proportions of legume in swards are complex (Schwinning and Parsons, 1996) and the legume/grass balance fluctuates, with consequent changes in fixation. Field-based measurements of fixation are essential (Ledgard and Peoples, 1988) to establish effects of different managements and cultural practices on N flows.

Many methods have been developed but none is completely satisfactory and most cannot be undertaken routinely. The review of Ledgard and Peoples (1988) provided a critical description of the principal methods, and their advantages and drawbacks; Danso and Ahmad (1995) provided a review for tropical legumes. The four main approaches are as follows:

- *N balance/difference* estimates differences in N yields between fixing legumes and neighbouring non-fixing plants in the same soil. This simple method depends only on being able to measure plant N, but requires comparison with a suitable non-fixing plant and assumes that both crops absorb the same amounts of N from the same soil pools. A more simplistic approach is to base estimates on proportions of legume present (Cowling, 1982) or to develop relationships between fixation and dry matter yields (Watson and Goss, 1997).
- *Acetylene reduction assays* depend upon nitrogenase not only reducing N_2 to ammonia (NH_3) but also catalysing ethylene production from acetylene (Turner and Gibson, 1980). Measurement of acetylene then provides a means, with a suitable conversion ratio, of determining fixation. The method is inexpensive and sensitive but is indirect; it provides only short-term estimates and requires confidence in the conversion factor. A further disadvantage is that there is auto-inhibition of nitrogenase by acetylene (Witty *et al.*, 1988), making the method unacceptable for research (Peoples *et al.*, 1989).
- *Xylem solute methods* rely on changing patterns of mobile nitrogenous solutes, especially ureides, varying with fixation rate and being determined in the transpiration stream (Aveline *et al.*, 1995). Although simple and relatively inexpensive, they provide only instantaneous measurements, are indirect, need to be calibrated and are restricted to legumes that are ureide exporters (Danso and Ahmad, 1995).
- *Stable isotopic methods* depend upon determining ^{15}N and ^{14}N by mass spectrometry after enriched sources are added to soil in which fixing and non-fixing plants are growing. It is assumed that this added N and the N present in native soil pools are taken up in the same proportions by both plants, and that fixation 'dilutes' the enrichment, allowing proportions of fixed N in the legume to be calculated by difference. Potentially, this is an accurate method that gives an integrated

measure of fixation (Zanetti *et al.*, 1996). Enriched sources of ^{15}N are expensive and analysis depends on the availability of sophisticated equipment.

Recently, natural abundance ^{15}N methods have been used for pastures (Sanford *et al.*, 1995), legume monocultures (Gault *et al.*, 1995; Peoples *et al.*, 1996) and depend on natural fractionation of ^{14}N and ^{15}N during biological transformations. This results in small increases in ^{15}N abundance of soil compared with that of atmospheric N_2. Plants fixing atmospheric N_2 will therefore have different natural abundance [15]N 'signatures' than plants using soil or fertilizer N. This difference is used to calculate fixation, assuming that no fractionation occurs within the plants. The main advantage is that this process does not require added enriched N, and does not disturb natural equilibria, but it requires great care in sample preparation and demands instrumentation with high precision. Analytical equipment is relatively expensive and the method is insensitive if natural abundance levels do not differ substantially from those of the atmosphere. There is also substantial variability between 'non-fixing' plants.

Recycling of N and P

Internal and external recycling

Perennial plants reabsorb N and P from senescent and dying tissue for translocation to new growth and this is especially important under extensive forms of management. Internal recycling is usually quantified by either balance approaches or, more precisely, with isotopic tracers; both require detailed and labour-intensive measurements.

External recycling of nutrients from residues and dung is important in grasslands and requires biological decomposition before N or P can be reused. As management intensifies, there is a shift from internal towards external cycling. Hutchinson *et al.* (1990) calculated that the ratio of internal : external recycled P in plants decreased from 1.86 to 0.18 as grazing sheep numbers increased from 0 to 30 ha^{-1}.

Estimates of the amounts of P and N returned in excreta can be made from measurements of herbage consumed and P and N concentrations. Generally, $> 95\%$ of P is excreted in dung and $< 5\%$ in urine. A greater proportion of N ($> 50\%$) is excreted in urine and this increases as N intake increases. Distribution of excreta in pastures is heterogeneous and influenced by animal behaviour and so quantification of N and P returns requires stratified and random sampling to take account of areas where animals congregate. Haynes and Williams (1993) reviewed nutrient recycling from dung pats and Harrison (1987) reviewed mineralization of organic P in dung, residues and soil.

N and P in manures

Recycling in stored manures and slurries, accumulated during housing, is tremendously important in overall N and P economies of intensive systems. Manures vary in N concentrations but less in P. Reasonably accurate estimates of mean P concentrations of dung, manure and slurries can be made from known concentrations of P in diets, using correction factors to adjust for retention and dilution of slurries by cleaning and rain waters. Barnett (1994) developed a method for measuring P fractions in manures. Inorganic P generally represents 35–60% of the total P, but this increases with age of manure.

Nitrogen is more complicated because substantial proportions are inorganic and available for uptake by plants and/or loss. There is a major need to have reliable, easy-to-use on-farm methods for NH_4^+ analysis of slurries and manures, and protocols for their use to provide information on fertilizer N equivalents and potential for generating losses. Methods available (D. Chadwick, B. Pain and B. Chambers, IGER, North Wyke, personal communication) include N meters relying on conversion of available NH_4^+ into NH_3, conductivity and ion-specific electrodes, NH_4^+ test strips used with a reflectometer and hydrometers. Whilst a number of these methods work reasonably well with slurries, none provides robust information for solid manures. There is a clear need for further technological development.

Mineralization and immobilization of soil N

Understanding of mineralization and the release of NH_4^+, and immobilization of inorganic N by soil microbes, remains fragmentary. There is normally *net* mineralization in long-term productive grassland soils, indicating a positive balance of gross mineralization against immobilization. There has been increased interest in developing methods to determine mineralization (Jarvis *et al.*, 1996b) because of needs to improve fertilizer recommendations, reduce losses and improve prediction.

Agricultural soils hold substantial but variable amounts of organic N, reflecting the balance between inputs of plant and animal residues and their breakdown by mineralization. Undisturbed systems move towards steady states dependent upon soil and climatic/environmental conditions. Soil disturbance during cultivation upsets equilibria of the processes. Improved measurement of mineralization is one key to increasing efficiency of N and techniques for this can divided into groups (Jarvis *et al.*, 1996b) as follows:

- *N balance* data provide simple means of assessment of net mineralization by using plants without other inputs as sinks for N released. Fertilizer labelled with ^{15}N can be used to distinguish supplies from other sources, the unlabelled plant N plus the net change in unlabelled soil inorganic N providing a measure of net mineralization. Substantial differences between estimates with or without labelled N (Powlson *et al.*, 1992) have been shown which may be experimental artefacts (Hart *et al.*, 1986). Whilst balance methods provide useful information, care is needed in interpretation because neither N released and partitioned into non-harvested parts nor losses are accounted for. There may be direct effects of plants on the processes, and soil inorganic N should be measured at beginning and end of the experiment. A further elaboration, requiring many measurements, is to construct a complete N balance (Powlson *et al.*, 1992) of crop uptake, soil inorganic N, organic pools and losses so that release can be calculated.

- *Laboratory methods* provide a potential release rate. One method incubates soil over a defined period under standard conditions to determine increases in inorganic N. This can be under aerobic (Stanford and Smith, 1972) or anaerobic conditions (Lober and Reeder, 1993), where only NH_4^+ is measured, to provide indices of release. Rates determined in this way often differ from field measurements, because mineralization is greatly influenced by soil pre-treatment. Although reasonable agreements have sometimes been found (Campbell *et al.*, 1988), overestimates of 67–343% often occur with laboratory methods (Cabrera and Kissel, 1988). Incubation methods enable greater understanding of the processes/mechanisms but, to be of practical value, development and standardization of a simple rapid method that can be used for prediction is required (Clough *et al.*, 1998).

  The second approach relies on chemical extractants for labile N, or by total soil N or organic matter determinations. Extractants are a rapid, convenient means of providing an index of N release and range in severity from hot water to strong salt solutions. Results have been variable and no method has been adequately tested in a wide range of field conditions (Jarvis *et al.*, 1996b). Other techniques include extraction of 'labile' N by, for example, electro-ultrafiltration (Linden *et al.*, 1993), but these are unlikely to have general applicability. Total soil organic N, measured directly or by applying a factor to soil organic matter contents, may be a good general indicator of release (Hadas *et al.*, 1986) but it is unlikely that simple relationships can be defined for widespread use (Freytag *et al.*, 1989). Physical fractionation of soil organic matter has also been used to predict N mineralization (Hassink, 1995).

- *Field measurements* include simple approaches to observe changes in soil NH_4^+ and NO_3^-. This is unlikely to be useful because these pools are spatially and temporally variable, especially in grazed pastures where the dynamics of inorganic N flows will not be known because uptakes vary through the year and soils periodically accumulate large amounts of N from excreta (Jarvis *et al.*, 1995).

A more realistic approach is to use field incubation techniques. These range from using soils in polythene bags, or intact cores to minimize disturbance, with or without exchange resins to trap NO_3^- (Di Stefano and Gholz, 1986) and acetylene to limit denitrification (Hatch *et al.*, 1990), so that changes in inorganic N can be determined accurately. A recent refinement (Hatch *et al.*, 1998) includes resin and acetylene, which, in appropriate combinations, can be used to quantify nitrification, denitrification, leaching and mineralization simultaneously.

- *Gross mineralization* measurements provide information on mineralization and immobilization processes rather than net rates, which are indicative of supply for plant uptake or loss; stable N isotopes have been used for this. Adding ^{15}N of known enrichment and observing its dilution is used to estimate changes in pools of inorganic N and rates of gross mineralization and nitrification (Barraclough and Smith 1987), for example, under different forms of management (Ledgard *et al.*, 1998).

Mineralization and immobilization of soil P

The balance between mineralization and immobilization of soil P is also important (Cole *et al.*, 1977). In contrast to N, inorganic soil P pools are often as large as soil organic pools, especially in intensively fertilized soils. As a consequence, changes in the balance of mineralization and immobilization of soil P cannot be measured easily or accurately and most methods require incubation of samples followed by extraction of P. Litterbag techniques remain the standard means for estimating apparent mineralization rates of litter and residues, although some biases are inherent (Hutchinson *et al.*, 1990). The technique is used in both short (4–8 weeks) and long terms (1–4 years) in laboratory or field incubations and it measures net loss rather than total mineralization by fractionating soil P before and after incubation. Microbial immobilization may be at least as large as uptake by higher plants. The usual method of estimating microbial P is to measure the difference in extractable P with 0.5 M HCO_3 (pH 8.5) before and after fumigation with chloroform ($CHCl_3$) (Harrison, 1987). The standard method for fractionating biologically meaningful soil P pools (Hedley and Stewart, 1982) includes extraction with 0.5 M $NaHCO_3$, treatment with $CHCl_3$, extractions with 0.5 M $NaHCO_3$, 0.1 M NaOH and 1 M HCL and, finally, oxidation (H_2O_2) and acid digestion of the residue. To improve precision, labile inorganic P content should be reduced by resin extraction prior to measuring microbial biomass (Hedley and Steward, 1982).

The sensitivity and precision of immobilization and mineralization estimates can be increased by using ^{32}P-labelled phosphate (McLaughlin *et al.*, 1988) which is only incorporated into organic matter by biological activity and not through physicochemical reactions. However, ^{32}P isotopes have short half-lives and cannot be used in long-term studies.

Mineralization of organic P is affected by the action of phosphatase and Harrison (1987) has reviewed factors (soil type, pH, roots, temperature, drying/wetting, and cultivation) that influence this enzyme.

P precipitation–dissolution and sorption/desorption processes

The solubility of P in soils is low and is controlled by precipitation and dissolution reactions and sorption/desorption processes. These can be examined directly by observations of solid phases, or indirectly from the composition of soil solutions (e.g. Frossard *et al.*, 1995). Electron microscopy, X-ray diffraction, high-resolution solid state ^{31}P nuclear magnetic resonance, infrared spectroscopy and/or sequential extractions are used for solid phases. Quantifying the composition of soil solutions and calculating chemical equilibria of P species will give information on the degree of saturation. Sorption/desorption studies are conducted by incubating soil samples in solutes with a range of P concentrations, ionic strength, etc. P concentration in solution is measured and plotted against amounts of P sorbed by the soil to give information on reactivity of applied fertilizers and availability of added P for uptake or leaching.

Four approaches are used to estimate the quantity of P, which is available for plant uptake (Frossard *et al.*, 1995):

- *Chemical extractants* are currently used in Europe to mimic the plant available P in topsoils. Tunney *et al.* (1997) described the range used currently and how the information obtained can be used for developing sustainable fertilizer strategies.
- *Water extraction* removes only small proportions of sorbed P, although increasing soil : solution ratio and desorption time increases the amount. P extracted appears to be a sensitive indicator of that directly available to plants and of the potential for eutrophication of surrounding surface waters (Sharpley and Rekolainen, 1997).
- *P sinks*, such as anionic resins or iron oxide as coated filters or in dialysis bags, are used in incubations to determine desorption.
- *Isotopic exchange* between radioactive ^{32}P introduced in solution and that located on solid phases of the soil (Frossard *et al.*, 1995) is also used to assess amounts and rates of desorbable P.

All four methods have advantages and disadvantages. Those that use extractants are simple, but do not provide information on the kinetics of release and do not necessarily extract homogeneous P pools. Sinks provide information on the kinetics of P release, but applicability of this information to field conditions is still uncertain. Isotopic exchange methods are claimed to identify homogeneous P pools (e.g. Frossard *et al.*, 1995) and provide information on the kinetics of release.

Soil N and P Pools

Soil N

Soil provides one of the major N pools within grassland systems. Much of it is unavailable in the short term but knowledge of total amounts is important and, with protocols for overcoming spatial variability, total contents can be determined by classical means, usually in association with C to make judgements about soil organic matter quality. In the short term, 'available' N (NO_3^- and NH_4^+) is of most importance and measurement is relatively easy (Chapter 12). Inorganic N in the profile at critical times has been used to aid fertilizer advice for cereal crops, but is not used extensively for grassland because of difficulties in relating simple tests to perennial swards with multiple harvests by grazing or cutting. A further complication is the recycled N in excreta and applied manures or slurries.

Consequently, most recommendation schemes for grasslands do not use inorganic N data but rely on more general 'broad-brush' knowledge of factors which may influence N pools (e.g. MAFF, 1994). Differentiation between cutting and grazing, established and new swards, background/ previous cropping history and categorization of the soil/site (e.g. texture/ rainfall) can be made. Because of needs to increase N use efficiency and reduce losses, alternatives to conventional response curves and economic optima have been developed. One approach is to prevent soil inorganic N from accumulating during the growing season, limiting it to a pre-determined level. This level is sustained by 'tactical' fertilization in relation to amounts in the soil as determined with a rapid field-based kit (Scholefield and Titchen, 1995); this method can then be used to achieve particular production or environmental goals. Currently, this approach is being developed so that model prediction can be coupled with soil analysis to target specific yields or losses (Scholefield *et al.*, 1997). Similar approaches have been developed in The Netherlands, where models are used with laboratory tests of inorganic N supply (Vellinga *et al.*, 1996). These methods demonstrate trends to use discrete measurements of soil N with models. For practical use, this approach will require only minimal data inputs.

Soil P

Total soil P ranges between 200 and 2000 mg kg^{-1}, equivalent to *c.* 400–4000 kg ha^{-1} in the top 20 cm. To improve understanding of soil P and its availability, fractionation schemes and tests are used to study transformations of fertilizer P and long-term effects after land use changes and to interpret soil P test values (Kuo, 1996). Soil tests have been used to assess risks of P losses in relation to potential for eutrophication of waters (Sharpley and Withers, 1994). Tunney *et al.* (1997) compared European methods and concluded that, whilst values were optimal agronomically, they were high with respect to environmental risk. Most of the tests lack clear upper limits at which the risks of excess P became unacceptable.

Kuo (1996) reviewed methods for determining forms of soil P. The top 5–10 cm of soil contains most P and many pasture plants abstract their supplies from this layer. Depth gradients in pasture soils may be distinct (Haygarth *et al.*, 1998a) because P is strongly sorbed. In general, leaching losses are small in agronomic terms unless the sorption capacity has been exceeded (p. 312). Van der Zee *et al.* (1990) described methods for determining total sorption capacity of the soil and the degree of saturation; in carbonate-free, sandy soils this is related to the amount of oxalate-extractable aluminium and iron. A critical degree of P saturation (DPS) has been defined as the saturation percentage that should not be exceeded in order to prevent excessive transfer to ground or surface waters: the critical DPS for carbonate-free sandy soils in The Netherlands has been established as 25% (Van der Zee *et al.*, 1990).

Losses and Emissions from Grassland Systems

Nitrogen

All grassland systems leak N and the potential for loss increases with N inputs (Jarvis, 1998). The main pathways are nitrate leaching and gaseous N emissions.

Nitrate leaching
Extensive investigation of nitrate leaching has aided understanding of other aspects of the N cycle, improved accuracy of N budgets, improved models and encouraged more efficient use of N fertilizer. The easiest way to measure leaching is to determine NO_3^- in the soil profile but interpretation is difficult, because some knowledge of water and solute movement is needed. Secondly, only isolated measurements are obtained, which take no account of the dynamics involved and other interacting processes. Finally, the method is only applicable to sites where water movement is predominantly downwards. Nevertheless, this type of data has been used to highlight N loss and effects of grassland management (Ryden *et al.*, 1984).

Lysimeters (intact and hydrologically isolated columns of soil) allow quantitative and qualitative analysis of one-dimensional downward flow to some depth and have been used successfully for decades. Care must be taken to prevent edge flow (e.g. Cameron *et al.*, 1990), especially in small-scale laboratory cores, but also in larger outdoor lysimeters. Intact monoliths, usually *c.* 70 cm in diameter and > 1 m deep, have been much used (Cameron *et al.*, 1990) to provide information on leaching under natural conditions, to compare different soils or treatments and to develop models. They are most useful for simulated cutting regimes.

Under grazing, problems of measurement are made more difficult by excretal returns and the variability that they impose. For these circumstances, but also with cut grass, ceramic cup samplers are widely used. These consist of porous ceramic cups attached to tubing to which vacuums can be applied to obtain samples. Cups are inserted to depths at which root uptake is minimal, and soil solutions samples are taken at intervals and analysed for NO_3^- (Barraclough *et al.*, 1992). With information on drainage the data obtained are used to estimate leaching. Goulding and Webster (1992) concluded that, whilst lysimeters were the only method that gave reliable direct and total measures of water and NO_3^- loss, suction cups were acceptable in unstructured, freely draining soils. They are cheap and simple but drawbacks are that: (i) they modify chemical equilibria of soil solutions and do not sample representatively; (ii) insertion may change local mineralization rates and drainage flows; and (iii) care is required to overcome operational and sampling errors, particularly in grazed swards.

Lysimetry is therefore the most direct and accurate method for measuring NO_3^- losses. Although studies have used micro-lysimeters fitted with resin bags to capture NO_3^- in the field, the problems of spatial variability are acute. To overcome this, larger scale (*c.* 1 ha) hydrologically isolated plots have been used to measure leaching (Scholefield *et al.*, 1993). Drainage or runoff waters can be sampled to determine NO_3^- loss over different time scales in relation to N inputs, other N transformations, dry matter and animal production, drainage and hydrology. Whilst field plots have contributed much to understanding of N flows, they can only be used on soils that permit hydrological isolation, they are resource demanding and they can have only minimal replication. Increasingly, models are being used to estimate leaching losses.

Gaseous N emissions

Gaseous N emissions include ammonia (NH_3) and nitrous oxide (N_2O), which are important in influencing atmospheric chemistry and global warming, respectively. Intensively managed grasslands are major sources (Jarvis and Pain, 1997). These gases are difficult to measure because often only small increases above low background concentrations occur and there is considerable spatial and temporal variability. Ammonia is emitted from applied fertilizer (especially urea) and from excreta either at grazing, during housing, or from stored and spread manures and slurries. Each of these sources requires a different or modified measurement method. For many studies, flow-through methods (Lockyer, 1984) comprising semi-circular tunnels (*c.* 1 m long, usually transparent) are placed on a uniformly treated area and air is drawn through with a fan. The product of the difference between inlet and outlet NH_3 concentrations and wind speed is the amount of NH_3 volatilized. This approach has been used for volatilization from fertilizers (Van der Weerden and Jarvis, 1997) and excreta (Pain and Misselbrook, 1997) and can be used with small plots for a wide range of comparisons and information over short periods. Disadvantages are that it cannot be used for grazed pastures and it may modify the environment and thus not provide an absolute measure because volatilization is dependent on wind, temperature and moisture.

For measurements of volatilization under realistic conditions, micrometeorological methods are widely used (Denmead, 1997). For areas of several hectares, gradient diffusion methods, which depend on stable conditions, are used and require a long wind fetch. For smaller areas ($< 100 \text{ m}^2$), where these are distinct in terms of the volatilization potential from the background, the mass balance method is used and depends on differences in horizontal fluxes (wind speed $\times NH_3$ concentration integrated with height) across upwind and downwind boundaries of the plot. Measurements are required of NH_3 concentration profiles up to 3–4 m above the boundary layer and wind speed and, unless the plot is circular, wind direction to calculate fetch (which is constant in a circular plot). This method is one of the simplest for NH_3 and has been used for grazing (Jarvis et al., 1989), applied slurries (Pain et al., 1989) and slurry storage tanks (Sommer, 1996). A further simplification is the use of stability-dependent heights (ZINST) (Wilson et al., 1982) which allow an estimate of surface fluxes from single measurements (Pain et al., 1989).

Bubbling a known volume of air through acid solutions (Jarvis et al., 1989) is the usual method of trapping atmospheric NH_3. Alternatively, acid-impregnated filter packs (Allen et al., 1988) or denuder tubes (Ferm, 1979), which can integrate changes in NH_3 over time, are used. Other investigations of fluxes demand rapid, sensitive on-line measurements of NH_3. Denmead (1997) reviewed the application of new techniques for increased sensitivity, reduced sampling time or direct measurements.

Passive methods such as simple badges which need wind data, or those which measure horizontal fluxes directly without the need to measure wind or the air volume sampled (Leuning et al., 1985), are also used. Air flow through the latter sampler is directly proportional to wind speed; the sampler tracks wind direction, and NH_3 is trapped on acid coatings on the internal surfaces. This type of sampler does not require power and can be used for long-term experiments in remote locations.

Denitrification is an important loss process in grassland soils and quantification of annual N losses requires a substantial effort with frequent, comprehensive measurements to overcome large temporal and spatial variations. Estimates of rates of denitrification are commonly determined with acetylene to stop the conversion of N_2O to N_2 with either incubated intact cores or cover boxes (Klemedtsson et al., 1988). Soil is exposed to acetylene for up to 48 h and evolved N_2O is determined. The method is most suitable for anoxic conditions with ample NO_3^- present and can be used confidently for potential rates under controlled conditions. For actual rates, the method has shortcomings when NO_3^- supply is dependent on nitrification; and, where incubation is used, problems may be caused by changing aeration of the cores (Smith and Arah, 1990). The method may underestimate denitrification in aerated soils because of reactions of NO with acetylene (McKenny et al., 1997).

^{15}N techniques can also be used but major disadvantages are the requirements for labelled N, the need for adequate incorporation into the soil and the complex calculations to correct for isotopic exchanges. An alternative is to use laboratory-based systems with flowing helium atmospheres (Scholefield and Hawkins, 1997) to purge intact soil blocks free of N_2 and then make simultaneous measurements of N_2 and N_2O by gas chromatography. This does not provide field rates, but can be used to examine denitrification and its products as functions of environmental and managerial conditions.

None of these methods integrates denitrification losses over large areas, which can only be obtained by generalization and aggregation of results; geostatistical methods (Velthof et al., 1996) may provide some help with this. Micrometeorological techniques also provide better integration of effects over large areas (Fowler and Duyzer, 1989), but these require large open areas with a long undisturbed wind fetch and can only be used to determine fluxes of N_2O and not N_2. Large enclosures have also been proposed (Smith et al., 1994).

Phosphorus

Excess P inputs are usually stored within the system because soils have large retention capacities. Losses are therefore generally small and associated with hydrological events; they may occur by surface runoff and erosion or by subsurface flow and tile drainage. These pathways are difficult to quantify because of large spatial and temporal variability. Generally, 10% of the area contributes to 90% of total losses, and 90% of annual losses may occur during one storm event (Pionke et al., 1997; Sharpley and Rekolainen, 1997). Quantification of loss requires understanding of the hydrology and P chemistry of the system. Consequently, only a few studies have quantified field losses (Haygarth et al., 1998a). Small-scale lysimeters or ordinary cup samplers are not practical, because of sampling problems, and P losses are therefore measured in larger lysimeters (e.g. Chardon et al., 1997), hydrologically isolated areas (Haygarth and Jarvis, 1997), or by system synthesis/modelling (Haygarth et al., 1998b).

Using lysimeters, Chardon et al. (1997) and Haygarth et al. (1998a) showed that dissolved organically bound P represented a significant fraction of total P in leachates and that both total P concentration and total downward loss varied with season. Hydrologically isolated fields, whether with artificial or natural drainage, allow the study of the three-dimensional movement of P in the catchment area. Special facilities are needed to collect runoff and for flow-proportional samples. Although permanent grassland soils have vegetative cover all year, the often P-rich top-soil plus dung returns increase potential for diffuse loss, especially on sloping land. Subsurface lateral flow is important in areas with shallow groundwater and special facilities are required to collect this flow in soils with an impermeable subsoil horizon. With artificial drainage, a sampling system connected to drains allows quantification of solute flow (De Vos, 1997).

Nguyen and Goh (1992) quantified P losses indirectly by using a budget approach and determined all inputs, outputs and internal P cycling over 35 years. They concluded that P losses were in the range of 2–5% of the total input in grazed grassland. Whilst losses are relatively small, surface waters are extremely sensitive to inputs of P and the diffuse loss of 1 kg P ha^{-1} year^{-1} could have substantial environmental impact (e.g. Sharpley and Rekolainen, 1997).

The Role of Models

Models of grassland nutrient cycling allow prediction and extrapolation. Models are much more developed for N than for P but the growing concern over diffuse sources of P loss will almost certainly stimulate improvements in P models. Modelling grassland systems is difficult and must accommodate wide ranges of soil types/conditions, management and climates. Models should contain three essential submodels – (i) the impact of the animal; (ii) sward dry matter production; and (iii) soil processes – and these should interact with other models, especially those that define hydrological impact and C fluxes. Particular requirements will depend on the spatial and temporal scales over which predictions are required and models exist for most, if not all, of the specific processes involved in nutrient cycling. One of the most comprehensive grassland soil models is CENTURY (Parton et al., 1988), which provides a mechanistic description for N and P and other major nutrients. The N model of Thornley and Verberne (1990), which contains the three submodelling components noted above, has a deterministic, mechanistic basis but has shortcomings in that it assumes that water is non-limiting and does not consider the effects of soil physical properties and conditions.

Other, empirically based N models have been used for a variety of objectives. Good examples are the mass balance models NCYCLE (Scholefield et al., 1991) and GRASMOD (Van de Ven, 1996) which can be used to describe the major components of managed grasslands. Both define annual product outputs and losses to the environment and provide information on key internal cycling processes. The future development of models such as these, over shorter time steps and in relation to production demands (Scholefield *et al.*, 1997), will have an important part to play in the improvement of decision support systems.

As this occurs, there will be a requirement for improved prediction of specific process, e.g. mineralization. Most models of N flows incorporate some consideration of these and improved prediction of all processes is needed for the development of good, efficient agricultural practices that minimize losses. For example, although CENTURY shows good potential for prediction of mineralization in grasslands, it is cumbersome and simpler approaches such as that based on soil thermal units, as suggested by Clough *et al.* (1998), may be more useful practically. Other equally simple approaches are required for other components of the cycle.

Increasingly, as the need to upscale information grows, models used in conjunction with appropriate on-site measurements will be used to extrapolate information so that rational decisions can be made to allow sustainable grassland management with minimal environmental risk.

References

Allen, A.G., Harrison, R.M. and Wake, M.T. (1988) A meso-scale study of the behaviour of atmospheric ammonia and ammonium. *Atmospheric Environment* 27, 1347–1357.

Aveline, A., Crozat, Y., Pinochet, X., Domenach, A.M. and Cleyet-Marel, J.C. (1995) Early remobilization: a possible source of error in the ureide assay method for N_2 fixation measurement by early maturing soyabean. *Soil Science and Plant Nutrition* 1, 737–751.

Barnett, G.M. (1994) Manure P fractionation. *Bioresource Technology* 49, 149–155.

Barraclough, D. and Smith, M.J. (1987) The estimation of mineralization, immobilization and nitrification in ^{15}N field experiments using computer simulation. *Journal of Soil Science* 38, 519–530.

Barraclough, D., Jarvis, S.C., Davies, G.P. and Williams, J. (1992) The relationship between fertilizer nitrogen applications and nitrate leaching from grazed grassland. *Soil Use and Management* 8, 51–56.

Brouwer, F.M. and Hellegers, P. (1997) Nitrogen flows at farm level across European Union agriculture. In: Romstad, E., Simonsen, J. and Vatn, A. (eds) *Controlling Mineral Emissions in European Agriculture: Economics, Policies and the Environment.* CAB International, Wallingford, UK, pp. 11–26.

Cabrera, M.L. and Kissel, D.E. (1988) Evaluation of a method to predict nitrogen mineralized from soil organic matter under field conditions. *Soil Science Society America Journal* 52, 1027–1031.

Cameron, K.C., Harrison, D.F., Smith, N.P. and McLay, C.D.A.M. (1990) A method to prevent edge flow in undisturbed soil cores and lysimeters. *Australian Journal of Soil Research* 28, 879–886.

Campbell, C.A., Jame, Y.W. and De Jong, R. (1988) Predicting net nitrogen mineralization over a growing season: model verification. *Canadian Journal of Soil Science* 68, 537–552.

Chardon, W.J., Oenema, O., Del Castilho, P., Vriesema, R., Japenga, J. and Blaauw, D. (1997) Organic phosphorus in solutions and leachates from soils treated with animal slurries. *Journal of Environmental Quality* 26, 372–378.

Clough, T.J., Jarvis, S.C. and Hatch, D.J. (1998) Relationships between soil thermal units, nitrogen mineralization and dry matter production in pastures. *Soil Use and Management* 14, 65–69.

Cole, C.V., Innis, G.S. and Stewart, J.W.B. (1977) Simulation of phosphorus cycling in semi-arid grasslands. *Ecology* 58, 1–15.

Cowling, D.W. (1982) Biological nitrogen fixation and grassland production in the United Kingdom. *Philosophical Transactions of the Royal Society, London, Series B* 296, 397–404.

Danso, S.K.A. and Ahmad, N. (1995) Assessment of biological nitrogen fixation. *Fertilizer Research* 42, 33–41.

De Vos, J.A. (1997) Water flow and nutrient transport in a layered silt loam soil. PhD thesis, Agricultural University, Wageningen, The Netherlands, 287 pp.

Denmead, O.T. (1997) Progress and challenges in measuring and modelling gaseous nitrogen emissions from grasslands: an overview. In: Jarvis, S.C. and Pain, B.F. (eds) *Gaseous Nitrogen Emissions from Grasslands.* CAB International, Wallingford, UK, pp. 423–438.

Di Stefano, J.F. and Gholz, H.L. (1986) A proposed use of ion exchange resins to measure mineralization and nitrification in intact cores. *Communications in Soil Science and Plant Analysis* 17, 989–998.

Ferm, M. (1979) Method for the determination of atmospheric ammonia. *Atmospheric Environment* 13, 1385–1393.

Fowler, D. and Duyzer, J.H. (1989) Micrometeorological techniques for the measurements of trace gas exchange. In: Andrea, M.O. and Schmiel, D.S. (eds) *Exchange of Trace Gases between Terrestrial Ecosystems and the Atmosphere.* John Wiley & Sons, Chichester, UK, pp. 189–207.

Freytag, H.E., Ramsch, H. and Luttich, M. (1989) Determination of nitrogen mineralization potentials from nitrogen contents of soils. *Archi fuer Acker- und Pflanzenbau und Bodenkunde* 33, 741–746.

Frossard, E., Brossard, M., Hedley, M.J. and Metherell, A. (1995) Reactions controlling the cycle of P in soils. In: Tiessen, H. (ed.) *Phosphorus in the Global Environment, Transfers, Cycles and Management.* John Wiley & Sons, New York, pp. 107–137.

Gault, R.R., Peoples, M.B., Turner, G.L., Lilley, D.M., Brockwell, J. and Bergersen, F.J. (1995) Nitrogen fixation by irrigated lucerne during the first three years after establishment. *Australian Journal of Agricultural Research* 46, 1401–1425.

Goulding, K.W.T. and Webster, C.P. (1992) Methods for measuring nitrate leaching. *Aspects of Applied Biology* 30, 63–69.

Hadas, A., Feigenbaum, S., Feigin, A. and Portnoy, R. (1986) Distribution of nitrogen forms and availability indices in profiles of differently managed soil types. *Soil Science Society America Journal* 50, 308–313.

Harrison, A.F. (1987) *Soil Organic Phosphorus, a Review of World Literature.* CAB International, Wallingford, UK, 257 pp.

Hart, P.B.S., Rayner, J.H. and Jenkinson, D.S. (1986) Influence of pool substitution on the interpretation of fertilizer experiments with [15]N. *Journal of Soil Science* 37, 389–403.

Hassink, J. (1995) Density fractions of soil macroorganic matter and microbial biomass as predictors of C and N mineralization. *Soil Biology and Biochemistry* 27, 1099–1108.

Hatch, D.J., Jarvis, S.C. and Phillips, L. (1990) Field measurement of nitrogen mineralization using soil core incubation and acetylene inhibition of nitrification. *Plant and Soil* 124, 97–107.

Hatch, D.J., Jarvis, S.C. and Parkinson, R.J. (1998) Concurrent measurements of net mineralization, nitrification and leaching from field incubated soil cores. *Biology and Fertility of Soils* 26, 323–330.

Haygarth, P.M. and Jarvis, S.C. (1997) Soil derived phosphorus in surface runoff from grazed grassland lysimeters. *Water Research* 31, 140–148.

Haygarth, P.M., Hepworth, L. and Jarvis, S.C. (1998a) Forms of phosphorus transfer in hydrological pathways from soil under grazed grassland. *European Journal of Soil Science* 49, 65–72.

Haygarth, P.M., Jarvis, S.C., Chapman, P.J. and Smith, R.V. (1998b) Mass balances of phosphorus in grassland systems and potential for transfer to waters. *Soil Use and Management* 14, 160–167.

Haynes, R.J. and Williams, P.H. (1993) Nutrient cycling and soil fertility in the grazed pasture ecosystem. *Advances in Agronomy* 49, 119–197.

Hedley, M.J. and Stewart, J.W.B. (1982) Method to measure microbial phosphate in soils. *Soil Biology and Biochemistry* 14, 377–385.

Hutchinson, K.J., King, K.L., Nicol, G.R. and Wilkinson, D.R. (1990) Methods for evaluating the role of residues in the nutrient cycling economy of pastures. In: Harrison, A.F. and Ineson, P. (eds) *Nutrient Cycling in Terrestrial Ecosystems: Field Methods, Applications and Interpretations.* Elsevier Applied Science, London, pp. 291–314.

Jarvis, S.C. (1999) Nitrogen dynamics in natural and agricultural ecosystems. In: Wilson, W.S., Ball, A.S. and Hinton, R.H. (eds) *Managing Risks of Nitrates to Humans and the Environment.* Royal Society of Chemistry, Cambridge, pp. 2–20.

Jarvis, S.C. and Pain, B.F. (eds) (1997) *Gaseous Nitrogen Emissions from Grasslands.* CAB International, Wallingford, UK, 452 pp.

Jarvis, S.C., Hatch, D.J. and Roberts, D.H. (1989) The effects of grassland management on nitrogen losses from grazed swards through ammonia volatilization: the relationship to excretal N returns from cattle. *Journal of Agricultural Science, Cambridge* 112, 205–216.

Jarvis, S.C., Scholefield, D. and Pain, B.F. (1995) Nitrogen cycling in grazing systems. In: Bacon, P.E. (ed.) *Nitrogen Fertilization in the Environment.* Marcel Dekker, New York, pp. 381–419.

Jarvis, S.C., Wilkins, R.J. and Pain, B.F. (1996a) Opportunities for reducing the environmental impact of dairy farming managements: a systems approach. *Grass and Forage Science* 51, 21–23.

Jarvis, S.C., Stockdale, E.A., Shepherd, M.A. and Powlson, D.S. (1996b) Nitrogen mineralization in temperate agricultural soils: processes and measurements. *Advances in Agronomy* 57, 187–235.

Klemedtsson, L., Svensson, B.H. and Rosswall, T. (1988) A method of selective inhibition to distinguish between nitrification and denitrification as sources of nitrous oxide in soil. *Biology and Fertility of Soils* 6, 112–119.

Kuo, S. (1996) Phosphorus. In: Sparks, D.L., Page, A.L., Helmke, P.A., Loeppert, L.H., Soltanpour, P.N., Tabatabai, M.A., Johnson, C.T. and Sumner, M.E. (eds) *Methods of Soil Analysis, Part 3: Chemical Methods.* Soil Science Society of America/American Society of Agronomy, Madison, Wisconsin, pp. 869–919.

Ledgard, S.F. and Peoples, M.B. (1998) Measurement of nitrogen fixation in the field. In: Wilson, J.R. (ed.) *Advances in Nitrogen Cycling in Agricultural Ecosystems.* CAB International, Wallingford, UK, pp. 351–376.

Ledgard, S.F., Jarvis, S.C. and Hatch, D.J. (1998) Short-term nitrogen fluxes in grassland soils under different long-term nitrogen management regimes. *Soil Biology and Biochemistry* 30, 1233–1241.

Leuning, R., Freney, J.R., Denmead, O.T. and Simpson, J.R. (1985) A sampler for measuring atmospheric ammonia flux. *Atmospheric Environment* 19, 1117–1124.

Linden, B., Lyngstrad, I., Sippola, J., Nielsen, J.D., Soegaard, K. and Kjellerup, V. (1993) Evaluation of the ability of three laboratory methods to estimate net nitrogen mineralization during the growing season. *Swedish Journal of Agricultural Research* 23, 161–170.

Lober, R.W. and Reeder, J.D. (1993) Modified water logged incubation method for assessing mineralization in soils and soil aggregates. *Soil Science Society America Journal* 57, 400–403.

Lockyer, D.R. (1984) A system for the measurement in the field of losses of ammonia through volatilisation. *Journal of the Science of Food and Agriculture* 35, 837–848.

MAFF (1994) *Fertiliser Recommendations for Agricultural and Horticultural Crops (RB209).* HMSO, London, 112 pp.

McKenny, D.J., Drury, C.F. and Wang, S.W. (1997) Reaction of nitric oxide with acetylene and oxygen: implications for denitrification assays. *Soil Science Society America Journal* 61, 1370–1375.

McLaughlin, M.J., Alston, A.M. and Martin, J.K. (1988) Phosphorus cycling in wheat pasture rotations. III. Organic phosphorus turnover and phosphorus cycling. *Australian Journal of Soil Research* 26, 343–353.

Nguyen, M.L. and Goh, K.M. (1992) Nutrient cycling and losses based on a mass balance model in grazed pasture receiving long-term superphosphate applications in New Zealand. I. Phosphorus. *Journal of Agricultural Science, Cambridge* 119, 89–106.

Pain, B.F. and Misselbrook, T.H. (1997) Sources of variation in ammonia emission factors for manure applications to grassland. In: Jarvis, S.C. and Pain, B.F. (eds) *Gaseous Nitrogen Emissions from Grasslands.* CAB International, Wallingford, UK, pp. 293–301.

Pain, B.F., Phillips, V.R., Clarkson, C.R. and Klarenbeek, J.V. (1989) Loss of nitrogen through ammonia volatilisation during and following the application of pig or cattle slurry to grassland. *Journal of the Science of Food and Agriculture* 47, 1–12.

Parton, W.J., Stewart, J.W.B. and Cole, C.V. (1988) Dynamics of C, N, P and S in grassland soils: a model. *Biogeochemistry* 5, 109–131.

Peoples, M.B., Faizah, A.W., Rerkasem, B. and Herridge, D.F. (1989) *Methods for Evaluating Nitrogen Fixation by Nodulated Legumes in the Field.* Monograph no. 11, Australian Centre for International Agricultural Research, Canberra, 76 pp.

Peoples, M.B., Palmer, B., Lilley, D.M., Lam-Mink-Duc and Herridge, D.F. (1996) Application of ^{15}N and xylem ureide methods for assessing N_2 fixation of three shrub legumes periodically pruned for forage. *Plant and Soil* 182, 125–137.

Pionke, H.B., Gburek, W.J., Sharpley, A.N. and Zollweg, J.A. (1997) Hydrological and chemical controls on phosphorus loss from catchments. In: Tunney, H., Carton, O.T., Brookes, P.C. and Johnston, A.E. (eds) *Phosphorus Loss from Soil to Water*. CAB International, Wallingford, UK, pp. 225–242.

Powlson, D.S., Hart, P.B.S., Poulton, P.R., Johnston, A.E. and Jenkinson, D.S. (1992) Influence of soil type, crop management and weather on the recovery of ^{15}N labelled fertilizer applied to winter wheat in spring. *Journal of Agricultural Science, Cambridge* 118, 83–100.

Romsted, E., Simonsen, J. and Vatn, A. (eds) (1997) *Controlling Mineral Emissions in European Agriculture: Economics, Policies and the Environment*. CAB International, Wallingford, UK, 292 pp.

Rowland, A.P. and Grimshaw, H.M. (1989) Analysis of waters. In: Allen, S.E. (ed.) *Chemical Analysis of Ecological Materials*. Blackwell Scientific Publications, Oxford, UK, pp. 62–80.

Ryden, J.C., Ball, P.R. and Garwood, E.A. (1984) Nitrate leaching from grassland. *Nature* 311, 50–53.

Sanford, P., Pate, J.S., Unkovich, M.J. and Thompson, A.N. (1995) Nitrogen fixation in grazed and ungrazed subterranean clover pasture in south west Australia assessed by the ^{15}N natural abundance technique. *Australian Journal of Agricultural Research* 46, 1427–1443.

Scholefield, D. and Hawkins, J.M.B. (1997) Determination of controls over denitrification using a helium atmosphere system. In: Jarvis, S.C. and Pain, B.F. (eds) *Gaseous Nitrogen Emissions from Grasslands*. CAB International, Wallingford, UK, pp. 27–35.

Scholefield, D. and Titchen, N.M. (1995) Development of a rapid field test for soil mineral nitrogen and its approach to grazed grassland. *Soil Use and Management* 11, 33–43.

Scholefield, D., Lockyer, D.R., Whitehead, D.C. and Tyson, K.C. (1991) A model to predict transformation and losses of nitrogen in UK pastures grazed by beef cattle. *Plant and Soil* 132, 165–177.

Scholefield, D., Tyson, K.C., Garwood, E.A., Armstrong, A.C., Hawkins, J. and Stone, A.C. (1993) Nitrate leaching from grazed grassland lysimeters: effect of fertilizer input, field drainage, age of sward and patterns of weather. *Journal of Soil Science* 44, 601–613.

Scholefield, D., Brown, L., Jewkes, E.C. and Preedy, N. (1997) Integration of soil testing and modelling as a basis for fertilizer recommendations for grassland. In: Lemaire, G. and Burns, I.G. (eds) *Diagnostic Procedures for Crop N Management*. INRA, Paris, pp. 138–147.

Schwinning, S. and Parsons, A.J. (1996) Analysis of the coexistence mechanisms for grasses and legumes in grazing systems. *Journal of Ecology* 84, 799–814.

Sharpley, A.N. and Rekolainen, S. (1997) Phosphorus in agriculture and its environmental implications. In: Tunney, H., Carton, O.T., Brookes, P.C. and Johnston, A.E. (eds) *Phosphorus Loss from Soil to Water*. CAB International, Wallingford, UK, pp. 1–53.

Sharpley, A.N. and Withers, P.J.A. (1994) The environmentally-sound management of agricultural phosphorus. *Fertilizer Research* 39, 133–146.

Smaling, E.M.A. and Fresco, L.O. (1993) A decision support model for monitoring nutrient balances under agricultural land use (NUTMON). *Geoderma* 60, 235–256.

Smaling, E.M.A. and Oenema, O. (1997) Estimating nutrient balances in agro-ecosystems at different spatial scales. In: Lal, L., Blum, W.H., Valentine, C. and Stewart, B.A. (eds) *Methods of Assessment of Soil Degradation. Advances in Soil Science.* CRC Press, New York, pp. 229–252.

Smith, K.A. and Arah, J.R.M. (1990) Losses of nitrogen by denitrification and emissions of nitrogen oxides from soils. *Proceedings of the Fertilizer Society* 299, 1–34.

Smith, K.A., Clayton, H., Arah, J.R.M., Christensen, S., Ambus, P., Fowler, D., Hargreaves, K.J., Skiba, U., Harris, G.W., Wienhold, F.G., Klemedtsson, L. and Galle, B. (1994) Micrometeorological and chamber methods for measurement of nitrous oxide fluxes between soils and the atmosphere: overview and conclusions. *Journal of Geophysical Research* 99, 16541–16548.

Sommer, S.G. (1996) Ammonia volatilization from farm tanks containing anaerobically digested animal slurry. *Atmospheric Environment* 31, 863–868.

Stanford, G. and Smith, S.J. (1972) Nitrogen mineralization potential of soil. *Soil Science Society America Proceedings* 38, 103–107.

Thornley, J.H.M. and Verberne, E.L. (1990) A model of nitrogen flows in grassland. *Plant Cell Environment* 12, 863–886.

Tunney, H., Breeuwsma, A., Withers, P.J.A. and Ehlert, P.A.I. (1997) Phosphorus fertilizer strategies: present and future. In: Tunney, H., Carton, O.T., Brookes, P.C. and Johnston, A.E. (eds) *Phosphorus Loss from Soil to Water.* CAB International, Wallingford, UK, pp. 177–204.

Turner, G.L. and Gibson, A.H. (1980) Measurement of nitrogen fixation by indirect means. In: Bergersen, F.J. (ed.) *Methods for Evaluating Biological Nitrogen Fixation.* John Wiley & Sons, Chichester, UK, pp. 111–138.

Van de Ven, G.W.J. (1996) A mathematical approach to comparing environmental and economic goals in dairy farming on sandy soils in the Netherlands. PhD thesis, Agricultural University, Wageningen, The Netherlands, 239 pp.

Van der Weerden, T.J. and Jarvis, S.C. (1997) Ammonia emission factors for N fertilizers applied to two contrasting grassland soils. *Environmental Pollution* 95, 205–211.

Van der Zee, S.E.A.T.M., Van Riemsdijk, W.H. and De Haan, F.A.M. (1990) *Protocol for Phosphate Saturated Soils.* Agricultural University, Wageningen, The Netherlands, 69 pp (in Dutch).

Vellinga, T.V., Wouters, A.P. and Hofstede, R.G.M. (1996) System of adjusted nitrogen supply (SANS) for fertilization of grassland. In: Cleemput, O. van (ed.) *Progress in Nitrogen Cycling Studies.* Kluwer Academic Press, Dordrecht, The Netherlands, pp. 381–385.

Velthof, G.L., Jarvis, S.C., Stein, A., Allen, A.G. and Oenema, O. (1996) Spatial variability of nitrous oxide fluxes in mown and grazed grasslands on a poorly drained clay soil. *Soil Biology and Biochemistry* 28, 1215–1225.

Watson, C.A. and Goss, M.J. (1997) Estimation of N_2-fixation by grass–white clover mixtures in cut or grazed swards. *Soil Use and Management* 13, 165–167.

Wilson, J.D., Thurtell, G.W., Kidd, G.E. and Beauchamp, E.G. (1982) Estimation of the rate of gaseous mass transfer from a surface plot to the atmosphere. *Atmospheric Environment* 16, 1861–1867.

Witty, J.F., Minchin, F.R. and Beck, D.P. (1988) Measurement of nitrogen fixation by the acetylene reduction assay; myths and mysteries. *Developments in Plant and Soil Science* 32, 331–343.

Zanetti, S., Hartung, U.A., Luscher, A., Hobeisen, T., Frehner, M., Fisher, B.U., Hendrey, G.R., Blum, H. and Nösberger, J. (1996) Stimulation of symbiotic N_2 fixation in *Trifolium repens* L. under elevated atmosphere pCO_2 in a grassland ecosystem. *Plant Physiology* 112, 575–583.

Designing Animal Production Studies

D.I. Bransby[1] and A.R. Maclaurin[2]

[1]Department of Agronomy and Soils, Auburn University, Alabama, USA; [2]University of Zimbabwe, Mount Pleasant, Harare, Zimbabwe

Introduction

Animal production is the main management goal on a very large proportion of the world's grasslands. Within the context of 'animal production', specific goals vary widely, from maximizing economic returns as a result of selling livestock products in free market economies, to supporting animals for their religious significance in parts of Asia, and to indirect benefits such as hunting and tourism on game ranches and wildlife reserves in Africa. In western European countries large herbivores are also used to graze national parks or nature reserves to maintain a grassland vegetation or to encourage heterogeneity in woodlands. Furthermore, especially in economically developed countries, grassland managers are being required more than ever before to pursue these goals in an environmentally sustainable manner, and with particular concern for animal welfare. With this wide range of goals and constraints in mind, the purpose of this chapter is to assist researchers to design and conduct effective studies on animal production from grasslands, which include both rangeland and improved pastures.

The great diversity of management goals related to animal production from grasslands has led to an enormous volume of literature on this topic. Rather than reviewing all this information, the focus of this chapter is on general principles and guidelines, using selected case studies to help to make informed choices on experimental design and procedures. Some philosophical issues and as yet unpublished ideas are also presented in the hope that they might stimulate advances in this field.

©CAB *International* 2000. *Field and Laboratory Methods for Grassland and Animal Production Research* (eds L. 't Mannetje and R.M. Jones)

As with any technological research, the ultimate goal of studies on animal production from grasslands should be to benefit society. Unless the results of a study are ultimately used by the producer, or by an animal custodian, it is highly questionable whether the research was justified, especially in times of restricted or shrinking research budgets. Research must not be viewed as an end in itself, but as a means to an end, that end being successful technology transfer to those who use grasslands to support or produce animals. Unfortunately, too many investigators consider their work to be complete with publication of results in a scientific journal. While this is an important step in the generation and documentation of new information, it is of relatively little value if the information does not reach an end user. Morley (1978) expressed some of these sentiments, yet little progress seems to have been made on a global scale in increasing the practical value of research on animal production. In order to design relevant animal production studies, investigators need to be cognizant of the technological and socioeconomic context of their research. If this is neglected there is a high risk of wasting considerable time and funds on futile studies, especially when engaged in research for foreign countries and unfamiliar cultures. There is an obvious need for research to be participative with extension services and producers, the target groups of agricultural and animal production research (Chapter 16).

Advances in computer technology have vastly expanded research capability in many fields of science. Grassland and animal production research are no exceptions: the potential to use computers to collect, store and process data has offered many new opportunities. There is great potential for using computer modelling as an adjunct to, or possibly a partial replacement for, field experiments on animal production from grassland (see Chapter 3; also Jones *et al.*, 1995). Advances in mass media offer many new opportunities to improve technology transfer, yet relatively few of these opportunities are being exploited in the field of animal production. However, as most of the published research on animal production from grasslands has involved formal grazing experiments, this is where most of the ensuing discussion is focused.

Terminology

In any field of science, technological terms are needed to report results of research and to convey new ideas and concepts. As grazing technology has expanded, especially the numerous variations of rotational stocking, many new terms have evolved. A thorough examination of these terms reveals that many are not well defined, or are nebulous, or new terms for old concepts, thus causing more confusion instead of facilitating greater clarity. To address this problem, the Forage and Grazing Terminology Committee (1991) assembled a list of terms and definitions related to grazing lands and grazing animals. Although this committee was based essentially in the US, it comprised an extremely diverse membership, consulted a wide range of international literature, and solicited personal contributions from Australia and New Zealand.

The resulting publication contains one of the most comprehensive lists of terms and definitions on grazing lands and grazing animals, which should be helpful in achieving unambiguous communication at an international level. In contrast to similar publications, this list contains not only terms that were considered 'acceptable', but also those that were 'not acceptable', and an intermediate category of terms that were 'not recommended'. Furthermore, explanations were provided for why terms were classified as unacceptable or not recommended. Despite this, certain terms warrant further discussion.

Continuous stocking is defined as 'a method of grazing livestock on a specific unit of land where animals have unrestricted and uninterrupted access throughout the time period when grazing is allowed'. The more common term for this concept, *continuous grazing*, was not recommended 'because animals do not graze continuously'. However, it was recognized that continuous grazing, if used, is synonymous with continuous stocking.

Rotational stocking is defined as 'a grazing method that utilizes recurring periods of grazing and rest among two or more paddocks in a grazing management unit throughout the period when grazing is allowed'. Again, the more commonly used term for this concept, *rotational grazing*, was not recommended, although some investigators may choose to use it as synonymous with rotational stocking. A qualification to this definition was that the lengths of the grazing and rest periods should be specified. Furthermore, it was noted that words such as 'controlled' or 'intensive' were sometimes used in an attempt to describe the degree of grazing management, but that these words should not be used as synonymous with rotational stocking. In addition, *short duration grazing* was classified as an unacceptable term.

Regardless of attempts to define the concept of rotational stocking, it must be recognized that the number of subdivisions, the frequency and sequence of livestock movement among subdivisions, and the fence layout are all variables within the overall concept. This means that virtually an infinite number of potential rotational stocking systems exists, and results from any study that evaluates rotational stocking could be influenced by the particular design and management details chosen. Therefore, in designing and conducting rotational stocking studies and in reporting results, it is very important to describe precisely how the system was laid out and managed.

Stocking rate is defined as 'the relationship between the number of animals and the grazing management unit utilized over a specified time period', expressed as animal units over a described time period/area of land. In contrast, *stocking density* is 'the relationship between the number of animals and the specific unit of land being grazed at any one point in time', expressed as animal units at a specific time/area of land. Clearly, the difference between the terms is that stocking rate refers to a period of time, while stocking density refers to a point in time. Numerically, these two variables are identical for continuous stocking, but different for rotational stocking.

Set stocking is defined as 'the practice of allowing a fixed number of animals on a fixed area of land during the time when grazing is allowed', while *variable stocking* is 'the practice of allowing a variable number of animals on a fixed area of land during the time when grazing is allowed'. It is important to note that set stocking is not synonymous with continuous stocking, which is a broader concept that may involve either set or variable stocking. *Fixed stocking* is sometimes used synonymously with set stocking, but was not recommended. *Put-and-take stocking* is defined as 'the use of variable animal numbers during a stocking period or stocking season, with a periodic adjustment in animal numbers in an attempt to maintain desired sward management criteria, i.e. a desired quantity of forage, degree of defoliation, or grazing pressure'. The difference between variable and put-and-take stocking is that the former is considered to be a feasible practice on farms while the latter refers mostly to a research procedure that is discussed in a later section.

Planning Animal Production Studies

Animal production from grasslands involves complex biological and socioeconomic systems. Therefore, designing studies that ensure efficient use of resources requires extensive and very careful planning, which should include the following: (i) clear identification of the problem to be addressed; (ii) a thorough literature review of the topic; (iii) a clear statement of specific objectives, including socioeconomic goals; (iv) an assessment of the potential for results to benefit end users; (v) identification of participants; (vi) development of an appropriate experimental design; (vii) identification of variables to be measured and procedures to measure them; and (viii) a strategy for technology transfer. The importance of careful planning cannot be overemphasized. Items (i)–(v) above are dealt with briefly in this section, while items (vi)–(viii) are addressed in separate sections later.

If the general goal of a study is simply to determine the outcome of several predetermined treatments, the process may be relatively straightforward. However, studies that not only determine outcomes but also are able to explain why those outcomes were obtained are usually much more valuable. In particular, they offer greater opportunity for designing effective follow-up research, aid in extrapolation of results and provide more suitable data for developing computer models that could be used in the future (Jameson, 1989; Loewer, 1989). Therefore, they may contribute substantially to accelerated progress in pursuing a particular objective, when compared with experiments that identify only site- and time-specific outcomes without the capability of explaining results.

A clear statement of the problem to be addressed facilitates a focused literature review. Once the literature review is complete, research objectives need to be developed and clearly stated. These three steps (identification of the problem; literature review; statement of objectives) are critically important in planning the study, because they strongly influence subsequent decisions and choices.

At this stage of planning it is often useful to attempt an assessment of the potential for results from a study to benefit end users. This assessment may involve a study of potential technological, economic or sociological barriers to application of research results, communication with potential end users, or surveys (Chapter 16). Results of such assessments may lead an investigator to modify or change objectives, or in some cases to abandon the study completely if there is clearly no hope that the results will be used.

An example of a preliminary assessment is a survey among Alabama cattle producers (D.I. Bransby, 1987, unpublished data) conducted prior to establishing a grazing research programme. This survey established the following points, which strongly influenced the direction of the new research:

- Cattlemen were generally unwilling to replace existing perennial pastures with new species or forages.
- Persistence is considered a more important trait than yield and quality in perennial forage species.
- Most cattlemen were part-time producers, and owned fewer than 40 cows.
- Most calves were sold at weaning, very few being grazed on pasture in the region prior to entering the feedlot.

Informal surveys of the production and social environment in rural areas under subsistence agriculture in many African countries will reveal that livestock provide food, are a means of storing wealth, have religious significance, and are often grazed on communal grazing lands. In many cases, simple stocking rate experiments can demonstrate that a reduction in stock numbers would substantially reduce current rangeland degradation and improve range condition in these areas. However, the necessary reduction in stocking rate is often difficult, and sometimes impossible to achieve in practice due to sociological constraints and to the fact that livestock are generally kept for concurrent multiple reasons other than, or including, food production (e.g. draught, manure, transport, financial security, etc.). In such cases, grazing studies may be justified more for their demonstration value than for providing new scientific information, and focus should be more on how to encourage questioning of sociological barriers that limit use of improved practices, rather than on generating enormous files of data that may have little practical or scientific value. Procedures for participatory research are discussed in Chapter 16.

Identification of participants for animal production studies also may seem a simple matter but it is often neglected, resulting in relatively inefficient use of resources and restricted data sets that can be difficult to interpret. It is important to recognize that grassland ecosystems supporting animals are complex, and they can usually be more effectively studied by a team with members of diverse expertise, rather than by one or two individuals. Furthermore, additional participants with diverse expertise can collect a wider range of data that will substantially increase the value of the research at relatively little extra cost (Jones *et al.*, 1995). It is best to assemble such a team as early as possible in the planning phase, because the needs of each member may require certain design features that should be established well in advance. It is always desirable to have a grassland ecologist or management specialist and an animal nutritionist cooperating in animal production studies on grassland. Serious consideration should also be given to inclusion of other participants such as animal parasitologists, plant pathologists, soil scientists, economists, sociologists, computer modellers and, especially, statisticians. In addition, involvement of extension specialists and producers, or end users, should increase practical relevance of the work and the chance of effective technology transfer.

Development of an Appropriate Experimental Design

Experimental design is a key element of animal production studies from grasslands, because it strongly influences analysis, interpretation and application of results. For the purpose of this chapter, experimental design is assumed to include choice of treatments, replication and experimental layout, and only formal grazing experiments are considered. In most grazing experiments several animals and the area of land to which they are confined usually constitute the experimental unit. Drane (1989) made a case for using individual animals as experimental units, but it is difficult to accept this as a valid approach if it is recognized that valid statistical analysis requires independence among experimental units. Because each experimental unit in a grazing study involves a relatively large area of land, when compared with small plot cutting studies, the number of experimental units that is feasible in any particular grazing experiment is usually restricted. Furthermore, it is more likely that inherent variation among the units will be greater than in a set of contiguous small plots that cover only a fraction of the area. It is also important to recognize that the inherent variation among animals is often high. Because of the tendency for high experimental error in grazing experiments, it is not uncommon for treatment differences that could be biologically and economically meaningful to be statistically non-significant. The net result of this is that control of experimental error and the compromise between treatments and replication require special attention in animal production studies on grassland.

Clearly, this problem is not as severe with smaller animals such as sheep and goats, as compared with cattle, because more smaller animals can be stocked on a given area of land.

Control of experimental error

At the design stage it is very important to ensure the provision of a valid error term with adequate power for testing biologically and/or economically meaningful differences among treatments, and for determining confidence limits. This will determine the reliability of results and the level of confidence with which inferences can be made about the population under study. In this regard, randomization, number of error degrees of freedom, number of paddocks, number of animals per paddock and length of the experimental period are important considerations. Implications of these factors relative to analytical procedures and control of experimental error have been mostly documented (e.g. Mott and Lucas, 1952; Petersen and Lucas, 1960; Owen and Ridgeman, 1968; Matches, 1970). Unintentional confounding of important variables in grazing trials should be minimized, but is nearly impossible to avoid completely. Scarnecchia (1988) provided a helpful discussion on this topic. If the variables that will be confounded in a particular design are identified, the effects and implications of such confounding can be estimated. Although this estimation is largely a value judgement, it will often lead to clear acceptance or rejection of a particular design.

Total error degrees of freedom

In analysis of variance, the general principle behind tests of significance is that if variation that can be accounted for (e.g. treatment differences) is large relative to variation that cannot be explained (experimental error, or inherent variation among experimental units), then statistical significance is indicated. In the formula to calculate the variance ratio (F-test) statistic, for example, the size of the error term, or denominator, is determined largely by the number of error degrees of freedom offered by the experimental design: the greater this number, the smaller the error term will be, and the greater will be the chance of detecting statistical significance. The total number of error degrees of freedom in an experiment is determined mainly by the total number of experimental units in the study. Therefore, increasing the total number of error degrees of freedom by maximizing the total number of experimental units is a standard strategy for reducing experimental error in agricultural experiments. However, the relatively large size of experimental units often restricts the number of units that is feasible in any particular grazing study. This option, therefore, offers somewhat limited opportunity to reduce experimental error in grazing experiments, but still deserves some comment.

Bransby (1989b) pointed out that increasing error degrees of freedom from 2 to 3, and from 5 to 6, results in reduction of the error term by 52% and 12%, respectively. Because of the extreme sensitivity of the error term at the lower end of the range of error degrees of freedom, implications for grazing experiments that have very few experimental units are critical. For example, if a six-paddock grazing facility is to be used for an experiment with three treatments and two replicates, a randomized complete block design will result in only 2 error degrees of freedom, but a completely random design offers 3 error degrees of freedom. In this case, if the randomized block design is used and the block effect is small, considerable power is lost relative to a completely random design. Furthermore, it may not be possible to predict block effects with any reasonable accuracy prior to the experiment. In such a situation the best way to minimize experimental error may be to use a completely random design with long, narrow paddocks oriented in the direction of known or expected variation. Recognizing the severe restriction conferred on power of statistical tests by a limited number of error degrees of freedom, grazing experiments with fewer than eight paddocks and 4 error degrees of freedom may be hard to justify, regardless of design, and serious consideration should always be given to the compromise between size and number of experimental units. The value of obtaining pre-trial data from experimental animals also should not be overlooked.

Experimental site and animals

Selection of a relatively uniform experimental site (Fig. 14.1) is another obvious way to minimize experimental error, but uniform sites are often not available. Where heterogeneity is expected or unknown, data such as soil characteristics, forage yield and forage species composition collected prior to initiation of a grazing experiment can also be helpful in controlling experimental error. First, this information can be used to orientate long narrow paddocks in the direction of inherent variation in the site, thus reducing variability among these paddocks. A second option would be to block treatments according to site variability, and to remove some of this inherent variation by means of the block effect in the analysis. Thirdly, especially in cases where paddocks already exist, pre-trial data can be used as a covariant in an analysis of covariance to remove inherent variation, and in many cases this may be the preferred option. The value of obtaining pre-trial data (such as pre-trial weight gain while all animals are on the same diet) from experimental animals also should not be overlooked.

Finally, animal selection and assignment to experimental units and the length of the experimental period are also critically important factors in controlling experimental error in grazing experiments. Uniformity among experimental animals can present a conflict between statistical needs and practical value. Morley (1978) pointed out that wide variation among animals is likely to increase extrapolation value of results when compared

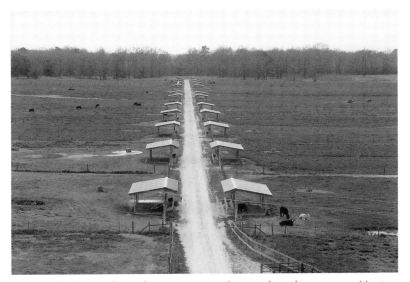

Fig. 14.1. Selection of a uniform experimental site such as this one near Montgomery, Alabama, is one of the most effective means of reducing experimental error in grazing experiments. Note also, the efficient layout of these 24 contiguous 0.8-ha paddocks, each with shade over a feed bunk (for supplemental feeding experiments), water, and easy access to a central lane leading to handling facilities. This minimizes stress on animals when they need to be weighed.

with a group of animals with a narrow genetic origin. However, wide variation among animals is also likely to increase the error term in grazing experiments, and thus reduce the likelihood of detecting statistical differences. Clearly, genetic uniformity can be achieved by obtaining animals from a single herd in which there is likely to be a large proportion of half siblings. Regardless of the level of uniformity among animals, it is probably reasonable to assume that there should be at least three animals in each experimental unit; more than this is preferable, but the number of animals per experimental unit must always be considered in relation to the total number of experimental units in the experiment.

Once these factors have been established, animals are usually assigned to experimental units by one of two procedures, in an attempt to minimize inherent variation without violating the assumptions of statistical analysis. Firstly, all animals can be stratified into relatively uniform groups and randomly assigned to experimental units from within these groups. For example, in an experiment with 12 paddocks and three animals per paddock, the 36 head could be stratified into three weight classes (heavy, medium and light) with 12 animals in each. From within each of these three groups, animals would then be assigned randomly to the 12 paddocks. Alternatively, animals can be subjectively assigned to the required number of groups (12), maximizing uniformity among groups, and then the groups are assigned randomly to paddocks. If the number of animals per experimental unit is relatively low, this procedure may be more effective in reducing experimental error than the stratification process.

Over the past decade in particular, animal welfare has become a major concern. Therefore, researchers need to pay special attention to the humane treatment of experimental animals. In many countries research agencies and institutions are required by law to have an animal welfare committee that reviews and approves the protocol for all experiments that involve vertebrate animals prior to initiation of the work. Cases of particular concern in animal production studies on grassland are those in which animals require surgery, such as that required to install oesophageal or rumen fistulae.

Other factors

In general, experimental error in measuring liveweight gain decreases as the length of the measurement period increases, because gut fill can cause major changes in animal weight over short periods of time. Consequently, it is preferable to conduct grazing studies in which animal weight gain is a response variable for at least 60 days, but periods of 90 days and longer will usually provide more precise results. Some researchers use the average of several animal weights taken on consecutive days at the beginning and end of a grazing study, in an attempt to reduce experimental error, while others use 'shrunk' weights after a period during which feed and water are withheld from animals to reduce uncontrolled effects of gut fill (Chapter 15). Effectiveness of these procedures for reducing experimental error varies, but is likely to be of most value in experiments that are conducted for a relatively short period of time (Stuedemann and Matches, 1989). Jameson (1989) pointed out that repeated measures analysis (discussed later), which uses intermediate weights together with beginning and end weights of animals, may reduce experimental error by increasing the error degrees of freedom, as compared with use of only initial and end weights.

Another option for control of experimental error and improved efficiency in grazing experiments is the use of specialized designs. For example, the change-over, cross-over or switch-back design is appropriate for dairy studies in which individual animals are the experimental units, but it is important that certain assumptions are met in order to ensure the validity of the design. Unfortunately, in many cases it is not possible to predict ahead of time whether the assumptions hold (Morley, 1978). Matches *et al.* (1974) described another efficient, specialized experimental design that used multiple assignment tester animals to evaluate a wide range of pasture systems, which involved grazing several pasture species in sequence with relatively few animals.

Treatments and replication

The matter of balance between the number of treatments and replicates in grazing experiments is usually one of compromise, also forced by the restriction on the total number of experimental units available (Bransby, 1989b). The final choice is influenced by biological, practical and statistical considerations. As the number of treatments in an experiment increases from two to three, and then to four, the number of comparisons between individual treatments increases from one to three, and then to six. In a way, the number of treatment comparisons reflects the amount of information that will be provided by an experiment. Furthermore, it is clear that the benefit in terms of additional treatment comparisons is relatively greater for each treatment added. However, for a fixed number of paddocks in a grazing research facility, treatments can be added only at the expense of replicates.

Stocking rate

In any grassland ecosystem that supports animals, stocking rate is probably the most important variable under the control of the manager, because of its profound effect on both animals and vegetation. Therefore, regardless of what the other treatments might be in a study, serious consideration should always be given to including stocking rate as a variable in grazing experiments, even at the expense of replication. Mott and Lucas (1952) made the observation that 'in many types of work it may be necessary to test all treatments at three or more stocking levels. This allows the optimum stocking rate to be ascertained for each treatment, and the several treatments to be compared at their optimum.' They also indicated that failure to compare treatments at the optimum stocking rate may result in biased comparisons. Burns *et al.* (1970), Matches (1970) and others have made similar statements. Additional advantages of grazing each treatment at several stocking rates include the following:

- Treatment × stocking rate interactions, which are quite common (Bransby *et al.*, 1988), can be detected.
- Confounding of pasture canopy conditions among treatments can be reduced by ensuring that a certain range in pasture canopy conditions (resulting from a spread of stocking rates) is common to all treatments.
- The heavy stocking rate provides an indication of pasture persistence under heavy grazing. This information is often just as important as results at the optimum stocking rate.
- Economic optimum stocking rates can be determined, even though they may vary with treatment, market conditions and other factors (Bransby, 1989a).
- Data provided by multiple stocking rate experiments are well suited to modelling.

If stocking rate is included as a variable in a grazing experiment it is important to achieve both heavy and light grazing. It does not matter if these stocking rates are slightly outside the range of economic importance, because the extremes are important in maximizing the precision of estimated response functions. In addition, it may be appropriate to impose a different range of stocking rates on different treatments if different levels of forage production are expected, such as in an experiment in which treatments are different levels of nitrogen fertilizer (Mears and Humphries, 1974). Different stocking rates can be created in a grazing experiment by keeping land area constant and varying animal numbers, keeping animal numbers constant and varying land area, or by varying both. Confounding is clearly inevitable. In general, varying animal numbers on equal land area results in heterogeneous variance among animals within pastures, whereas varying land area will result in heterogeneous variance among paddocks. Some statistical implications of each strategy are discussed by Petersen and Lucas (1960). Varying land area usually minimizes land and animal require-ments, and is therefore cost-effective, but will preclude re-randomization if the site is used for several experiments in sequence. From this point of view, equal paddock size is desirable. With equal paddock size the problem of heterogeneous variance among animals can be overcome by using the tester and grazer concept even if fixed stocking is employed. An equal number of tester animals from each stocking rate can be used to calculate average production per animal, while grazer or filler animals are used only to create the different stocking rates.

Thus, the ideal grazing experiment should include several treatments, each grazed at several stocking rates which should be replicated. However, the number of paddocks necessary to accommodate this type of design is often not available. In some cases this forces a choice between replication and stocking rate, and there is a difference of opinion on which option is better. Furthermore, this dilemma seems to be at least partly the incentive for the development of the put-and-take procedure (Mott and Lucas, 1952) for stocking grazing experiments.

Riewe (1961) appears to have been the first to recognize that the relationship between average daily gain (ADG) of animals and stocking rate is close to linear over the range in stocking rates that is of economic importance, and therefore, that stocking rate can be used as a covariant in an analysis of covariance. This linear relationship was subsequently confirmed in many other studies (e.g. Cowlishaw, 1969; Hart, 1972; Jones and Sandland, 1974; Sandland and Jones, 1975; Hart, 1978; Bransby *et al.*, 1988). Consequently, it is statistically valid to conduct a grazing experiment with, say, three treatments each grazed at four stocking rates, but with no formal replication. In such a case, pooled deviations from regression is the appropriate error term (Steele and Torrie, 1960; Draper and Smith, 1966; Zar, 1984). In a sense, treatments are replicated, with replicates deliberately but randomly confounded with treatment. Results can be expressed as three ADG–stocking rate regression lines, which can be considered as two-dimensional means. While differences among stocking rates cannot be tested without formal replication, a significant stocking rate effect is indicated if the slope of the regression line is significant, and a treatment × stocking rate interaction is indicated by a significant difference in slopes among regression lines for different treatments. Significant main effects are indicated by significantly different intercepts of parallel lines fitted to data from all treatments (Bransby *et al.*, 1988). Despite the statistical validity of this approach if the relationship between animal gain and stocking rate is linear, this is not always assured. Jones (1981) pointed out that non-linear relationships are more likely for mixed grass–legume pastures, where legume yield and thus N input will often vary with stocking rate. In these cases it would be best if stocking rates were replicated.

Stocking method

Development of the put-and-take procedure for the stocking of grazing experiments (Mott and Lucas, 1952; Mott, 1960; Petersen and Lucas, 1968; Matches, 1970; Matches and Mott, 1975) seems to have been an attempt to ensure formal replication and eliminate the need to stock each treatment at multiple stocking rates. The put-and-take procedure is implemented by adjusting animal numbers among treatments and replicates over time, in an attempt to ensure that each paddock is constantly stocked at a perceived optimum level of utilization. In contrast, fixed stocking experiments hold animal numbers constant over time, and allow the level of pasture utilization to vary (Wheeler, 1962). The relative merit of the two procedures has been the subject of strong debate in the past. Morley and Spedding (1968) and Morley (1978) were highly critical of the put-and-take approach, primarily on the grounds that it did not represent farm or ranch practice. Wheeler *et al.* (1973) provided an analysis of both fixed and variable methods of stocking, and attempted to list research conditions under which each would be most appropriately used. Two studies (Burns *et al.*, 1970; Marten and Jordan, 1972) indicated that results from variable and fixed stocking experiments may be very similar, provided several levels of stocking are used for each treatment.

Bransby (1989b) pointed out some additional weaknesses of put-and-take, including the following:

- The optimal sward condition or level of utilization (which is the basis for adjustment of animal numbers) cannot be known unless this factor is varied experimentally.
- The economic optimum stocking rate and associated level of pasture utilization may vary widely with market conditions.
- Treatment × stocking rate interactions cannot be detected.
- If treatment × stocking rate interactions exist, results will have very narrow application.

- The level of pasture utilization cannot be perfectly measured or replicated.
- If utilization level is confounded with replicates and treatments in put-and-take grazing experiments, existence of true replication is questionable and results can be biased.

Examples of experiments in which this last difficulty was experienced were reported by Burns *et al.* (1984), Read and Camp (1986) and Sollenberger *et al.* (1988). In these experiments animal numbers were adjusted in an attempt to keep herbage mass ha^{-1} equal among treatments and replicates over time, yet herbage mass still varied by 500–1300 kg ha^{-1}, and this could have had a profound effect on results.

Rotational vs. continuous stocking

Although the general approach in this chapter has been to focus on principles that have broad application, rather than on specific details or experiments, grazing studies in which continuous and rotational stocking are compared deserve special comment. As Morley (1978) correctly pointed out:

> Subdivision (of land) is necessary for the grazing management of livestock, but whether subdivision of an area grazed by a given group is necessary, or even desirable, is by no means clear. Evidence based on animal production data is especially lacking, most experiments finding no advantage and some even disadvantages. The protagonists of subdivision can always fall back on the arguments that the grazing cycle was too long or too short, or that insufficient subdivisions were used. There is an inexhaustible supply of such rationalizations . . .

Some 20 years later the state of knowledge on this topic seems to have advanced very little, despite intensified interest in this type of management in many countries. Morley (1978) continued by pointing out that investigators need to take great care in designing experiments that are, as far as possible, not vulnerable to the type of arguments cited above. He then proceeded to outline several approaches for doing this. However, most of these options would involve extremely large and unwieldy experiments that would exceed the resources available to the majority of investigators.

While it is true that there is an almost infinite number of variations of rotational stocking, it is possible to narrow these down to a relatively small range that would have the greatest chance of being superior to continuous stocking. Although it is recognized that movement of animals among subdivisions in a rotational stocking system is best done on a flexible basis, to simplify this discussion a fixed pattern of livestock movement is assumed. Besides stocking rate, the most important features in a rotational stocking system are the number of subdivisions and the length of the stocking and recovery periods, which together form the cycle length. In most situations it would be reasonable to make the recovery period long enough to accumulate a grazable forage canopy, without sacrificing too much in forage quality as a result of excessive plant maturity. This means that the length of the recovery period and the cycle length will be determined primarily by the rate of pasture growth: if pasture growth is fast, such as with improved pastures in high rainfall regions, the recovery period should be relatively short (perhaps 2–4 weeks), but if pasture growth is slow or intermittent, such as with arid rangeland, the recovery period needs to be longer (several months). If this principle is accepted, the only other major decision concerns the number of subdivisions.

Once the cycle length has been set (assume 28 days for this example), the most important influence of the number of subdivisions is through the effect on the relative length of the stocking and recovery periods. It seems reasonable to assume that stocking periods should preferably be short enough to prevent plants that have been grazed from producing enough regrowth to allow further grazing in the same stocking period. Recovery periods should be long enough to allow a reasonable accumulation of forage without plants becoming too mature. Hence, within a given cycle length it is desirable to have a short stocking period and a long recovery period. If this is accepted, data in Table 14.1 indicate that there is very little benefit in using more than six to eight subdivisions. This is because there is very little change in the length of the grazing and recovery periods for subdivisions added beyond a total of eight, and relatively little change in the length of these periods even beyond a total of four.

Given the rationale outlined here, a grazing experiment that compares rotational and continuous stocking should preferably use six or more sub-divisions for rotational stocking, and a cycle length related to plant growth rate. This should result in a system that falls within a range of options that offers rotational stocking the best chance of prevailing over continuous stocking. Ideally, both rotational and continuous stocking should be implemented at several stocking rates. Such an experiment should be relatively impervious to the almost endless list of excuses (Morley, 1978) offered by protagonists of rotational stocking in cases where it is not superior to continuous stocking. Unfortunately, few such experiments have been reported in the literature. However, Fourie and Bransby (1996) com-pared rotational stocking with six subdivisions and continuous stocking, each grazed at four stocking rates over 8 years on semiarid rangeland in South Africa, but found no difference in animal production.

Table 14.1. Relationship between the number of subdivisions for rotational stocking and the length of stocking and recovery periods, assuming a cycle length of 28 days.

Number of subdivisions	2	4	6	8	10	12	14	16
Length of stocking period (days)	14	7	4.7	3.5	2.8	2.3	2.0	1.8
Length of recovery period (days)	14	21	23.3	24.5	25.2	25.7	26.0	26.2

Confounding is another important issue that needs careful attention in experiments that compare rotational and continuous stocking. Many factors in these experiments, such as paddock size, stocking density, animal distribution over time, and quality and quantity of herbage available to livestock over time, differ among treatments. Therefore, if the experiment is not carefully designed in relation to objectives, separate effects of these variables will remain obscure. In an apparently unique experiment, Hart *et al.* (1993) addressed this type of problem by comparing rotational stocking among eight subdivisions with continuous stocking in paddocks that were either the same size as the subdivisions in the rotational stocking treatment, or much larger. Here, one of the objectives was to separate the effects of subdivision and paddock size from the effects of moving livestock among the subdivisions in the rotational stocking treatment. In general, the conclusion from this experiment was that movement of livestock among subdivisions provided little benefit, but smaller paddocks resulted in more uniform herbage utilization and greater animal weight gain. Therefore, these findings partially supported the contention of Morley (1978) that subdivision of land is necessary for the grazing management of livestock, but that subdivision of the area grazed by a given group, and movement of animals among subdivisions, may not provide any clear benefit.

Variables to be Measured

The value of animal production studies on grassland depends largely on what variables are measured, and with what precision they are measured. Therefore, the choice of variables to be measured in grazing studies is extremely important. Precision of measurements for any particular variable under study depends largely on what methods are used to make the measurements or estimates, which depend largely on the objectives for measuring the variable. Because this is the subject of other chapters, it is not discussed here, but methods to be used in collecting data in grazing studies need to be given very careful consideration at the design or planning stage. The first step is to decide what variables are to be measured, and what the logistical and scientific implications are of either measuring them or not.

Variables in grazing studies can be divided into treatment variables, controlled variables and response variables. Treatment variables are those that form the treatments in an experiment, such as method of stocking (e.g. rotational vs. continuous), forage species, stocking rate and level of fertilization. If any of these is a continuous variable, such as stocking rate or level of fertilizer, care should be taken to apply the variable as uniformly as possible across replicates. It must be recognized that replicates are defined as experimental units treated exactly alike, and any heterogeneity in applying treatment variables to replicates may increase experimental error and reduce power of statistical tests. Controlled variables can be defined as variables that are neither treatment nor response variables, but are kept equal across all treatments and replicates in an experiment. For example, if an experiment is conducted at only one stocking rate and one fertilizer level, these are controlled variables that need to be applied as uniformly as possible across all experimental units. Again, failure to do this could increase experimental error. This is a particular problem with the put-and-take or variable stocking method of conducting grazing experiments, because sward-related factors such as the amount of herbage present are controlled variables in these studies but in many cases they can be neither precisely measured nor controlled.

In contrast to many other types of agricultural research, there are many potential response variables that could be measured in grazing experiments, and it is often logistically impossible to measure even those that are most important. Once again, this makes it necessary to prioritize and compromise. Animal response variables include weight gain, reproductive performance, milk production or wool production, forage selection and consumption, time spent grazing and distance travelled while grazing (Chapter15). Pasture responses include botanical composition (Chapter 4), herbage quality (Chapter 11), sward structure (Chapter 5), plant demography (Chapter 6) and quantity of herbage per unit area (Chapter 7). Furthermore, depending on treatments and objectives, it may be necessary to measure soil responses, such as changes in nutrient distribution and soil loss (Chapter 12). Obviously, prioritization of response variables to be measured will be determined primarily by the objectives of the experiment and available resources. However, care should always be taken to make maximum use of opportunities to collect useful additional information that may not be directly related to objectives.

Animal production variables

Animal production is usually at the top of the priority list of potential variables to be measured, because it constitutes the primary response to treatments and the variable on which any economic analysis will be performed. This variable will also have a major influence on the number of animals required for an experiment, and the length of the experimental period. For example, experiments that evaluate the response of reproductive performance (such as calving or lambing percentage) to treatments require a large number of animals and need to run for several years in order to provide reliable results. In contrast, dairy experiments aimed at determining responses of milk production to treatments can be conducted over relatively short periods of time with relatively few animals, because milk production can be measured precisely and responds quickly to differences in diet. Experiments in which animal weight gain is the response variable are intermediate.

Regardless of which animal production variable is of interest, several other considerations are necessary. Although animal production is measured on individual animals, animal production per unit area is a variable of primary interest in grassland studies. Economic theory states that profit is maximized when return to the most limiting factor of production is maximized, and land is frequently the most limiting factor in animal production systems on grassland. Total animal production per unit area ($P\,\text{ha}^{-1}$) has three components and is calculated as follows:

$$P\,\text{ha}^{-1} = P/\text{an} \times SR \times T$$

where P/an is daily production per animal, SR is stocking rate and T is time in days.

Ideally, for an unbiased evaluation of treatments in a grazing experiment in terms of production per unit area, all treatments should be grazed at several stocking rates and both production per animal and time should be response variables. Unfortunately, in many grazing experiments only one stocking rate is used, and time is a controlled variable that is kept equal across all treatments. In such experiments, differences in production per unit area among treatments are a result of only differences among treatments in production per animal, with stocking rate and time having no influence on the outcome. The relatively few experiments that have involved grazing two or more treatments at several stocking rates (e.g. Mears and Humphries, 1974; Bransby et al., 1988; Mannetje and Jones, 1990) provided data with much greater utility. However, despite the importance of time in calculating production per unit area, and in many cases the probability of differences among treatments in the length of time that they could support animal production, the option to use time as a response variable in grazing experiments seems to have been almost completely overlooked in experiments measuring liveweight gain, though 'length of lactation' has often been measured as a response variable in dairy cows. Therefore, this possibility is discussed in a separate section.

Plant variables

Animal production is a function of the quantity and quality of feed consumed and so measurements of these variables may help to explain why specific differences in animal production occur among treatments. However, under normal grazing conditions their measurement involves sophisticated, labour-intensive methodology, and estimates are often subject to high variation, making it difficult to detect significant differences among treatments. Many components of animal behaviour are easier to monitor, but less valuable in explaining differences among treatments in animal production.

Because the quantity and quality of forage consumed strongly influence animal production and are difficult to measure, measurement of sward factors that are related to these variables can be useful alternatives, but should not be considered as direct substitutes. Stocking rate affects animal production through its effect on the quantity and quality of herbage present, and the effect of these variables on the quality and quantity of forage consumed. If the amount of herbage present per unit area is measured in multiple stocking rate trials, it is possible to develop relationships that describe changes in production per animal and per unit area with both stocking rate and the amount of herbage present. Relationships between the amount of herbage present per unit area and stocking rate can also be compared across treatments.

Development and comparison of these relationships among treatments substantially increases meaningful interpretation of data, compared with examination of the relationship between animal production and stocking rate only (Bransby *et al.*, 1988). Therefore, measurement of the amount of herbage present should receive high priority among pasture canopy variables that can be measured. In some cases, the amount of leaf or green material present per unit area has been a better predictor of animal production than the total amount of herbage present (Mannetje, 1974; Mannetje and Ebersohn, 1980). Because of the difficulty in simulating animal selection, quality of herbage present is likely to be less useful.

Botanical composition in rangeland and mixed-species improved pasture will often strongly affect animal production, especially if legumes are a component of the sward. Therefore, high priority should also be given to quantifying botanical composition in grazing studies, preferably by estimating the weight of herbage contributed by different species, rather than by estimates of plant frequency (Chapter 4).

Soil variables

Although soil-related variables have been measured in relatively few grazing experiments, increasing concern about the effects of animals on the environment are an incentive to serious consideration of measurement of at least some of these in grazing studies. Soil loss and excessive accumulation and leaching of nutrients are among the most serious concerns of environmentalists, relative to animal production systems on grasslands (Chapters 12 and 13). It is well established that soil loss is strongly associated with pasture canopy cover, which can be estimated more readily. Hence, measurement of canopy cover can partially reflect the potential for soil loss in grazing treatments, and may be especially useful if combined with measurement of other related variables, such as ground litter and basal cover.

Accumulation and leaching of nutrients are of greatest concern in animal production systems on grassland where large quantities of nutrients are being imported, especially in the form of animal wastes for fertilizer, or as supplemental feed. Nitrogen and phosphorus are among the nutrients that cause the greatest concern. These two nutrients should be monitored closely in experiments that include treatments that could cause excessive nutrient accumulation and leaching (Chapter 13). On the positive side, grasslands are known to contribute significantly to carbon sequestration (Bransby *et al.*, 1998), which is a process that is considered to have many environmental benefits.

Weather data

Precipitation records are usually essential to define the experimental conditions and to relate the conditions experienced during the experiment to long-term conditions at that site. If the experimental data are to be used to help in development of models, or used in conjunction with models, it is essential to have records of on-site precipitation (preferably daily) temperature (as close as practicable to the site) and occurrence of frosts, snow and ice where relevant (preferably on the site). It is also highly desirable to have information on evaporation, whether directly from a pan or through indirect variables such as temperature, humidity and wind speed, and on the water-holding capacity of the soil and depth of rooting.

Time as a Factor in Grazing Experiments

Duration of experiments

In designing grazing studies, time needs to be considered from several points of view. First, the most appropriate duration of a grazing experiment should be estimated at the design stage. Where perennial grasslands are under study and treatments are expected to have cumulative effects over time, long-term experiments are particularly valuable. Jones *et al.* (1995) offered an excellent discussion on some of the advantages of long-term trials, with special reference to changes in botanical composition. They pointed out that botanical changes may take place only after several years, often in relation to rainfall variability, changing soil fertility, longevity of individual plants and cumulative effects of stocking rate, and these shifts in botanical composition may lead to changes in animal production. Although botanical change is an important component of sustainability, which is currently assigned high priority, funding for long-term studies is often difficult to obtain.

Time as a response or treatment variable

Earlier in this chapter it was indicated that time within a grazing season could be treated as a response variable in grazing studies. Typically, grazing is initiated and terminated at the same time on all treatments in grazing experiments, regardless of how well the treatments are synchronized relative to the optimum length of the grazing season. Since length of the grazing season may substantially affect total animal production per unit area, this approach may result in biased comparisons among treatments. Therefore, it could be better to treat time as either a response or treatment variable, instead of as a controlled variable, and to start and end grazing on different treatments at different times, based on some objective criterion. For example, grazing could be initiated on each treatment when the pasture canopy reached a predetermined condition or height, and terminated on a similar sward-related basis, or when plant or animal production dropped to a certain level (Bransby, 1989b). The point in time at which the latter condition occurred could be determined by allowing grazing to continue slightly beyond this point, and then using a regression relationship between production and time to predict the exact cut-off date and production for each treatment. Alternatively, different dates for starting and terminating grazing could be imposed on several treatments in a factorial design, in the same way that multiple stocking rate experiments are conducted and analysed. For experiments in which forage production among treatments is somewhat out of phase, this approach would probably provide more meaningful data than if a fixed period of grazing were applied to all treatments. It is also possible that, when feed is limited, rotational stocking could provide a slightly longer period of animal production than continuous stocking. However, there appears to be no evidence of such studies in the literature.

Repeated measures analysis

Analysis of data over time within a grazing season is another important time-related issue in grazing research that seems to have been largely overlooked. Typically, results of grazing trials are reported as total production, or an average for each treatment over the entire grazing period, even though milk production is recorded daily and animal weight may be measured every few weeks. This amounts to loss of important information, because animal production often changes within and among treatments over time, and markets for animal products are also dynamic systems (Kouka *et al.*, 1994). For example, it may be extremely important to know if treatment differences were detected in the first 60 to 90 days of a 150-day experiment, or whether they became evident only in the last

30 days. Restriction of data analysis to total seasonal production will not provide this information.

Correlation among repeated measures made on the same experimental unit over time is an aspect of statistical analysis that requires special attention. Agricultural data collected in this way have most commonly been processed by means of a split plot in time analysis. This option uses the experimental unit or paddock as the whole plot, and the measurement on that unit at a particular point in time or in a particular year as the sub-plot. The approach is mostly valid from a statistical point of view if the interest is in relatively long intervals, such as differences in treatments over consecutive years, but it may often be invalid if measurements are taken frequently, such as every few days or at intervals of up to several weeks. Littell *et al.* (1998) indicated that considerable advances have been made over the past two decades in developing more appropriate procedures and software to analyse repeated measurements data sets. In particular, mixed model analyses were implemented previously by adapting fixed-effect methods to models with random effects. More recent procedures implement random effects in the statistical model and permit modelling of the covariance structure of the data, thereby computing efficient estimates of fixed effects and valid standard errors of the estimates. Burns *et al.* (1983) also described a useful experimental design in which some treatments are retained over time, while others are changed, and this added considerably to the efficiency of the experiment. Greater use of these procedures to analyse and present changes in treatment responses over time would enhance the value of data collected in many grazing studies.

Technology Transfer

In a sense, grazing research cannot be considered complete until successful technology transfer is at least under way, and in many cases this can be more difficult than conducting the research. Therefore, it should be given special attention from the very beginning of the project. Earlier in this chapter it was suggested that extension personnel and one or more livestock producers should be involved in planning grazing experiments. If even greater involvement of such individuals is feasible, it will increase the chance of successful technology transfer (Chapter 16). For example, extension personnel could help to collect, analyse and report data, while selected livestock producers may be asked to test one or more of the best treatments from an experiment on a commercial or larger scale, even before the experiment is terminated. As for research, technology transfer needs to be different for large commercial operations and smallholders.

If the community in which the research is being conducted is economically driven, livestock production will depend largely on economics. Therefore, economic analysis of data will substantially increase the probability of successful technology transfer and, if appropriate, such analyses should be incorporated into the plan at the design stage (Jacobs, 1974; Bransby, 1989a).

It is well established that visual evidence of successful new technology can contribute substantially to successful technology transfer. In this regard, visual differences in some cases can be even more powerful than economic differences. Grazing experiments often provide excellent visual differences among treatments. If distinct visual differences among treatments are evident, technology transfer can be enhanced considerably by holding regular field days for producers to review the experiment at first hand. These differences should also be recorded throughout the duration of the experiment by means of good photographs and on video tape. As well as submission of articles to scientific journals, results should be published in farm magazines, bulletins and even newspaper articles, and included in television and radio programmes.

Smallholders often keep animals for many purposes, including meat, milk, fibre, manure, fuel and financial security, and for customary, social and religious reasons. The animals are usually maintained on crop residues and rangeland, which is managed communally by the community and which is often stocked with more than one species of domestic livestock, and sometimes accessible also to wildlife. To be meaningful under such situations, research and technology transfer need to take into account the type of farming system under consideration, and the livestock holders' circumstances, desires and inclinations. If this is not done, especially in smallholder communities, the entire research–technology transfer process may be ineffective.

References

Bransby, D.I. (1989a) Justification for grazing intensity experiments: economic analysis. *Journal of Range Management* 42, 425–430.

Bransby, D.I. (1989b) Compromises in the design and conduct of grazing experiments. In: Marten, G.C. (ed.) *Grazing Research: Design, Methodology, and Analysis.* Crop Science Society of America, Madison, Wisconsin, pp. 53–68.

Bransby, D.I., Conrad, B.E., Dicks, H.M. and Drane J.W. (1988) Justification for grazing intensity experiments: analyzing and interpreting grazing data. *Journal of Range Management* 41, 274–279.

Bransby, D.I., McLaughlin, S.B. and Parrish, D.J. (1998) A review of carbon and nitrogen balances in switchgrass grown for energy. *Biomass and Bioenergy* 14, 379–384.

Burns, J.C., Mochrie, R.D., Gross, H.D., Lucas, H.L. and Teichman, R. (1970) Comparison of set-stocked and put-and-take systems with growing heifers grazing Coastal bermudagrass (*Cynodon dactylon* L. Pers.). In: Norman, M.J.T. (ed.) *Proceedings of the 11th International Grassland Conference.* University of Queensland Press, St Lucia, Queensland, pp. 904–909.

Burns, J.C., Giesbrecht, F.G., Harvey, R.W. and Linnerud, A.C. (1983) Central Appalachian hill land evaluation using cows and calves. I. Analysis of an unbalanced grazing experiment. *Agronomy Journal* 75, 865–871.

Burns, J.C., Mochrie, R.D. and Timothy, D.H. (1984) Steer performance from two perennial *Pennisetum* species, switchgrass, and a fescue-Coastal bermudagrass system. *Agronomy Journal* 76, 795–800.

Cook, C.W. and Stubbendieck, J. (1986) *Range Research: Basic Problems and Techniques*, revised edn. Society for Range Management, Denver, Colorado.

Cowlishaw, S.J. (1969) The carrying capacity of pastures. *Journal of the British Grassland Society* 24, 207–214.

Drane, J.W. (1989) Compromises and statistical designs for grazing experiments. In: Marten, G.C. (ed.) *Grazing Research: Design, Methodology, and Analysis*. Crop Science Society of America, Madison, Wisconsin, pp. 69–84.

Draper, M.R. and Smith, H. (1966) *Applied Regression Analysis*, 1st edn. John Wiley & Sons, New York, 372 pp.

Forage and Grazing Terminology Committee (1991) *Terminology for Grazing Lands and Grazing Animals*. Pocahontas Press, Blacksburg, Virginia, 38 pp.

Fourie, J.H. and Bransby, D.I. (1996) Effects of stocking rate and continuous and rotational stocking on steers grazing semi-arid rangeland in South Africa. In: West, N.E. (ed.) *Proceedings of the 5th International Rangeland Congress*. Society for Range Management, Denver, Colorado, pp. 157–158.

Hart, R.H. (1972) Forage yield, stocking rate, and beef gains on pasture. *Herbage Abstracts* 42, 345–353.

Hart, R.H. (1978) Stocking rate theory and its application to grazing on rangelands. In: Hyder, D.N. (ed.) *Proceedings of the 1st International Rangeland Conference*. Society for Range Management, Denver, Colorado, pp. 547–550.

Hart, R.H., Bissio, J., Samuel, M.J. and Waggoner, J.W. Jr (1993) Grazing systems, pasture size and cattle grazing behavior, distribution and gains. *Journal of Range Management* 46, 81–87.

Jacobs, V.E. (1974) Needed: systems outlook in forage-animal research. In: Keuren, R.W. van (ed.) *Crop Science Society of America Special Publication 6*. Crop Science Society of America, Madison, Wisconsin, pp. 33–48.

Jameson, D.A. (1989) Time series, dynamic models and adaptive sequential decisions in grazing research. In: Marten, G.C. (ed.) *Grazing Research: Design, Methodology and Analysis*. Crop Science Society of America, Madison, Wisconsin, pp. 97–108.

Jones, R.J. (1981) Interpreting fixed stocking rate experiments. In: Wheeler, J.L. and Mochrie, R.D. (eds) *Forage Evaluation: Concepts and Techniques*. AFGC/CSIRO, Melbourne, pp. 419–430.

Jones, R.J. and Sandland, R.L. (1974) The relation between animal gain and stocking rate. *Journal of Agricultural Science* 83, 606–611.

Jones, R.M., Jones, R.J. and McDonald, C.K. (1995) Some advantages of long-term grazing trials, with particular reference to changes in botanical composition. *Australian Journal of Experimental Agriculture* 35, 1029–1038.

Kouka, P.-J., Bransby, D.I. and Duffy, P.A. (1994) Profitability of cattle production from rye, oats, and a rye + ryegrass mixture grazed at different stocking rates. *Journal of Production Agriculture* 7, 417–421.

Littell, R.C., Henry, P.R. and Ammerman, C.B. (1998) Statistical analysis of repeated measures data using SAS procedures. *Journal of Animal Science* 76, 1216–1231.

Loewer, O.J. (1989) Issues on modeling grazing systems. In: Marten, G.C. (ed.) *Grazing Research: Design, Methodology, and Analysis.* Crop Science Society of America, Madison, Wisconsin, pp. 127–136.

Mannetje, L. 't (1974) Relations between pasture attributes and liveweight gains on a subtropical pasture. *Proceedings 12th International Grassland Congress.* Moscow Vol. 3, pp. 299–304.

Mannetje, L. 't and Ebersohn, J.P. (1980) Relation between sward characteristics and animal production. *Tropical Grasslands* 14, 273–280.

Mannetje, L. 't and Jones, R.M. (1990) Pasture and animal productivity of buffel grass with Siratro, lucerne or nitrogen fertilizer. *Tropical Grasslands* 24, 269–281.

Marten, G.C. and Jordan, R.M. (1972) Put-and-take vs. fixed stocking for defining three grazing levels by lambs on alfalfa–orchardgrass pastures. *Agronomy Journal* 64, 69–72.

Matches, A.G. (1970) Pasture research methods. In: Barnes, R.F. *et al.* (eds) *Proceedings of the National Conference on Forage Quality Evaluation.* Nebraska Center for Continuing Education, Lincoln, Nebraska, pp. 1–32.

Matches, A.G. and Mott, G.O. (1975) Estimation of the parameters associated with grazing systems. In: Reid (ed.) *Proceedings of the Third World Conference on Animal Production.* Sydney University Press, Sydney, pp. 203–208.

Matches, A.G., Martz, F.A. and Thompson, G.B. (1974) Multiple assignment tester animals for pasture systems. *Agronomy Journal* 65, 719–722.

Mears, P.T. and Humphries, L.R. (1974) Nitrogen rate and stocking rate of *Pennisetum clandestinum* pastures. II. Cattle growth. *Journal of Agricultural Science* 83, 469–478.

Morley, F.H.W. (1978) Animal production studies on grassland. In: Mannetje, L. 't (ed.) *Measurement of Grassland Vegetation and Animal Production.* Commonwealth Agricultural Bureaux, Farnham Royal, UK, pp. 103–162.

Morley, F.H.W. and Spedding, C.R.W. (1968) Agricultural systems and grazing experiments. *Herbage Abstracts* 38, 279–287.

Mott, G.O. (1960) Grazing pressure and the measurement of pasture production. In: *Proceedings of the 8th International Grassland Conference.* Alden Press, Oxford, pp. 606–611.

Mott, G.O. and Lucas, H.L. (1952) The design, conduct and interpretation of grazing trials on cultivated and improved pastures. In: *Proceedings of the 6th International Grassland Conference.* Pennsylvania State University, State College, Pennsylvania, pp. 1380–1385.

Owen, J.B. and Ridgeman, W.J. (1968) The design and interpretation of experiments to study animal production from grazed pasture. *Journal of Agricultural Science* 71, 327–335.

Petersen, R.G. and Lucas, H.L. (1960) Experimental errors in grazing trials. In: *Proceedings of the 8th International Grassland Congress.* Alden Press, Oxford, pp. 747–750.

Petersen, R.G. and Lucas, H.L. (1968) Computing methods for evaluating pastures by means of animal response. *Agronomy Journal* 60, 682–687.

Read, J.C. and Camp, B.J. (1986) The effect of the fungal endophyte, *Acremoneum coenophialum* in tall fescue on animal performance, toxicity and stand maintenance. *Agronomy Journal* 78, 848–850.

Riewe, M.E. (1961) Use of the relationship of stocking rate to gain of cattle in an experimental design for grazing trials. *Agronomy Journal* 53, 309–313.

Sandland, R.L. and Jones, R.J. (1975) The relation between animal gain and stocking rate in grazing trials: an examination of published theoretical models. *Journal of Agricultural Science* 85, 123–128.

Scarnecchia, D.L. (1988) Minimizing confounding in case studies of agricultural systems. *Agricultural Systems* 26, 89–97.

Sollenberger, L.E., Ocumpaugh, W.R., Euclides, V.P.B., Moore, J.E., Quesenberry, K.J. and Jones, C.S. Jr (1988) Animal performance on continuously stocked 'Pensacola' bahiagrass and 'Floralta' limpograss pastures. *Journal of Production Agriculture* 1, 216–220.

Steele, R.G.D. and Torrie, J.H. (1960) *Principles and Procedures of Statistics*, 1st edn. Mcgraw-Hill, New York, 481 pp.

Stuedemann, J.A. and Matches, A.J. (1989) Measurement of animal response in grazing research. In: Marten, G.C. (ed.) *Grazing Research: Design, Methodology, and Analysis*. Crop Science Society of America, Madison, Wisconsin, pp. 21–36.

Wheeler, J.L. (1962) Experimentation in grazing management. *Herbage Abstracts* 32, 1–7.

Wheeler, J.L., Burns, J.C., Mochrie, R.D. and Gross, H.D. (1973) The choice of fixed or variable stocking rates in grazing experiments. *Experimental Agriculture* 9, 289–302.

Zar, J.H. (1984) *Biostatistical Analysis*, 2nd edn. Prentice-Hall, Englewood Cliffs, New Jersey, 718 pp.

Measuring Animal Performance

15

D.B. Coates[1] and P. Penning[2]

[1]CSIRO, Davies Laboratory, Aitkenvale, Australia; [2]Institute of Grassland and Environmental Research, North Wyke, Okehampton, Devon, UK

Introduction

A clear concept and definition of the objectives of an experiment, covering both purpose and context in which the results are to be applied, is absolutely necessary if measurements of animal performance are to be relevant and useful. Many factors must be considered, including the desired output (e.g. meat, milk, fibre, offspring) and market considerations in relation to the output (age, weight and condition of live animals; carcase quality; milk quality and composition; fleece weight and quality). Decisions must be made about the most appropriate experimental animals (species, sex, age, weight, uniformity and temperament) and the agronomic practices to be applied (e.g. fertilizer type and rate). Also to be taken into account are animal husbandry procedures for the control of diseases and parasites, the grazing system that would be most appropriate and, very importantly, the time frame required to produce meaningful results (e.g. for annual forages or permanent pastures). All the above factors will determine treatment variables to be applied, what measurements should be made and how they should be made. Good techniques in measuring animal performance will be of limited value unless they are coupled with appropriate experimental design.

The effort and resources expended in measuring animal performance will also be wasted if the results are confounded by factors that are unidentified or uncontrolled and that are outside the scope of the work being conducted. Of particular importance are the effects of infective disease, external and internal parasites, mineral deficiencies or toxicities,

©CAB *International* 2000. *Field and Laboratory Methods for Grassland and Animal Production Research* (eds L. 't Mannetje and R.M. Jones)

and in some cases anti-nutritive factors arising from infected (bacterial or fungal) plant material. While it is impossible to identify and control all such factors, appropriate preventive measures, monitoring procedures or other safeguards should be put in place to minimize the risk of compromising the experimental results.

This chapter will deal with ruminant livestock only. Although most of the reference material will be drawn from work with cattle and sheep, the principles will generally apply to other ruminants though many techniques will be inappropriate for wild ruminants. Corbett (1978) provided a good overview of techniques used in the measurement of animal performance to that time and we recommend it be read in conjunction with this review, particularly the section on animal management not covered here. We have paid greatest attention to useful techniques developed during the last 20 years.

Growth and Body Composition

Liveweight and liveweight change

Liveweight (LW) is measured both as a stand-alone measurement or to determine LW change when sequential weights are taken. With appropriate equipment LW can be measured accurately. The problem lies in what that weight means in relation to the status of the animal at that particular time and the purpose for which the measurement is to be used. This is because LW can vary substantially over short periods without any change in the gross energy content of the animal. Such variation is due to changes in gut fill, which can account for over 20% of LW (Kennedy, 1995), and to changes in body water volume. Since many factors can affect gut fill and body water content, procedures must minimize variation within and between treatment groups and between successive weighings (Hughes, 1976).

Daily herbage intake usually ranges between 10 and 30 g dry matter (DM) kg^{-1} LW (1–3% of LW) but in hot climates the intake of water (including water in herbage) may exceed 20% of LW. Thus, substantial within-day variation in LW may be associated with the daily pattern of grazing, drinking, urinating and defecating. Consequently, a set routine where animals are mustered and weighed at the same time of day is recommended to reduce variation in gut fill between animals and between weighing occasions. The order in which the animals are mustered and weighed becomes important in large grazing experiments, where the whole process may take many hours.

Fasting animals overnight is often practised to reduce variation in gut fill. Water is also usually withheld during the overnight fast but there may be circumstances where it is inadvisable to do this. Overnight fasting may be practised with lactating as well as dry stock but the offspring should remain with their dams to allow normal suckling. In a subtropical environment, weight losses in steers subjected to a 16 h overnight fast (feed and water) averaged around 8% of their unfasted weight (L. 't Mannetje and D.B. Coates, unpublished data). The difference between full and fasted weight has implications in comparing results across experiments because liveweight gain (LWG) will be around 8% lower and dressing percentage around 4% higher when fasted rather than full LW is recorded.

Various factors can influence an animal's intake of herbage and water and therefore affect LW in relation to time of weighing (within or between days). These factors include the often cyclical nature of daily DM intake, reduced intake during oestrus in females, loss of appetite that may occur with transient illness or current weather conditions, especially rain. These effects are only temporary and will generally have no significant effect on longer-term LW change but they may confound LW change over periods of a month or less.

Gut fill is also affected by herbage quality, being least when herbage is lush and highly digestible and increasing as herbage becomes more fibrous. Thus, gut fill is likely to increase progressively as the pasture matures and its quality declines. In some cases, LW maintenance may be associated with a reduction in tissue weight and gross energy content. Conversely, in seasonally dry environments, rapid reductions in gut fill occur when diet quality changes from poor fibrous material at the end of the dry season to high quality green leaf at the break of the growing season. On these occasions, apparent LW losses may occur when animals are gaining in tissue weight and gross energy content. Such losses can be substantial (10% of LW; D.B. Coates, unpublished data) but highly variable between animals and treatments. Obviously these LW changes do not reflect changes in tissue or carcase weight and cannot be considered as reliable indicators of treatment differences. Since LWs recorded at the beginning and end of grazing periods have the greatest influence on the experimental results and treatment comparisons, it is important that special efforts be made to minimize errors or biases at these times. This includes taking a series of measurements at the beginning and the end of a grazing period. In grazing trials where experimental animals are periodically replaced, the change-over should not coincide with the transition season. For a more detailed discussion see McLean et al. (1983).

The limitations mentioned above generally decrease in relative importance as the cumulative LWG increases. Conversely, LW changes over short periods can be very misleading.

The usefulness of LW change as a measure of animal performance is also limited by the variation in the chemical composition of LW gain or loss, or indeed, changes that occur in the chemical composition of the entire animal. Corbett (1978) stated that a threefold variation in energy value is

possible between unit gain made at low LW by young lean animals and that
of heavy, fat animals. Differences in the energy value of gain may also occur
between early and late maturing animals of the same age and similar LW,
due to differences in partitioning of net energy for growth between muscle
and fat. Given the same increase in energy accretion, late maturing animals
will record higher LWG than early maturing animals. Hence, when treatment effects on pasture productivity are being investigated, differences in
maturity type may be important when allocating animals across treatments.
A mixture of breeds that vary in maturity type is acceptable provided each
breed is equally represented in each experimental unit. Variation in the
chemical composition of LWG is one of many factors that should be
considered when comparing animal performance between experiments.
Additionally, it may warrant consideration when experiments are subjected
to economic analysis.

LW change during pregnancy is a special case where the relative
increase in gross energy content of the dam is well below the relative
increase in LW due to the amount of fluid associated with the developing
fetus. LWG during pregnancy may therefore mask a significant deterioration in nutritional status of the dam, though LW can be adjusted for
pregnancy in cows (Silvey and Haydock, 1978).

Where the availability of animal scales is limited, LW can be estimated
from heart girth measurements (the girth measurement immediately
behind the forelegs and avoiding the hump). Relationships between LW
and heart girth (HG) first need to be developed for the species and
breed of animal in question. Reports on the accuracy of LW estimates
from HG measurements vary from being acceptable for cattle (e.g. Young,
1972; Berge, 1977) and sheep (Warriss and Edwards, 1995) to poor (e.g.
Spurling, 1974).

Measuring body composition

Pasture productivity as measured by economic output in meat-producing
enterprises is determined by the quality of the product as well as by LWG.
This increases the need for rapid, low-cost and accurate measurements of
body composition in both live and slaughtered animals. Body composition
can be measured in terms of water, protein, fat and ash in the whole
animal or carcass or in terms of the amount and distribution of muscle
and fat. Much of the early work involved the physical dissection of carcasses,
or alternatively, determining whole-carcass chemical composition and
developing predictive relationships between portions of the carcase
(e.g. 9–11 rib cut) and the whole carcase (e.g. Ledger et al., 1973).
Other relationships were developed to predict carcase composition from
simple physical measurements such as the thickness of fat over the eye

muscle at the 11th rib (Johnson and Charles, 1976) or rib-eye area as an indicator of muscling. Charles (1974) also developed regression relationships between the thickness of the anal or caudal fold in live cattle and the percentage of muscle and fat, and between anal fold thickness and dressing percentage.

Various methods have been developed for estimating chemical composition in the live animal. The early methods were based on measurements of total body water (TBW) relative to LW using the principle that the proportions of water, protein and ash in the fat-free empty body tend to be constant for a given species. TBW is estimated by measuring the dilution of an injected marker substance and the methodology has been described by Corbett (1978). Tritiated water and deuterium oxide (Lunt *et al.*, 1985) have both been used as marker substances, the latter having the advantage of being non-radioactive but having the disadvantage of a time-consuming assay. Urea has also been used successfully as a marker substance (Kock and Preston, 1979; Rule *et al.*, 1986). Urea shows even and rapid distribution throughout the body water; it is non-toxic, is not foreign to the body, does not cause any physiological disturbances, can be accurately and easily measured in either whole blood or plasma (Kock and Preston, 1979) and poses no health risk to humans.

Dilution techniques and other indirect methods for estimating the chemical composition of live animals all depend on developing regression equations relating indirect measurements on a sample of live animals to the results obtained from chemical or physicochemical analyses of the animals after slaughter. Rule *et al.* (1986) concluded that equations should be tested with a subsample of cattle from the population for which its use is intended, before using published prediction equations for calculating body composition *in vivo*.

Ultrasonic techniques (Busk, 1989; Fisher, 1997) are now commonly used to evaluate carcase conformation and composition in live animals. Earlier techniques relied on ultrasound imaging at specific locations (e.g. at the 13th thoracic vertebra) to determine subcutaneous fat depth and eye muscle area as indices of carcase composition. More recently the velocity of ultrasound (VOS) has shown advantages over other ultrasound techniques (Fisher, 1997). Characteristics of the ultrasonic techniques include relatively low capital and operating costs, portability and useful accuracy, objectivity in the case of VOS, and the ability to assess large numbers of animals in a relatively short time.

A suite of other emerging technologies, such as video image analysis (Kuchida *et al.*, 1995), bioelectrical impedance analysis (Berg and Marchello, 1994), magnetic resonance imaging (Baulain, 1997), fast neutron activation analysis (Wolff *et al.*, 1996), and X-ray computerized tomography (Sehested, 1984) have been tested experimentally for estimating body composition.

Livestock units

One of the key factors under the control of management in grazed pastures is stocking rate but, because of the variation in animal size both within and between species, stocking rate may be difficult to interpret in terms of grazing pressure. Expressing stocking rate in terms of livestock units (LUs) or livestock equivalents per unit area has been used to compare productivity of pastures grazed by different classes of livestock more appropriately. In principle, LU attempts to quantify the grazing animals at pasture on the basis of equivalent forage intakes.

LUs can be defined as a nominal LW regardless of the animal species or physiological status. For example, if a 500 kg animal represents 1 LU then a 250 kg animal represents 0.5 LU. The nominal LW selected for the LU is usually arbitrary but representative of a typical mature animal of a certain species, such as a medium-sized mature, dry cow or ewe, though the tropical livestock unit (TLU) of 250 kg LW is intermediate between large and small ruminants. There will, however, be substantial variation in forage intake for an LU based purely on LW because intake per unit of LW varies with animal species, body size and physiological status. Within a species, the effect of body size can be eliminated by expressing intake relative to metabolic weight. It has been extensively demonstrated that intake is constant over a wide range of LWs when it is expressed as kg $LW^{0.75}$. In addition to the effect of body size there are species differences in intake per unit metabolic weight when fed the same forage. Ternouth *et al.* (1979) showed that intakes of mature sheep and cattle were the same when expressed in relation to LW to the power 0.9. Minson and Whiteman (1989) recommended a standard livestock unit (SLU) for defining stocking rate in grazing studies where 1 SLU equates to the intake of a non-lactating bovine of 500 kg LW. A virtually identical SLU or animal unit (AU) was defined by Allen (1991) as the equivalent of one mature non-lactating bovine weighing 500 kg and fed at maintenance level. It was assumed that a DM intake of 8 kg day^{-1} equates with 1 AU.

The problem with an SLU calculated from LW is that it becomes outdated as soon as there is a change in LW. Roberts (1980) proposed a method for overcoming the main impact of changing LW by using the minimum (W^{min}) and maximum (W^{max}) LWs recorded during the grazing period (e.g. a year) in the calculation of an Effective Stocking Rate (SR) for cattle, where:

$$\text{Effective SR} = ((W^{min} + W^{max}) / 2)^{0.75} \times \text{Nominal SR}$$

Mature Animal Equivalents can be determined as (Effective SR/100) where one Mature Animal Equivalent is the equivalent of a mean metabolic weight of 100 kg (i.e. a mean LW of 464 kg). The principles advocated by Roberts (1980) and Minson and Whiteman (1989) could be combined.

Reproduction

General principles

Obtaining data on reproductive performance is relatively simple for many traits, but results can be very misleading unless precautions are heeded, especially precautions to minimize confounding effects. Silvey (1977) described a range of problems associated with experiments using reproducing females. In addition, animal husbandry (e.g. time and duration of mating) and other procedures should be relevant to the context in which the experimental findings are to be applied. Policies on culling and replacement of females need to be defined at the outset. Generally speaking, a female that fails to conceive in two successive mating seasons may be deemed barren (Coates and Mannetje, 1990). Similarly, protocols in response to animal health and calving problems or use of supplementary feed need to be established.

Appropriate procedures should minimize non-treatment effects that may confound treatment differences. This is particularly important with reproducing females because of the binomial nature of data for oestrus, conception, calving and weaning and because a single, short-term event can have long-term consequences on reproduction. The following recommendations are made on the understanding that the issues being addressed are not components of the investigation. Firstly, all females should be structurally sound and functionally fertile. It is sometimes appropriate, therefore, to use pregnant females when experiments are first stocked. Alternatively, visual appraisal and the palpation of the reproductive organs by experienced operators will help in assessing functional fertility. Diseases and parasites need to be controlled. Reproductive diseases such as vibriosis, trichomoniasis and brucellosis are particularly important, as outbreaks can ruin experiments. Other diseases that may cause abortion or temporary infertility, such as leptospirosis and ephemeral fever, can seriously affect research outcomes.

Sire fertility and functional ability are potential problems in experiments on female reproduction. All sires must be functionally fertile. Visual appraisal for structural and genital soundness, measures of potential fertility using indicators such as scrotal circumference and semen volume and quality (Andersson and Alanko, 1992) and the assessment of serving capacity (Blockey, 1989) may be used. Appraisals of male fertility and soundness should be made before each mating period. Since the probability of sub-fertility or sterility increases with age, young sires are recommended. Sires should be clear of venereal infections and, where possible, protected by vaccination. Temporary or permanent infertility can occur during the mating period as the result of disease or injury. Preventive measures should be taken where risks are known (e.g. vaccination against ephemeral fever) and sires should be regularly inspected during the mating period. Rotating sires among the groups of breeding females at intervals of 1–2 weeks during mating can alleviate the problem of confounding female reproductive performance with sire effects. However, where paddock sizes are large, sires may take time to 'settle down' in a new paddock to become familiar with their territory and with other animals. Consequently, the interchange of sires during mating may not be advantageous (Coates and Mannetje, 1990).

Artificial insemination (AI) can avoid the practical and technical problems associated with using sires in paddock matings and eliminate sire effects on treatment differences. The quality of the prepared semen needs to be assured, as does the technical proficiency of the inseminator. A period of paddock mating after the insemination programme has been completed may be desirable in some situations.

Female reproductive performance

Different measures or indicators of reproductive performance are covered briefly below. The fertility parameters measured and the methodology adopted will depend on the experimental objectives.

Number or proportion of females cycling
Oestrus cycling is readily detected by successive blood progesterone assays, usually 10 days apart (Entwistle, 1986). Herd status may be determined at a particular time or it may be monitored by blood sampling according to a pre-arranged schedule. The occurrence of oestrus can be determined by attaching marker devices (crayon markers for rams: Radford et al., 1960; or chin-ball harnesses for bulls: Lang et al., 1968) to entire or vasectomized males and observing the females on a regular basis for evidence of mounting. Alternatively, oestrus can be detected by applying heat-mount detector pads to the backs of cows (Baker, 1965). Determining the oestrus status of females may be warranted in experiments concerned with growth and development, in screening animals for some specific purpose (e.g. inclusion in an AI programme or where an experiment demands functional females) or where data on post-partum return to oestrus are required.

Number or proportion of females served
Detecting the number of females served relies on evidence of mounting. The marker devices described above are used for this purpose and it has to be assumed that marked females have been served and impregnated. However, heat-mount detector pads can be triggered without cows being served, as when cows crowd together under shelter during inclement weather. The same detection devices may be used to determine the number of matings (number of separate oestrus events where a female is served) per conception. Data on the number of females served may be required for

calculating other indices such as the percentage of pregnancies or successful parturitions relative to females served.

Number of cows pregnant

Pregnancy status of cows can be determined by manual palpation of the
ovaries and uterus. Proficient operators can detect pregnancy after 6–7
weeks and determine fetal age to the nearest month. Ultrasound imaging
can detect pregnancy in sheep (White and Russel, 1987) and cattle. Progesterone assays of milk can detect early pregnancy (Sasser and Ruder, 1987)
and are particularly useful in AI programmes.

Time and number of embryonic losses

Data on mating events can provide evidence of early embryonic loss.
Successive matings at the normal oestrus interval would indicate an
unsuccessful mating whereas a delayed return to service would indicate
conception followed by early embryonic death. Determining pregnancy
status, including fetal age, at set intervals can provide information on fetal
losses but care needs to be taken that the testing does not itself contribute
to fetal loss. In cattle, regular weighing may identify fetal losses late in
pregnancy.

Calving or lambing rate and neonatal mortalities

If accurate information on the number of live and dead offspring born is
required then the herd or flock must be monitored daily. Still-births can be
identified by lungs that have never been inflated. Whether offspring
have suckled before dying can be determined by inspecting the intestines
for evidence of milk. Offspring should be identified by ear tagging or by
recording identifying characteristics until permanent identification can
be applied. Less precise data for calculating calving or lambing rates can be
obtained by mustering or inspecting herds at set intervals (weekly, fortnightly or monthly) or at the conclusion of the calving or lambing season.
Given accurate pregnancy diagnosis, the number of pregnant females
failing to produce live offspring at a certain time (e.g. end of calving or
lambing season) can be accurately determined but the losses cannot be
classified into pre-natal, peri-natal and post-natal categories. With small
ruminants, where multiple births are common, reproductive rates can be
described in various ways to account for the frequency and litter size of multiple births. Thus, calculated calving and lambing rates can vary depending
on the method of assessment and it is therefore essential that the basis of
calculation be clearly defined.

Incidence of dystocia

Morning and afternoon inspections of the herd will be required to obtain
accurate information on the incidence of dystocia or to minimize deaths of

both dam and offspring where it occurs. Unfortunately, there is evidence suggesting that too much interference prior to and during parturition may increase the incidence of dystocia (Dufty, 1972).

Weaning rate

Calculating weaning rate presents fewer difficulties than calculating calving or lambing rate because the number of offspring weaned (numerator) is accurately known. However, a clear definition of the number of dams used in the calculation (denominator) is required. Weaning rate is usually based on the number of females mated, regardless of subsequent mortalities, though common sense needs to be exercised in cases where female mortalities are unrelated to the treatment being investigated.

Birth dates and weights

Information on birth dates may be required as one indicator of herd fertility status during the previous mating period, to calculate intervals between successive parturitions or as a factor in statistical models for analysing female fertility and progeny growth rate (Coates *et al.*, 1987a). Daily inspections are necessary for accurate determinations of birth weight.

Growth rate and weaning weight

While acquiring raw data on growth rate and weaning weight of suckling calves or lambs is straightforward, the data must be standardized with respect to sex of progeny and age-of-dam effects for valid comparisons. Entire males grow faster than castrates, which grow faster than female progeny. Adjustment for age of dam is necessary because mothering ability or milk supply increases as females mature. Published differences due to age of dam and gender of offspring vary considerably for sheep (e.g. Wilson *et al.*, 1985; Killedar *et al.*, 1987) and cattle (e.g. Brinks *et al.*, 1961; Winks *et al.*, 1978). Different adjustment factors are applicable for temperate and tropical regions. The most suitable adjustment factors are those derived for local conditions (genotype and plane of nutrition). In sheep, birth weight and growth to weaning is affected by litter size (Snowder and Glimp, 1991). Growth rate to weaning may be expressed either as weight per day of age or as average daily gain (ADG). The former requires a knowledge of the birth date but no initial weight is required. Date of birth may also influence growth rate due to seasonal changes in the nutritional status of pasture. Therefore, many statistical models include birth date as a factor for the analysis of growth rate and weaning weight (Coates *et al.*, 1987a). When it is desirable to concentrate births within a narrow time period it is possible to synchronize oestrus by hormone therapy (Fitzpatrick and Finlay, 1993; Frisch and O'Neill, 1996).

Dam LW, LW change and body condition
LW is intimately linked with reproductive performance through its effect on fertility and milk yield and, in harsh environments, with survival. Thus, condition scoring and measuring LW, as outlined above in the section 'Growth and Body Composition', either at regular intervals or at critical times through the reproductive cycle, are integral to interpreting reproductive performance *per se* and to identifying causes of poor performance.

Reproductive indices
Female reproductive performance has various components (fertility, fecundity, mortality and mothering ability) but performance in each of these areas can be integrated in reproductive indices such as weight of weaned progeny per female mated or per unit area. These indices can be useful for overall treatment or system comparisons. If necessary, the gain or loss of LW (including loss by death) of the breeding females can be included in an index of total productivity.

Male reproductive performance

An evaluation of likely male reproductive performance can be made by means of visual appraisal for structural soundness, an assessment of the quantity and quality of semen produced and an assessment of libido. Structural soundness must include not only the anatomical soundness of the genital organs but also skeletal soundness and mobility. The assessment of semen quantity and quality is made on samples of semen collected by electro-ejaculation or by using an artificial vagina in association with a teaser animal (Moore, 1985). Scrotal circumference is a simple but effective indicator of male fertility (Andersson and Alanko, 1992). Serving capacity has been recommended as a useful measure of libido and fertility in bulls and rams (Blockey and Wilkins, 1984) and positive relationships between serving capacity and fertility of sires have been reported but there have been reservations about the effectiveness of the serving capacity test with respect to *Bos indicus* bulls and tropical environments (Blockey, 1989). Male reproductive performance can be determined directly from test matings provided satisfactory safeguards are in place to minimize the confounding of male reproductive performance with female fertility and disease. However, there are obvious practical limitations to measuring the potential reproductive capacity of males. Unsatisfactory male reproductive performance can be readily detected in single-sire mating groups, while reproductive performance of sires in multiple-sire mating groups can be assessed by using blood group analyses of sires, dams and progeny or DNA marking.

Milk

Milk yield

For animals that are milked daily it is relatively easy to measure milk production directly. Milking systems, linked to computers, can automatically record milk yields of individual animals and take milk samples for the determination of composition. For suckling animals, estimating milk yield and composition is more difficult. Essentially, there are four basic techniques: (i) weighing animals before and after suckling; (ii) body-water dilution techniques; (iii) estimating milk secretion rates; and (iv) calculations based on weight gain of the offspring. The methods of measuring milk production described by Corbett (1978) are still in use with only minor modifications.

Suckling and weighing offspring

The weigh–suckle–weigh technique has been used commonly for non-dairy sheep (Owen, 1957) and cattle (Neville, 1962). A typical routine with cattle would be to remove the calf from the cow for 8 h and then allow a preliminary suckling. Calf weight changes at three consecutive sucklings at 8 h intervals are then measured and summed to give estimates of 24 h milk yield. Alternatively, a suckling during darkness can be avoided by timing the preliminary suckling for the late afternoon and then measuring calf weight changes at sucklings on the following morning and again in the late afternoon (Neville, 1962). More frequent measurements are required for sheep (Owen, 1957). The development of electronic balances to weigh animals accurately has improved the precision of this technique. Losses of faeces and urine during suckling must be prevented to avoid underestimates of milk production. With grazing animals, labour inputs for handling, separating and weighing offspring are considerable and may unacceptably interfere with grazing behaviour (Le Du et al., 1979). These difficulties have led to the development of alternative techniques, such as the estimation of milk secretion rates.

Milk secretion rates

With non-dairy sheep, less than one-half of the milk available to the suckled lamb can be extracted by hand milking (Peart, 1982). This led to development of techniques for estimating milk yield using oxytocin (Doney et al., 1979; Le Du et al., 1979). It involves injecting a dose of oxytocin into the jugular vein, waiting for about 60 s, followed by hand or machine milking until milk flow ceases. A second dose is then injected and the udder stripped of milk. Offspring are prevented from suckling for 4–6 h. The milking procedure is then repeated, the milk weighed and the time between milkings recorded. This enables 24 h secretion rate to be estimated. Excellent agreement between the oxytocin technique and the calf suckling technique was reported by Le Du *et al.* (1979), though Le Du *et al.* (1978) found that milk fat was overestimated. They suggested that the oxytocin technique required less labour and caused less disturbance to animals. Gibb and Treacher (1980) compared milk yields estimated using oxytocin with those calculated from the LW gain of young. They concluded that measuring secretion rate over a 4 h period once per week overestimated milk yield. They also calculated that weekly use of the oxytocin technique deprived lambs of 5% of their mothers' milk production and cautioned against making more frequent measurements.

Calculations of milk yield from LW gain of young

Weight gains of suckled animals are measured over several weeks. Known energy values for body weight gain, efficiency of energy utilization and energy values for milk (ARC, 1980; AFRC, 1993) are then used to estimate milk intakes. Gibb and Treacher (1980) used data from Penning and Gibb (1979) to calculate a direct relationship between milk intake (MI g) and lamb growth rate (GR g day^{-1}) during the first 4 weeks of life:

$$MI = 70.16 + 4.467 \, GR$$

This technique assumes that milk is the only food eaten and therefore can only be applied during the first weeks of life before animals begin to graze. Penning and Gibb (1979) showed how the onset of herbage intake was related to milk intake (lambs with low milk intakes started to consume herbage earlier than those with high milk intakes) and how herbage intake increased with age. Therefore, this technique has only limited application in the grazing situation unless herbage intake can be allowed for.

Body water dilution techniques

This method is based on water dilution in the offspring due to intake of water from the milk. It offers potential advantages over other techniques in that animals do not need to be milked and disturbance is minimized (Peart, 1982). One version of this method is to inject tritiated water into the young animal and, after allowing 2–6 h for equilibration, take a blood sample to determine the level of radiation. Comparison of results of this assay with one made 7–14 days later provides an estimate of water turnover rate, which was found to agree closely with actual milk intake (Corbett, 1978). However, this technique suffers the serious disadvantage that it cannot take into account water derived from other sources (Peart, 1982), leading to overestimates of milk production (Wright *et al.*, 1974). Double isotope methods (Wright and Wolff, 1976) have been used to overcome this problem, with dam and offspring receiving different isotopes. The ratio of these isotopes, in samples of blood from the young animal, can be used to correct for water intake arising from sources other than milk, but in some countries there are strict regulations on the use of radioactive materials and considerable work is required to carry out the isotope analyses. In addition, costs will be high since treated animals must be removed from the food chain unless stable isotopes can be used. Stable isotopes are also expensive and analysis requires relatively sophisticated equipment.

All the above techniques have some disadvantages and experimenters should carefully consider whether estimating milk yield is essential. Furthermore, in some cases dams are capable of producing more milk than the young can consume so that comparisons of milk yields *per se* may not be strictly valid (Peart, 1982; Penning *et al.*, 1996).

Milk composition

The nutritional value of milk depends on its composition and routine analytical procedures have been developed to measure various fractions and other attributes of importance such as fat, solids not fat (SNF), protein, lactose, urea, mineral concentrations and somatic cell count. Most of the procedures have been developed for application in the dairy industry and there is usually a choice of available tests for any one fraction.

Wool and Animal Fibre

The biology of wool growth has been reviewed by Reis and Sahlu (1994). Techniques to measure wool growth and yield outlined by Corbett (1978) are still in use with only minor modifications. The two main methods used for measuring wool growth are the patch method (Moule, 1965) and dye banding (Chapman and Wheeler, 1963). Corbett (1978) preferred dye banding because it is quicker, simpler and probably more reliable. McCloghry (1997) improved the dye banding technique by using non-toxic hair-dye cream to mark the fleece. Measuring wool production (fleece weight) is straightforward but it is important to distinguish between production as estimated by greasy fleece weight and the amount of clean wool produced, since the percentage of clean wool, or yield, varies with breed and environmental conditions. Near-infrared reflectance spectroscopy (NIRS) has been used as an alternative to scouring for estimating clean fleece weight (Scott and Roberts, 1978).

Wool quality is determined largely by fibre diameter and length. Andrews *et al.* (1987) compared five different methods for measuring fibre diameter: the airflow method, sonic fineness tester, liquid scintillation spectrometer, fibre fineness distribution analyser and the projection micro-scope, the latter method being accepted as the benchmark procedure. They concluded that the projection microscope was the least preferred because of cost, in spite of the biases exhibited by the other methods. Subsequently, the Optical Fibre Diameter Analyser (OFDA) was developed to provide a rapid, accurate measurement of average fibre diameter and diameter distribution (Baxter *et al.*, 1991; Qi *et al.*, 1994). The OFDA combines the attributes of the projection microscope with automatic image analysis technology. Qi *et al.* (1995) described an upgraded imaging system capable of measuring average fibre diameter and average staple length with their standard deviations, mechanical yield, fibre medullation and colour of scoured fibres. Computer-assisted image analysis can also be used to measure wool follicle density and fibre diameter in skin sections (McCloghry *et al.*, 1997). Nagorcka *et al.* (1995) described a non-destructive and inexpensive technique for quantifying and characterizing the density of fibres and follicles in skin.

Important textile industries have been based on cashmere and mohair production from goats (Lupton, 1996) and fibre production from South American camelids (Russel, 1994). The techniques outlined above may be suitable for measuring fibre production and quality in these animals.

Measurement of Selectively Grazed Herbage

Background

In the absence of supplementation, the productivity of grazing animals is directly related to the quantity and quality of the herbage consumed. Knowledge of the quantitative and qualitative attributes of ruminant diets is therefore necessary to fully understand pasture–animal relationships and to manage grassland systems effectively. The dietary attributes that have received most attention are botanical composition, chemical composition, digestibility and intake.

Botanical composition

Holechek *et al.* (1982) identified direct observation, utilization techniques, stomach analysis, oesophageal fistula sampling and microhistological examination of faeces (faecal MHE) as procedures for estimating botanical composition of range herbivore diets. Direct observation, utilization techniques and stomach analysis have serious limitations regarding quantitative assessments of diet composition but faecal MHE (where fragments of the cuticularized epidermis from the ingested plant species are identified in the faeces) and oesophageal sampling have been widely used. Faecal MHE is particularly useful in studying diet selection in wild herbivores, while oesophageal sampling is used primarily in domestic ruminants. Accurate estimation of botanical composition using faecal MHE is a problem because the proportion of species in the faeces is often different from that consumed. Also, it is difficult to make quantitative estimates from microscopic examination, because some plant material may become unidentifiable in the faeces and because procedures of sample collection and processing may bias results (Slater and Jones, 1971).

Accurate measurement of botanical composition is less of a problem in extrusa samples from oesophageal fistulated animals than in faecal samples. Although manual separation of extrusa into major groups, individual species, or plant parts within species, is time consuming and low in precision (Hoehne *et al.*, 1967), various procedures using microscopic examination have been successfully applied (e.g. Hamilton and Hall, 1975). NIRS may be used for predicting botanical components in extrusa once calibration equations have been developed (Volesky and Coleman, 1996).

The major shortcoming of oesophageal sampling is that extrusa does not necessarily represent the diet of test (resident) animals (Coates *et al.*, 1987b; Jones and Lascano, 1992; Clements *et al.*, 1996). This may arise from differences in preference between the oesophageal fistulated animals and the test animals or merely from herbage selected over a short grazing time (15–30 min) being different from that consumed over a full day or longer. For example, ruminants can have up to eight to ten grazing periods per day (Arnold, 1962) and diet selection changes with increasing satiation and with subtle changes in the pasture and weather, so one or more extrusa samples may not reflect the total daily intake (McManus, 1980). Differences between samples collected in the morning and afternoon (Coates *et al.*, 1987b) clearly demonstrate how grazing preference may change during the course of a day. Previous grazing history and fasting may also affect dietary preference (Parsons *et al.*, 1994b). Another major disadvantage of the oesophageal fistula technique is the cost in labour and time in properly caring for fistulated animals.

A remote control system has been developed for collecting multiple oesophageal fistula samples from goats (Raats *et al.*, 1996). The fistula plug is not removed during sampling but incorporates a valve that can be operated by remote radio control. This allows the operator to collect samples throughout the day without disturbing the animal's normal feeding behaviour.

Dietary C_3 (cool season grasses and most dicot species) and C_4 (tropical grasses, sedges and rarely dicots) proportions can be calculated from the faecal $\delta^{13}C$ values of grazing animals (Jones *et al.*, 1979; Jones, 1981), where $\delta^{13}C$ is a measure of the ratio of the naturally occurring carbon isotopes ^{12}C and ^{13}C. When animals are on a constant diet, faecal $\delta^{13}C$ values are generally slightly more negative than the feed values and a good working approximation is faecal $\delta^{13}C$ = diet $\delta^{13}C - 1$ (Jones *et al.*, 1979). Values can be determined with great accuracy and precision using a mass spectrometer to measure the relative proportions of ^{12}C and ^{13}C (Le Feuvre and Jones, 1988) and single faecal values reliably reflect the integrated diet over a period of at least 3 days (Coates *et al.*, 1991). The faecal $\delta^{13}C$ technique is especially useful for diet selection studies in the warmer climates where all the grasses are C_4 species. This allows for the division of dietary components into grass (C_4) and non-grass (C_3), an important separation because of the contrasting chemical composition of the two fractions. The technique has been usefully applied to study diet selection in cattle grazing grass/legume pastures (Jones and Lascano, 1992; Clements et al., 1996; Coates, 1996) and to measure the contribution of forbs or browse in the diets of animals grazing C_4 grasslands.

The technique requires sampling of both faeces and component species within the test pasture, the former to obtain faecal $\delta^{13}C$ values and the latter for determining feed $\delta^{13}C$ values of the dietary C_3 and C_4 components. Because the C_3/C_4 composition of the faeces will be different from that of the diet if the two fractions differ in organic matter digestibility (OMD), estimates of OMD for the C_3 and C_4 dietary components should be determined so that appropriate adjustments can be calculated and applied where extra accuracy is warranted (Jones, 1981). Sampling and analysis protocols have been reported by Jones et al. (1979), Le Feuvre and Jones (1988) and Coates et al. (1991).

The technique has a number of advantages compared with the oesophageal technique:

- The estimate relates directly to target animals.
- Sampling is simple and the test animals do not have to be yarded or even disturbed; fresh, uncontaminated faecal samples can be collected direct from the paddock and as often as desired.
- The technique is objective, reliable and accurate.
- Estimates can be made for individual animals or for groups (bulk samples) as required.
- Unlike oesophageal sampling, there is no need to prepare and maintain special animals.
- Frozen or dried samples can be easily stored indefinitely and analysed when convenient.

The main disadvantages are as follows:

- The technique only allows for separation into C_3 and C_4 components, thus limiting its application.
- The $\delta^{13}C$ of plant species is subject to some seasonal variation (as much as one unit) and so component species need to be analysed for the determination of standard values at each faecal sampling or at least at regular intervals.
- Within both the C_3 and C_4 components there is some variation between species in $\delta^{13}C$ value.
- Equipment for preparation and analysis of samples is expensive and the analysis by mass spectometry requires considerable technical expertise.

Estimating the botanical composition of the diet by means of alkane analysis of herbage and faeces is described in a later section (p. 375).

NIRS of faecal samples (faecal NIRS) is emerging as a promising technology for estimating botanical composition. Like other applications of NIRS, predictions rely on developing relationships between laboratory reference values of the attribute under consideration and NIR spectral characteristics. The laboratory reference values are determined by standard analytical techniques. Usually the laboratory and NIR analyses are performed on the same substrate (e.g. forage sample). However, where faecal NIRS is used to predict dietary attributes, laboratory reference values are measured on samples identical or similar to the diet, while NIR analyses are performed on faecal material from animals receiving the matching diet (Lyons and Stuth, 1992). The application of faecal NIRS to estimate dietary botanical composition is in its infancy but useful applications could be developed, at least for broad groupings of components in specific situations such as grass vs. browse or legume. Work in north-east Queensland has demonstrated good prediction of dietary C_3/C_4 proportions using faecal NIRS (D.B. Coates, unpublished data). Once a reliable calibration equation has been developed, faecal NIRS offers a very quick and inexpensive means of obtaining quantitative estimates of dietary composition. The major disadvantages are the cost and effort involved in developing calibration equations and the initial cost of the NIR spectroscope and associated software.

Chemical composition and nutritive value of the diet

Selective grazing results in the diet often being quite different from the pasture on offer. Consequently, the major limitation in accurately estimating dietary chemical composition of grazing animals is obtaining samples that truly represent the diet. The problem is reduced where management minimizes selective grazing, such as in intensive strip grazing. The difficulty increases as species diversity, spatial heterogeneity and paddock size increase. The easiest situation occurs in monospecific swards of small area where, by carefully observing grazing animals, forage samples can be plucked to represent the plant parts consumed. At the other extreme are grasslands covering thousands of hectares, comprising hundreds of grass and forb species together with trees and shrubs, with a high degree of spatial heterogeneity in pasture composition, soil type and fertility, topography and soil moisture status. In such situations it is impossible to harvest manually samples of herbage that closely reflect the diet of the grazing animal and other techniques have to be employed.

Sampling with oesophageal fistulated animals

Obtaining samples of extrusa from oesophageal fistulated animals has long been regarded as an appropriate method to overcome problems of selective grazing (Van Dyne and Torell, 1964). Many early publications dealt with comparisons of the chemical composition of the extrusa relative to that of the herbage consumed because of differences that could arise from mastication, salivary contamination and the incomplete recovery of ingested herbage in the extruded boluses. These studies confirmed that, although urea is recirculated in saliva, the N concentration of extrusa provides a reliable estimate of the N concentration of herbage consumed (Langlands, 1966a; Little, 1972). Similarly, the Ca, S, Mg, Cu, Mn and Mo concentrations in extrusa can be used to predict the dietary levels (Little, 1975) but extrusa P and Na levels are elevated due to salivary contamination. Nevertheless, dietary P levels can be determined if oesophageal fistulated animals are injected with ^{32}P to label their salivary P (Little et $al.$, 1977). Excess saliva should not be discarded because of the substantial amount of forage P in the liquid fraction and adjustments also need to be made for salivary DM, especially when feed on offer is low in moisture (D.B. Coates, unpublished data).

Because the botanical composition of extrusa is often an unreliable predictor of the diet of resident animals, it can be concluded that the chemical composition of extrusa may not reliably reflect that of the diet. Nevertheless, corrections can be applied if relationships between chemical composition and botanical composition can be determined (Coates, 1999a). For example, in tropical grass/legume pastures there is usually a close correlation between N concentration and legume content of herbage consumed. The regression relationship between N concentration and the C_3 (legume) content of herbage can be determined on samples of extrusa; the dietary C_3 content of resident animals can be determined from faecal C ratios; and the dietary N concentration can be estimated by applying the regression formula. Such corrections can be made for any attribute that is correlated with the C_3 content of selected herbage. Similar corrections could be applied where animals graze temperate grass/legume pastures where alkane technology (p. 375) could be used to determine the grass/ legume proportions of extrusa and diet.

The most promising new development for predicting diet quality is based on faecal NIRS (Lyons and Stuth, 1992) where predictions are based on robust relationships between faecal NIR spectral characteristics and chemical composition of diet samples. Lyons and Stuth (1992) developed calibration equations for predicting crude protein (CP) and OMD levels in the diet of free grazing cattle from NIR analysis of their faeces. The calibration equations have been expanded by increasing the diversity and number of samples (both diet reference values and faecal spectra) in the calibration set to improve reliability of predictions. Similar technology is being developed in Australia for predicting diet quality attributes of cattle grazing tropical and subtropical pastures (Coates, 1999b). Although untested to date, there is scope for expanding the range of dietary attributes to include fibre fractions such as neutral and acid detergent fibre (NDF, ADF). Preliminary results from feeding experiments have indicated that useful predictions of digestible dry matter intake may be possible using faecal NIRS (D.B. Coates, unpublished).

Faecal NIRS equations have also been developed to assess diet quality of free-ranging goats (Leite and Stuth, 1995) and there is no logical reason why this approach could not be used to predict diet quality for any herbivore. The main advantages of faecal NIRS predictions of diet quality are as follows:

- In many situations there is no alternative means of measuring or estimating diet quality, especially at the landscape scale.
- The estimate is directly related to the target animals.
- Once appropriate calibration equations are developed, analysis is rapid and inexpensive.
- All attributes for which calibration equations exist can be predicted from a single faecal NIR analysis.

The main disadvantages are as follows:

- Developing robust calibration equations with reliable predictive ability is expensive and time consuming and instrumentation is expensive.
- Validation of calibration equations and routine checking of their accuracy is difficult compared with most other NIRS applications where chemical analyses and NIR spectra are obtained from the same sample.

Digestibility of grazed herbage

Definition

Digestibility is a measure of the proportion of the total intake of feed, or of a component of the feed, that has been digested and does not appear in faeces. The percentage digestibility (*D*) is calculated as:

$$D = (I - F) / I \times 100$$

where *I* equals intake and *F* is the output in faeces. However, this is in fact apparent digestibility. True digestibility is very difficult to measure because faeces also contain metabolic excretions (microbial and endogenous matter). Digestibility is expressed on a DM or OM basis and may also be calculated for the diet as a whole or for some dietary fraction such as protein or minerals.

Digestibility is a function of the diet (chemical and physical attributes) and the animal (e.g. species, age, intake and parasitic status). Therefore, the way in which digestibility estimates are determined and used in animal nutrition and grassland research requires a degree of caution.

Digestibility and intake of selected herbage are the main determinants of productivity in grazing ruminants, together determining intake of digestible energy. Thus, herbage digestibility is considered a key measure of

dietary nutritive value and tremendous effort has been directed at developing techniques for its measurement. The prediction of forage digestibility
by laboratory methods has been reviewed by Minson (1990) and Weiss
(1994) and of *in vivo* digestibility by Cochran and Galyean (1994).

In vitro *digestibility estimates on dietary samples*

The rumen liquor and acid–pepsin method of Tilley and Terry (1963) and
the pepsin–cellulase method (McLeod and Minson, 1978) are both widely
used. The main disadvantages of *in vitro* methods are as follows:

- Herbage samples, obtained either by plucking pasture, or by sampling
  with oesophageal fistulated animals, may not truly represent the diet of
  the grazing animal (p. 370).
- The correlation between *in vivo* and *in vitro* digestibility is not particularly strong. Clark and Beard (1977) reported RSDs of > ± 4 percentage
  units for regression equations relating *in vivo* DM digestibility to DM
  disappearance in the pepsin–cellulase and rumen liquor *in vitro* techniques. Comparable residual standard deviations reported by McLeod
  and Minson (1978) were lower at ± 3.3 (pepsin–cellulase) and ± 2.6
  (rumen liquor–pepsin) percentage units for a combined grass and
  legume set of 82 samples. The accuracy of predicted *in vivo* digestibility
  from *in vitro* analysis is likely to improve as the diversity of forage types
  in the regression relationship is restricted and where the standards of
  known *in vivo* digestibility are similar to the forages being analysed.
- Estimates of digestibility cannot be determined for individual grazing
  animals. True *in vivo* digestibility depends on animal factors as well as
  the properties of the plant material.

Other laboratory methods estimate *in vivo* digestibility using relationships with chemical components of forage samples, particularly fibrous
fractions such as crude fibre, NDF, ADF, hemicellulose, cellulose and lignin
(Van Soest, 1994). The predictive reliability of regression relationships
depends to a large extent on whether the standard forages used to develop
predictive equations represent the diversity of species and environmental
interactions characteristic of the forages to be tested. No individual fibre
fraction is closely correlated with digestibility over wide ranges of feeds and
forages. Therefore, reference forages should be selected from locations
similar to those of the forages to be tested (Van Soest, 1994) and the reference forages should also encompass environmental variation with respect
to growing conditions (e.g. temperature, moisture, soil fertility). ADF is
frequently used as the preferred predictor, being more closely correlated
with digestibility than NDF or lignin. However, lignin would be a more
accurate predictor of digestibility if differences in the lignin to cell wall
characteristics of different forages were accounted for. This has led to the
development of summative equations where the unlignified and wholly
digestible cell contents are treated separately from the cell wall fraction

(Goering and Van Soest, 1970). Summative systems provide more accurate predictions of digestibility when applied to forage mixtures but are of lesser benefit when applied within a single plant species (Van Soest, 1994).

Another alternative is the nylon bag technique, where samples of forage are enclosed in small sachets of indigestible fabric, such as nylon or dacron, and incubated in the rumen of fistulated animals (Weiss, 1994). Sample size, pore size of fabric, position of sample within the rumen, diet of the host fistulated animal and incubation time all affect DM disappearance. The technique may be used with or without a subsequent pepsin incubation. Reports on the predictive accuracy of this technique vary (e.g. Keyserlingk and Mathison, 1989).

The anaerobic digestion of animal feeds produces gaseous products (CO_2 and CH_4) and *in vivo* digestibility can be estimated by measuring *in vitro* gas production of feed samples incubated in buffered ruminal fluid (Menke *et al.*, 1979). Technical improvements such as computerized monitoring of gas production have been developed (Pell and Schofield, 1993). The method can also be used to estimate degradation rates and kinetics of fibre digestion by measuring and modelling gas production over time (Beuvink and Kogut, 1993; Schofield *et al.*, 1994).

Further discussion of laboratory and *in vivo* methods of measuring digestibility is given in Chapter 11.

Faecal index techniques

Faecal index techniques involve the development of quantitative relationships between a faecal characteristic and the variable under consideration. The most common index for estimating dietary digestibility is faecal N (Corbett, 1978). The technique has serious limitations because regression relationships between faecal N and digestibility are not constant and vary with pasture species, season, locality and even fertilizer treatment. Considering the effort required to develop regression relationships for accurately estimating digestibility in given situations, other techniques are preferred.

Plant marker techniques

The ideal plant marker for estimating digestibility is one that is completely indigestible, readily recovered and analysed in both feed and faeces, and uniformly distributed throughout above-ground plant parts. Lignin, silica and different plant pigments have been investigated but are not satisfactory (Corbett, 1978). More recently, plant alkanes (see below) have been used with considerable success.

Forage NIRS

NIR analysis of forage samples is used extensively for the routine measurement of forage digestibility but the accuracy of prediction depends on the accuracy of laboratory reference values used in calibration. Once calibration equations have been developed, rapid and inexpensive estimates of forage digestibility can be made. Calibration equations can be developed for predicting digestibility of fresh as well as dried and ground samples (e.g. Boever *et al.*, 1994).

Faecal NIRS

Reports by Lyons and Stuth (1992) and Leite and Stuth (1995) in the US, together with studies in Australia (Coates, 1999b), indicate that useful predictions of dietary digestibility in grazing ruminants may be made using faecal NIRS. The accuracy of the predictions will partly depend on the method used to determine laboratory reference values for matching with faecal NIR spectra in developing the calibration equations. If the reference values are determined by *in vitro* analysis of oesophageal extrusa samples, or even of forage samples fed in pens, then calibration equations will incorporate any bias in the relationship between laboratory estimated and true *in vivo* digestibility values of the calibration samples. Actual *in vivo* estimates of digestibility (by conventional feeding trials or by the alkane technique in grazing animals) made on the animals from which the faecal NIR spectra are obtained would be preferable, albeit often too costly or impractical.

Plant wax alkanes as marker substances

Recent developments with indigestible plant cuticular wax components, especially *n*-alkanes, have opened up new opportunities for accurately estimating herbage intake, digestibility and botanical composition of the selected diet in free grazing animals. The subject is covered by Dove and Mayes (1991) and Dove (1994) and in Chapter 11.

Measuring intake in grazing animals

The cuticular wax of pasture plants contains a mixture of alkanes of carbon chain length C25 to C35. The odd-numbered carbon chains predominate and concentrations of even-chain alkanes are low by comparison. Faecal recovery of plant alkanes is not complete, though it increases with increasing chain length. However, faecal recoveries of odd- and even-chain alkanes, of chain length n and $n - 1$ respectively, are similar and it has been shown that by dosing animals with synthetic even-chain alkanes such as C32 (assume dose rate of D_j mg day^{-1}) and measuring concentrations of the natural and dosed alkanes in herbage (H_i and H_j, respectively) and in faeces (F_i and F_j), herbage intake can be calculated by:

$$\text{INTAKE} = (F_i/F_j) \times D_j / (H_i - (F_i/F_j) \times H_j)$$

Because faecal recovery rates of a dosed and natural alkane pair (e.g. C32 and C33) are similar, incomplete faecal recovery of alkanes *per se* is of no consequence as the ratio F_i/F_j remains constant. Analytical accuracy in extracting and measuring alkane concentrations, obtaining a truly representative sample of the consumed herbage for measuring H_i and H_j, and accurate control of the dose rate of the even-chain alkane are all required for accurate measurement of herbage intake. Errors associated with obtaining a representative sample of herbage consumed is a major concern, because alkane concentrations differ not only between plant species but also between parts within plants. Herbage concentrations can be determined on plucked pasture or oesophageal extrusa. Dosing with synthetic even-chain alkane can be achieved by twice-daily administration of paper pellets (alkane impregnated into shredded paper) or gelatin capsules. Controlled-release devices, similar to those developed for chromic oxide, are now available and allow continuous release of synthetic alkane over a period of 14 days or more. Reliable techniques are available for extracting alkanes from plant and faecal material and alkane concentrations are determined using gas–liquid chromatography. Comparisons between alkane-estimated and actual herbage intakes confirm the accuracy of the technique when applied to temperate forages.

Botanical composition and digestibility

Differences between species in individual alkane concentrations enable the botanical composition of herbage mixtures to be calculated, whether these mixtures be harvested forage, extrusa samples, or diets of grazing animals as reflected in their faeces (Newman *et al.*, 1995). The latter application overcomes the main problems associated with the use of oesophageal fistulated animals for estimating dietary botanical composition, but the methodology is constrained by a number of limitations. Alkane concentrations need to be determined in both herbage and faecal samples and differences in alkane levels between plant parts (Dove *et al.*, 1996) will be a source of error if herbage samples harvested for analysis contain plant parts in different proportions from those consumed by grazing animals. This is of greater importance where calculations are dependent on actual concentrations of individual alkanes rather than on relative proportions of alkanes within a species. Another limitation is the incomplete faecal recovery of alkanes and corrections have to be made to overcome this problem. Faecal recovery rates based on direct measurement in housed animals may be applied, but the preferred technique is to dose test animals with a mixture of even-chain alkanes for calculation of faecal recovery rates relative to chain length. Dosing also enables intake to be quantified. Another constraint is that the number of species that can be separated is limited to the number of alkanes used in the estimate. Digestibility of individual dietary components is not needed to estimate botanical composition of the diet from faecal alkanes and the technique can be used to estimate digestibility of the whole diet.

Where test animals are dosed with a mixture of even-chain alkanes, analysis of faeces and hand-plucked herbage of individual component species allows the calculation of diet botanical composition, total herbage intake, intake by components and digestibility of the whole diet.

Dung, Urine and Methane Production

This section considers output of both dung and urine and some urinary metabolites used in animal production studies. Methane production has received attention because of concerns about the contribution of ruminants to greenhouse gas emissions and global warming.

Faecal output

Faecal output (FO) is frequently used to estimate forage intake (I):

$$I = FO/(1 - D)$$

where D is digestibility of the forage. Collecting, drying and weighing total FO is the most accurate method but there are difficulties involved in total collection and various marker techniques have been developed.

Total collection

Total collection of faeces from grazing animals requires specially designed harnesses so that faeces can be voided into a collection bag. In principle the method is simple but difficulties arise (Corbett, 1978). In particular, complete collection cannot be guaranteed and even when incomplete collection is known or suspected it cannot be quantified. The fresh weight of FO in cattle is substantial, sometimes exceeding 30 kg day^{-1} for a 500 kg animal. Therefore, bags need to be emptied at least twice a day and the implications for good harness design are obvious. Because of these problems, indirect estimates of FO are generally preferred in grazing animals. However, total collections are often used to check indirect estimates.

Faecal marker methods

The most common marker method for estimating FO relies on the use of an indigestible external marker (Kotb and Luckey, 1972). FO can then be calculated by relating the concentration of the marker in the faeces to a known marker dose. The technique depends on marker concentration in collected faecal samples being representative of the total FO. Effective marker dosing and faecal sampling protocols are therefore essential. The technique, up to the mid-1980s, was based on oral application of regular, discrete doses of marker ensuring an even distribution throughout the digestive tract (Corbett, 1978). Once-daily dosing generally results in diurnal fluctuations in faecal marker concentration but twice-daily dosing is usually satisfactory. Dosing should commence 1 week before faecal sampling, to reach an equilibrium state. Faecal sampling protocols aim to provide an estimate of mean marker concentration that represents that of total FO. Rectal grab samples can be taken when the marker is administered and faecal sampling should be maintained long enough to overcome errors due to short-term changes in voluntary intake and rate of passage of digesta. Collection periods will differ depending on the experimental objectives but generally lie within 5–14 days.

Chromic oxide (Cr_2O_3) is the most commonly used external marker for estimating FO but other markers, including ytterbium (Hatfield *et al.*, 1990), paraffin-coated magnesium ferrite (Bruckental *et al.*, 1987), dysprosium (Krysl *et al.*, 1988) and titanium oxide (Mayes *et al.*, 1995), have also been used. Morgan *et al.* (1976) recommended Cr EDTA as a better marker than Cr_2O_3 because it could be analysed more accurately and rapidly. However, there is variable absorption and urinary excretion of Cr EDTA and this can bias the estimates of FO. Cr EDTA is used primarily as a marker in digestive studies (site of digestion, digesta kinetics and digesta flows) rather than for estimating FO.

The limitation of frequent dosing of Cr_2O_3 was overcome by the development of intra-ruminal slow-release capsules or controlled-release devices (CRDs), which were designed to release a constant amount of marker into the rumen over a period of 3 weeks or more (Laby *et al.*, 1984; Furnival *et al.*, 1990b). Where regular yarding of test animals is impractical, faecal samples can be collected directly from the paddock but this will usually mean that individual estimates of FO cannot be made, due to difficulties in matching faecal samples with individual animals. Identification of paddock-collected faecal samples is possible if animals are dosed with different-coloured plastic particles (Minson *et al.*, 1960) but this also requires frequent dosing.

Unbiased estimates of FO using CRDs depend on a constant rate of release of the marker at the rate specified by the manufacturer. Given a uniform rate of release of Cr_2O_3 from the CRD, the actual release rate often varies from the specified rate due to both animal and pasture effects (Furnival *et al.*, 1990a, b; Doyle *et al.*, 1994). Unbiased estimates of FO also depend on full recovery of the marker during chemical analysis. Partial recovery leads to overestimation of FO. Therefore, faecal standards with known concentrations of marker should be included in all analytical runs (Costigan and Ellis, 1987). Conversely, natural or artificial contamination of pasture with Cr, the latter from previous marker studies, can lead to high faecal concentrations and underestimates of FO. Faecal samples collected from undosed animals grazing the same pasture as the test animals should therefore be included as controls when determining faecal marker concentrations.

Experiments evaluating CRDs have found cases of underestimation, overestimation and close agreement with FO determined by total collection, but most have reported overestimation. Overestimates are due either to incomplete recovery of the marker from faecal samples (analytical error) or to release of marker from the CRD being less than the specified rate. Either way, experimental procedures can be applied to take account of these sources of error. However, procedures to correct for differences between actual and specified marker release rates add considerably to the cost and inconvenience of the technique. Rumen fistulated animals can be used together with test animals to check on the rate of release of marker from the CRD (Furnival *et al.*, 1990b), or total faecal collection as well as marker estimated FO can be made on selected animals to derive correction factors (Hollingsworth *et al.*, 1995).

Marker concentration curves can be used as an alternative to the steady-state technique described above for estimating FO (Susmel *et al.*, 1996). The technique depends on characterizing the marker excretion curve following a single pulse dose of an external marker. Since marker excretion curves require frequent sampling, the technique does not lend itself to use with grazing animals.

Finally, any sampling procedure may disturb normal grazing behaviour, with possible reductions in forage intake and FO. The effect is likely to be more pronounced in animals that are not accustomed to the presence of humans or to frequent handling. Therefore, quietening and training of animals prior to experimental sampling will help to avoid bias.

Urinary output and urinary markers

Urine is an important excretory path for N, Na, K and sometimes P in ruminant animals, and estimation of urinary excretion of these substances is necessary for nutrient cycling and balance studies. In addition, the composition of urine can be used to detect dietary deficiencies or excesses (Langlands, 1966b). More recently, urinary metabolites are being investigated as markers for determining feed intake, diet composition and nutrient supply in grazing and browsing ruminants (Mayes *et al.*, 1995).

Measurement of total urinary output
Samples of urine from grazing animals of both sexes are easy to obtain when animals are constrained in a race or crush but total collection is difficult. Engels and Hugo (1969) and Betteridge and Andrews (1986) described equipment for total collection of urine from grazing sheep and steers, respectively. Animals have to be trained and accustomed to the equipment to minimize effects on grazing behaviour and intake. Situations in which animals may be harnessed with urine collection equipment are severely restricted.

Orr *et al.* (1995) measured urinary excretion in sheep without special equipment by collecting urine and faeces together in faecal bags containing a quantity of Na bentonite granules to absorb the urine. If animals are dosed with Cr_2O_3 then the nutrients in the total collection can be apportioned to faeces and urine by calculating the ratio of faecal nutrients to chromic oxide in faecal grab samples. This technique was simplified by White *et al.* (1997) using the ratio of faecal nutrients to ADF in faecal grab samples.

Where animals are confined in metabolism crates, difficulties in total collection of urine occur mainly with females where urine has to be separated from faeces. Appropriate separation and collection devices have been described (Magner *et al.*, 1988; Kowalczyk *et al.*, 1996).

An alternative to total collection of urine is to use an index substance for estimating urinary excretion of waste products. The technique depends on a constant quantitative relationship between the substance under investigation (e.g. urinary N) and the index substance, as well as a uniform daily excretion of the index substance. Creatinine, a waste product of muscle metabolism, is the most commonly used index substance. It is excreted in mammalian urine in approximately constant amounts daily for a given LW and is relatively little affected by diet. Langlands (1966b) described the technique and its shortcomings.

Urinary metabolite markers

Many metabolites are excreted in the urine. Currently there is interest in the aromatic and purine metabolites that are excreted in response to ingestion of feed, the aromatic metabolites being derived mainly from ruminal fermentation of lignocellulose, while purine derivatives originate mainly from microbial biomass synthesized in the rumen (Mayes *et al.*, 1995). These metabolites show considerable potential as urinary markers for estimating feed intake and microbial protein yield.

Methane production

Techniques for measuring methane (CH_4) emissions by grazing animals have been developed using portable polythene tunnels (polytunnels) over areas of sward being grazed by sheep or calves (Lockyer, 1997). Air is drawn through the tunnels by fans and CH_4 production is calculated from inlet and outlet concentrations of CH_4. Eating, ruminating and idling activity of animals in the tunnels were also measured simultaneously with measurements of CH_4 by D.L. Lockyer and R.A. Champion (IGER, UK, 1998, personal communication). They showed how the measurements were correlated and the diurnal fluctuations in gas production corresponded with circadian patterns of grazing behaviour. This has been taken further by P.H. Murray (IGER, UK, 1998, personal communication) who measured CO_2 and CH_4 production by grazing animals, allowing energy expenditure by the grazing animals to be estimated. An alternative technique was developed by Johnson *et al.* (1994) using sulphur hexafluoride (SF_6) as a tracer. Slow-release intra-ruminal boluses of SF_6 together with equipment for collecting methane and SF_6 into a container carried on the animal were developed for determining total daily production of CH_4.

Grazing Intake

In grazing animals, intake (I) is usually estimated by measuring both FO and D of the grazed herbage, i.e. $I = FO / (1 - D)$. The techniques for measuring digestibility and FO have already been described.

The faecal alkane technique offers the best potential for reliably estimating intake in grazing cattle but the technique has still to be validated for tropical pastures.

Alternative methods for estimating intake in grazing animals are: (i) estimating herbage mass before and after grazing; (ii) weighing animals before and after grazing (see next section); (iii) estimating bite mass and multiplying by total bites per 24 h (see next section); and (iv) using reverse feeding standards to calculate intake from energy retention and outputs and the metabolizable energy level of the diet.

The weighing and bite mass × total bite techniques require estimates of the water content of the herbage eaten to enable DM intake to be calculated. DM may vary between herbage species and plant parts, spatially and temporally (Orr *et al.*, 1997b) and so estimates of diet selection are also important in these techniques. Thus, accurate estimates of diet selection and its composition are vital to virtually all the techniques discussed but are notoriously difficult to make and may introduce major sources of error into the estimation of intake by grazing animals.

Estimating intake using reverse feeding standards requires the monitoring of animal production (LW change) and output (e.g. milk) over several weeks and the use of feeding standards to convert total production into metabolizable energy (ME) (AFRC, 1993). Estimates of ME concentration in the diet from pasture samples are also made so that herbage intake can be calculated (Baker, 1982). Minson and McDonald (1987) developed an equation for predicting the herbage intake of beef cattle from their LW and growth rate without the need for any laboratory analyses of the diet selected. Diet quality was estimated solely from the growth rate and weight of cattle.

Grazing Behaviour

This chapter can only consider some aspects of foraging and ingestive behaviour. Books on behaviour in cattle (Phillips, 1993) and sheep (Lynch *et al.*, 1992) contain more information.

Measurement of grazing behaviour takes many different aspects, depending on scale and purpose. Regarding scale, studies on highly productive, intensively managed temperate pastures in paddocks of a few hectares or less will obviously be concerned with different behavioural attributes than studies on extensively managed pastures in paddocks covering hundreds or thousands of hectares and incorporating broad-scale heterogeneity. Regarding purpose, measurements made and experimental design will vary depending on objectives.

Grazing behaviour is important because of the immediate effect on the animal's productivity and also because of the consequences of present grazing behaviour on future grazing opportunities, pasture composition and productivity. Ultimately, the purpose of studying grazing behaviour must be to assist livestock producers to manage pastures for improved productivity and/or sustainability.

This section gives a brief overview of the development and use of techniques for measuring the various components of ingestive behaviour that determine intake, the measurement of dietary preferences and some spatial aspects of grazing behaviour.

Ingestive components of grazing intake

Daily herbage DM intake (I) is the product of grazing time and intake rate (IR) (Allden and Whittaker, 1970). IR is the product of bite mass (BM) and biting rate (BR), while BM is the product of bite volume and density of herbage in the grazed horizon. Thus sward structure is the first immediate limiting factor to intake, while digestive, physical and metabolic controls of intake are considered to be longer-term control mechanisms.

Short-term measurements of BM and IR

Estimating intake of sheep by weighing them before and after grazing (Allden and Whittaker, 1970) was further developed by Penning and Hooper (1985) by using an electronic balance to weigh sheep to ± 10 g. The balance was controlled by a portable computer, which also recorded the weighings. Animals were fitted with bags to prevent loss of faeces and urine, weighed, allowed to graze for approximately 1 h and weighed again. Weight gains were adjusted for insensible weight loss and the adjusted increase in LW gave an estimate of fresh herbage intake. Representative samples of herbage were dried to give an estimate of DM content. Animals were also fitted with behaviour recorders (Penning *et al.*, 1984; Rutter *et al.*, 1997) to record grazing time and number of bites taken. This technique was later adapted for use with dairy cows (Gibb *et al.*, 1995). From these measurements it was possible to measure IR and BM over relatively short periods and relate these to sward structure.

Forage intake can be estimated by the alkane technique and, with daily recordings of behaviour, BM can be calculated. However, using the alkane approach may not be suitable when sward conditions are changing rapidly, because of the number of days required to estimate mean intake and because BM and short-term IR may vary in a non-linear manner in response to changes in sward structure (Penning *et al.*, 1994). Despite these reservations, Romney *et al.* (1996) found surprisingly good agreement between the two techniques for estimating intake.

Measuring jaw movements

Chacon *et al.* (1976) observed that when cattle are eating, 'counting' all jaw movements as bites overestimated biting, as some of the movements were associated with mastication. Overestimating BR resulted in an under-estimate of BM. The number of bites may be recorded by observing animals since a characteristic head jerk occurs as animals bite herbage from the sward (Hodgson, 1982) but it is very difficult to count and discriminate between jaw movements associated with biting, manipulation and mastica-tion. In practice, it is impossible for an observer to record these parameters continuously for long periods and for several animals simultaneously. This has led to sampling techniques where an observer estimates BR for about a minute over intervals throughout the day. Champion *et al.* (1994) showed that sheep have different rates of jaw movement depending on the time of day and night. Therefore, within-day variation in BR needs to be taken into account when designing intermittent sampling routines to estimate total daily jaw movements. These difficulties have led to the development of automatic recording systems (see 'Telemetry', p. 387). For example, Chambers *et al.* (1981) developed a system to distinguish bites from other jaw movements by using an accelerometer to measure and count head jerks associated with biting. The system described by Penning *et al.* (1984) could discriminate between bites and other jaw movements (mastications) during eating by sheep. It was demonstrated that, since there is a fixed maximum jaw movement rate, the allocation of jaw movements between biting and masticating provides a mechanism for IR control (e.g. Penning *et al.*, 1994). Rutter *et al.* (1997) developed an automatic recording system that can count and discriminate between different types of jaw movements for grazing cattle. These detailed recording techniques have led to major advances in our understanding of grazing behaviour.

Sward structure, BM and grazing jaw movements

BM is a function of bite depth, bite area and herbage density in the grazed horizon. In the field it is difficult to measure these parameters and several workers have used hand-constructed swards to facilitate detailed measure-ments (e.g. Laca *et al.*, 1992). Burlinson *et al.* (1991) used a modification of the short-term techniques and contained animals within crates placed on the sward. They were able to graze a limited area of prepared sward immediately in front of the crate. These techniques only permit measurements to be made over a few minutes and for a limited number of bites. Although providing valuable insights into the grazing process, results must be interpreted with caution since immediate previous diet and hunger status can influence diet selection and BM (Parsons *et al.*, 1994a). In addition, Penning *et al.* (1993b) showed that sheep kept as individuals may graze differently from those in groups and recommended a minimum group of four sheep as the experimental unit.

Techniques have been developed to measure bite depth and area in the field. For example, Wade *et al.* (1989) monitored marked tillers at frequent intervals and estimated bite depth from measurements before and after grazing. It was found that dairy cows consistently removed a third of tiller height, regardless of initial tiller height or whether the tillers had been previously grazed. Similar results were reported for hand-constructed swards (Laca *et al.*, 1992). Edwards *et al.* (1996) and Orr *et al.* (1997a) estimated bite area and bite depth by observing the number of bites taken from a sward by cattle or sheep, placing a mesh grid over the grazed area, and mapping the area on paper using the grid cells as a guide. Bite depth was measured as the difference between grazed and ungrazed areas of sward.

Using the mapping technique is difficult and somewhat subjective, as it is often very difficult to see where the animals have grazed. The coefficients of variation between observers in estimates of area grazed varied between 16 and 49% (A. Harvey, IGER, UK, 1998, personal communication), emphasizing the difficulties involved in discerning grazed from ungrazed areas.

BM also appears to be under behavioural control *per se*, as fasted animals have been shown subsequently to increase BM and BR (Newman *et al.*, 1994b). This suggests that normally animals do not eat at maximum possible rates. More detailed reviews of the grazing process are available (e.g. Parsons *et al.*, 1994a; Woodward, 1997).

Grazing time and meal patterns

Grazing time can be estimated by observing animals but this is tedious, and difficult at night. Several automatic systems that can be used to record grazing time are described in the telemetry section below. However, frequent observations (at least one per minute) are required. Forbes (1986) and Sibly *et al.* (1990) revealed two types of pauses during eating: those within an eating bout (intra-meal intervals) and those between eating bouts (inter-meal intervals). For grazing sheep, Penning *et al.* (1993a) showed that intra-meal intervals were of at least 6 min duration. This technique was used by Gibb *et al.* (1997) to determine the number and duration of meals taken by grazing dairy cows. IR during grazing is not constant but varies in relation to daily meal patterns (Orr *et al.*, 1997b) and within meals. Penning *et al.* (1993a) developed a method to examine IR within meals and found that the relationship between grazing time and IR was linear only if intra-meal intervals were removed, to give *eating time*. This has important implications in using the product of short-term IR and *grazing time* to estimate daily intake and it is recommended that the product of *eating time* × IR, rather than *grazing time* × IR, be used to estimate daily intake (Gibb, 1998).

Dietary preference and diet selection

Dietary preference may be defined as 'diet selection without environmental constraints' (after Hodgson, 1979). On the other hand, diet selection represents what the grazing animal actually consumes. It is the result of the interaction between the animal's dietary preferences for the various pasture components on offer, and the constraints associated with availability (relative amounts) and accessibility (ease of harvesting a desired component).

Techniques for determining dietary preferences vary from offering animals hand-made swards to providing animals with a choice of species growing as monocultures (e.g. Parsons *et al.*, 1994b). Preference ranking can be determined by direct observation or time-lapse video-recording (Parsons *et al.*, 1994b). The interpretation of results is critical since dietary preference can be influenced not only by the relative palatability of species on offer but also by: (i) previous dietary history, either in the immediate or long-term past (e.g. Parsons *et al.*, 1994b); (ii) time of day (e.g. Rutter *et al.*, 1998); (iii) hunger (Newman *et al.*, 1994a); (iv) dietary mineral deficiencies such as P (Coates and Le Feuvre, 1998); (v) duration of intake, since results from relatively long-term measurements may differ from short-duration tests; and (vi) other species present.

In mixed pastures, estimates of dietary preference have been based on the composition of the selected diet but the results are confounded by various constraints to uninhibited selection, including botanical composition and sward structure. Attempts have been made to overcome the problem of unequal proportions by calculating various selection or preference indices that make allowance for the proportion of a component in the pasture as well as in the diet. If X is the percentage of a component in the diet, and Y is the percentage of that component in the pasture, then the simplest index is the selection ratio (SR), where:

$$SR = X / Y.$$

Theoretically, SR can vary between 0 and almost infinity, with values of 0–1 representing selection against a component (lower proportion in the diet than in the pasture) and values of 1 to infinity representing selection for a component. To overcome the occurrence of absurdly high values for SR, the selection index (SI) may be preferred, where:

SI = $(X - Y) / (X + Y)$ (Winter, 1988).

SI values can only vary between −1 and +1; negative values indicate selection against, positive values selection for. An alternative to SI is the selection coefficient (θ), where:

$\theta = [X / (100 - X)] / [Y / (100 - Y)]$ (Ridout and Robson, 1991).

Krueger (1972) calculated relative preferences (RP) by incorporating frequency % as well as percentage composition in diet and pasture.

The problem with these indices is that the calculated value is still partly dependent on pasture composition and, as such, can be misleading as an indicator of preference ranking. It is important to note that animals will rarely, if ever, select one component to the exclusion of other components on offer. Coates (1996) maintains that when choice is not constrained by limitations of quantity and accessibility, cattle will develop a stable dietary composition where the different components are consumed in set proportions. Animals will endeavour to maintain these proportions even when choice is constrained, and the divergence from the desired proportions will increase as the constraints to free choice increase. This theory is supported by the results of Rutter *et al.* (1998) and Penning *et al.* (1997) where monocultures of ryegrass and clover were offered, in different proportions by area, to dairy cows and sheep, respectively. The preferred proportions will be subject to gradual and sometimes sudden changes as influenced by changes within the pastures and environmental factors.

Research on grazing and foraging behaviour addresses the underlying mechanisms and processes that affect diet selection. It includes such matters as the mechanisms of learning in diet selection, including the problem of dealing with phytotoxins (e.g. Provenza *et al.*, 1992), post-ingestive feedback mechanisms (Provenza, 1995), cognitive and non-cognitive mechanisms in relation to the selection of feeding sites and selection of herbage within feeding sites (e.g. Bailey *et al.*, 1996), social aspects such as gregarious tendencies and mob behaviour patterns with respect to temporal and spatial decisions in grazing (e.g. Bailey, 1995), and foraging models and foraging theory (Bailey *et al.*, 1996). The field is too broad to allow us to review the various techniques that have been used. In addition to the references above, we refer readers to a review by Gordon (1995) of animal-based techniques for grazing ecology research.

Spatial aspects of foraging behaviour

Spatial aspects of foraging behaviour are of special significance in extensive grazing situations where herbivores are confronted with heterogeneity in topography, soil type, vegetation, rainfall pattern and even predatory risk. The study of foraging behaviour is important at this scale because of the effect of grazing distribution and intensity on animal productivity and pasture condition. Techniques for studying livestock distribution and forage utilization patterns may be based on records of the actual physical presence of animals in specified locations or by inferring utilization patterns from other measurements or observations. The physical presence of livestock (numbers and location) may be determined by routine inspections from horseback (e.g. Hart *et al.*, 1991) or motorized conveyance. Locating animals may be assisted by fitting some animals with radio telemetry collars (Pinchak *et al.*, 1991) or using a global positioning system (GPS) (Roberts *et al.*, 1993). Decisions have to be made on the frequency of inspections needed to satisfy the experimental objectives (periods within years or seasons; days within periods; number of records within days) and on the data to be recorded for each observation (e.g. number of animals, location, animal activity, weather conditions, etc.) (Pinchak *et al.*, 1991). For large areas, observations may be made from the air (Low *et al.*, 1981), with obvious restrictions due to cost.

Grazing distribution and relative grazing intensities can also be estimated from ground surveys of the area. The paddock is divided and marked according to a predetermined grid or transect pattern and at each sampling point the pasture and the component species are rated or scored according to the level of utilization. Determining the level of utilization may present difficulties and require training, especially when the pasture is actively growing. Errors in the actual estimates of utilization can be tolerated in determining grazing distribution patterns, provided any bias is consistent across the paddock. Survey frequency is of obvious importance in determining spatial by temporal relationships. Faecal distribution patterns can also be used in the assessment of grazing distribution.

Finally, techniques have been developed where Landsat imagery can be used to estimate the spatial distribution of grazing livestock and the patterns of livestock movement in large paddocks in the arid zones (Pickup and Chewings, 1988; Pickup and Bastin, 1997).

Telemetry

In grazing systems we are mainly concerned with biotelemetry, defined as 'assessment or control of biological parameters from animals, subjects and patients with relatively little disturbance or constraint of the animal/patient, resulting in undisturbed and noise free measurement of physiological parameters' (Kimmich, 1980). Telemetry has an important role to play in monitoring ingestive behaviour and physiological processes of grazing ruminants that may roam over relatively large areas whilst grazing. Many telemetric systems have been designed, with varying degrees of success, to record grazing behaviour automatically. These systems may be described as 'storage telemetry', where the data from sensors are recorded and stored on devices carried by the animals; or 'radio telemetry', where the data are transmitted to a remote processing/storage device. Biotelemetry has been extensively reviewed by Amlaner and MacDonald (1980).

Storage telemetry

Storage telemetry involves sensors and some recording device being carried by animals. Canaway *et al.* (1955) were amongst the pioneers to use telemetry to record grazing behaviour but their equipment was bulky and data required lengthy manual processing. Stobbs and Cowper (1972) developed a compact recorder for measuring the time and duration of grazing and to record jaw movements during grazing and rumination.

Advances continued, with refinements to existing systems and development of new sensors and recording systems with advanced capabilities (e.g. Chambers *et al.*, 1981; Penning, 1983; Penning *et al.*, 1984). The system developed by Penning *et al.* (1984) provides accurate information on time spent eating, ruminating and idling, diurnal patterns of the activities, and jaw movement counts during eating (with the ability to distinguish between biting and masticating jaw movements) and ruminating. Baldock *et al.* (1987) made a further modification so that heart rate could be recorded. Existing sensors, recording systems and electronic technologies were combined and refined by Brun *et al.* (1984) for monitoring diurnal patterns of grazing, ruminating and idling in grazing cattle; information concerning this equipment is available from J.-P. Brun (INRA, Theix, France).

More recent developments incorporate solid-state recorders that utilize single-board computers and solid-state memory devices to record jaw movements (Rutter *et al.*, 1997). The equipment could also incorporate GPS that, with correction, could locate animals with an accuracy of approximately 5 m. Solid-state recorders with the ability to monitor grazing behaviour of cattle and sheep over several days and that can distinguish between biting and masticating jaw movements whilst animals are eating have been developed (Champion *et al.*, 1997; Rutter *et al.*, 1997). Further information on the availability and performance of this equipment is available from http://www.ultrasoundadvice.co.uk.

Finally, video recordings have been used by several workers. For example, Parsons *et al.* (1994b) described the use of twelve security CCT video cameras that were multiplexed and the signals recorded by a time-lapse video recorder. These were used in conjunction with behaviour recorders (Penning, 1983; Penning *et al.*, 1984) to measure dietary selection by grazing sheep. However, lengthy manual interpretation of the tapes was required and recordings could not be made at night.

Radio telemetry

Early development of radio telemetry for measuring grazing behaviour was limited by the type of equipment available and the manual interpretation of data but subsequently there has been significant progress in data collection and processing. For example, Coulter and O'Sullivan (1988) used radio telemetry to monitor grazing behaviour of cattle; they measured head position and counted total jaw movements and steps taken. The data were transmitted every 3 min to a receiving station and were stored on a PC for subsequent analysis.

One recent development described by Scheibe et al. (1998) is a combined storage telemetry and radio telemetry system, which is commercially available (Ethosys, IMF Electronic, GmbH, Frankfurt/Oder D10315, Germany). It monitors grazing behaviour from a collar that contains an accelerometer, head position sensor and movement sensor and all the electronics. Data are stored on the animal until it comes within range of a receiving station, which is usually near a point that animals frequently visit (e.g. water trough). The data are then automatically down-loaded and can be subsequently analysed. This system can be used on a wide range of domestic and wild animals and can run for long periods (several months) without having to be removed from animals. The data collected can be processed automatically by computer programs.

Conclusions

Many different technologies and techniques have been developed for measuring and understanding all aspects of animal performance. New techniques will continue to be developed in parallel with advances in other fields such as biochemistry, electronics, spectrophotometry/spectroscopy and computing. For many measurements the existing technologies are adequate and improvements may come by way of increased efficiency (cost, time, portability, etc.). For others, increased accuracy would be desirable. Making accurate estimates of digestibility and intake in grazing animals, the very factors that together determine animal productivity, still presents real difficulties in most situations and remains a challenge. Nevertheless, we conclude by stressing that the effective measurement of animal performance depends largely on choosing the most appropriate technique in relation to the prevailing circumstances and the purpose for which the measurements are to be used, together with the correct application of the chosen method.

References

AFRC (1993) *Energy and Protein Requirements of Ruminants. An Advisory Manual prepared by the AFRC Technical Committee on Responses to Nutrients.* CAB International, Wallingford, UK.

Allden, W.G. and Whittaker, I.A.McD. (1970) The determination of intake by grazing sheep: the interrelationship of factors influencing herbage intake and availability. *Australian Journal of Agricultural Research* 21, 755–766.

Allen, V.G. (1991) Terminology for grazing animals. In: *Proceedings, 2nd Grazing Livestock Nutrition Conference, 2–3 August, 1991.* Steamboat Springs, Colorado, pp. 94–100.

Amlaner, C.J. and MacDonald, D.W. (1980) *A Handbook on Biotelemetry and Radio Tracking.* Pergamon Press, Oxford, UK.

Andersson, M. and Alanko, M. (1992) Relationship between testicular measurements, body weight and semen quality in young dairy bulls. *Acta Veterinaria Scandinavica* 33, 15–20.

Andrews, R.N., Hawker, H. and Crosbie, S.F. (1987) Evaluation of five methods for measuring mean fibre diameter of fleece samples from New Zealand sheep. *New Zealand Journal of Experimental Agriculture* 15, 23–31.

ARC (1980) *The Nutrient Requirements of Ruminant Livestock. Technical Review by an Agricultural Research Council Working Party.* CAB, Farnham Royal, UK.

Arnold, G.W. (1962) The influence of several factors in determining the grazing behaviour of Border Leicester × Merino sheep. *Journal of the British Grassland Society* 17, 41–51.

Bailey, D.W. (1995) Daily selection of feeding areas by cattle in homogeneous and heterogeneous environments. *Applied Animal Behavioural Science* 45, 183–199.

Bailey, D.W., Gross, J.E., Laca, E.A., Rittenhouse, L.R., Coughenour, M.B., Swift, D.M. and Sims, P.L. (1996) Mechanisms that result in large herbivore grazing distribution patterns. *Journal of Range Management* 49, 386–400.

Baker, A.A. (1965) Comparison of heat mount detectors and classical methods for detecting heat in beef cattle. *Australian Veterinary Journal* 41, 360–361.

Baker, R.D. (1982) Estimating herbage intake from animal performance. In: Leaver, J.D. (ed.) *Herbage Intake Handbook.* British Grassland Society, Hurley, UK, pp. 77–93.

Baldock, N.M., Penning, P.D. and Sibly, R.M. (1987) A system for recording sheep ECG in the field using a miniature 24-hour tape recorder. *Computers and Electronics in Agriculture* 2, 57–66.

Baulain, U. (1997) Magnetic resonance imaging for the *in vivo* determination of body composition in animal science. *Computers and Electronics in Agriculture* 17, 189–203.

Baxter, B.P., Brims, M.A. and Taylor, T.B. (1991) *Description and Performance of the Optical Fibre Diameter Analyser (OFDA).* Report No. 8, IWTO Technical Committee Meeting, Nice, France.

Berg, E.P. and Marchello, M.J. (1994) Bioelectrical impedance analysis for the prediction of fat-free mass in lambs and lamb carcases. *Journal of Animal Science* 72, 322–329.

Berge, S. (1977) On the estimation of weight and increase of weight by means of the chest girth in Norwegian Red cattle at the Agricultural University at As, Norway in the years 1972 and 1974. *Acta Agriculturae Scandinavica* 27, 65–66.

Betteridge, K. and Andrews, W.G.K. (1986) A device for measuring and sampling urine output from free-grazing steers. *Journal of Agricultural Science, Cambridge* 106, 389–392.

Beuvink, J.M.W. and Kogut, J. (1993) Modeling gas production kinetics of grass silages incubated with buffered ruminal fluid. *Journal of Animal Science* 71, 1041–1046.

Blockey, M.A.deB. (1989) Relationship between serving capacity of beef bulls as predicted by the yard test and their fertility during paddock mating. *Australian Veterinary Journal* 69, 348–351.

Blockey, M.A.deB. and Wilkins, J.F. (1984) Field application of the ram serving capacity test. In: Lindsay, D.R. and Pearce, D.T. (eds) *Reproduction in Sheep.* Australian Academy of Science, Canberra, Australia, pp. 53–58.

Boever, J.L. de, Waes Jvan, Cottyn, B.G. and Boucque, C.V. (1994) The prediction of forage maize digestibility by near infrared reflection spectroscopy. *Netherlands Journal of Agricultural Science* 42, 105–113.

Brinks, J.S., Clark, R.T., Rice, F.J. and Kieffer, N.M. (1961) Adjusting birth weight, weaning weight, and preweaning gain for sex of calf in range Hereford cattle. *Journal of Animal Science* 20, 363–367.

Bruckental, I., Lehrer, A.R., Weitz, M., Bernard, J., Kennit, H. and Neumark, H. (1987) Faecal output and estimated voluntary dry-matter intake of grazing beef cows, relative to their live weight and to the digestibility of the pasture. *Animal Production* 45, 23–28.

Brun, J.-P., Prache, S. and Bechet, G. (1984) A portable device for eating behaviour studies. In: *Proceedings of the 5th European Grazing Workshop.* Edinburgh.

Burlinson, A.J., Hodgson, J. and Illius, A.W. (1991) Sward canopy structure and the bite dimensions and bite weight of grazing sheep. *Grass and Forage Science* 46, 29–38.

Busk, H. (1989) Applications of ultrasound imaging in animal science. In: Kallweit, E., Henning, M. and Groeneveld, E. (eds) *Application of NMR Techniques on the Body Composition of Live Animals.* Elsevier Applied Science, London, pp. 75–90.

Canaway, R.J., Raymond, W.F. and Tayler, J.C. (1955) The automatic recording of animal behaviour in the field. *Electronic Engineering, March* 1955, 102–105.

Chacon, E., Stobbs, T.H. and Sandland, R.L. (1976) Estimation of herbage consumption by grazing cattle using measurements of eating behaviour. *Journal of the British Grassland Society* 31, 81–87.

Chambers, A.R.M., Hodgson, J. and Milne, J.A. (1981) The development and use of equipment for the automatic recording of ingestive behaviour in sheep and cattle. *Grass and Forage Science* 36, 97–105.

Champion, R.A., Rutter, S.M., Penning, P.D. and Rook, A.J. (1994) Temporal variation in grazing behaviour of sheep and the reliability of sampling periods. *Applied Animal Behaviour Science* 42, 99–108.

Champion, R.A., Rutter, S.M. and Penning, P.D. (1997) An automatic system to monitor lying, standing and walking behaviour of grazed animals. *Applied Animal Behaviour Science* 54, 291–305.

Chapman, R.E. and Wheeler, J.L. (1963) Dye-banding: a technique for fleece growth studies. *Australian Journal of Science* 26, 53–54.

Charles, D.D. (1974) A method of estimating cascase components in cattle. *Research in Veterinary Science* 16, 89–94.

Clark, J. and Beard, J. (1977) Prediction of the digestibility of ruminant feeds from their solubility in enzyme solutions. *Animal Feed Science and Technology* 2, 153–159.

Clements, R.J., Jones, R.M., Valdes, L.R. and Bunch, G.A. (1996) Selection of *Chamaecrista rotundifolia* by cattle. *Tropical Grasslands* 30, 389–394.

Coates, D.B. (1996) Diet selection by cattle grazing *Stylosanthes*-grass pastures in the seasonally dry tropics: effect of year, season, stylo species and botanical composition. *Australian Journal of Experimental Agriculture* 36, 781–789.

Coates. D.B. (1999a) The use of faecal $\delta^{13}C$ values to improve the reliability of estimates of diet quality when sampling tropical pastures with oesophageal fistulated cattle. *Australian Journal of Experimental Agriculture* 39, 1–7.

Coates, D.B. (1999b) Faecal spectroscopy (NIRS) for nutritional profiling of grazing cattle. In: *Proceedings of the VIth International Rangeland Congress*, 19–23rd July 1999. Townsville, Queensland, Vol. 1, pp. 466–467.

Coates, D.B. and Le Feuvre, R. (1998) Diet composition of cattle grazing *Stylosanthes*-grass pastures in the seasonally dry tropics: the effect of phosphorus as fertiliser or supplement. *Australian Journal of Experimental Agriculture* 38, 7–15.

Coates, D.B. and Mannetje, L. 't (1990) Productivity of cows and calves on native and improved pasture in subcoastal, subtropical Queensland. *Tropical Grasslands* 24, 46–54.

Coates, D.B., Mannetje, L.'t and Seifert, G.W. (1987a) Reproductive performance and calf growth rate to weaning of Hereford and Belmont Red cattle in subtropical, subcoastal Queensland. *Australian Journal of Experimental Agriculture and Animal Husbandry* 27, 1–10.

Coates, D.B., Schachenmann, P. and Jones, R.J. (1987b) Reliability of extrusa samples collected from steers fistulated at the oesophagus to estimate the diet of resident animals in grazing experiments. *Australian Journal of Experimental Agriculture* 27, 739–745.

Coates, D.B., Van Der Weide, A.P.A. and Kerr, J.D. (1991) Changes in faecal $\delta^{13}C$ in response to changing proportions of legume (C_3) and grass (C_4) in the diet of sheep and cattle. *Journal of Agricultural Science, Cambridge* 116, 287–295.

Cochran, R.C. and Galyean, M.L. (1994) Measurement of *in vivo* forage digestion by ruminants. In: Fahey, G.C. Jr, Collins, M., Mertens, D.R. and Moser, L.E. (eds) *Forage Quality, Evaluation, and Utilization.* American Society of Agronomy/Crop Science Society of America/Soil Science Society of America, Madison, Wisconsin, pp. 613–643.

Corbett, J.L. (1978) Measuring animal performance. In: Mannetje, L.'t (ed.) *Measurement of Grassland Vegetation and Animal production.* Bulletin 52 Commonwealth Bureau of Pastures and Field Crops. CAB, Farnham Royal, UK, pp. 163–231.

Costigan, P. and Ellis, K.J. (1987) Analysis of faecal chromium derived from controlled release marker devices. *New Zealand Journal of Technology* 3, 89–92.

Coulter, B.S. and O'Sullivan, M. (1988) A remote monitor for animal behaviour using radio telemetry. In: *Proceedings 12th General Meeting of the European Grassland Federation, July, 1988*, Dublin, pp. 450–454.

Doney, J.M., Peart, J.N., Smith, W.F. and Louda, F. (1979) A consideration of the technique for estimating milk yield of suckled sheep and a comparison of estimates obtained by two methods in relation to the effects of breed, level of production and stage of lactation. *Journal of Agricultural Science, Cambridge* 92, 123–132.

Dove, H. (1994) Plant cuticular wax alkanes – a new technique for estimating diet selection and intake in the grazing animal. *Proceedings of the Australian Society of Animal Production* 20, 55–57.

Dove, H. and Mayes, R.W. (1991) The use of plant wax alkanes as marker substances in studies of the nutrition of herbivores: a review. *Australian Journal of Agricultural Research* 42, 913–952.

Dove, H., Mayes, R.W. and Freer, M. (1996) Effects of species, plant-part, and plant-age on n-alkane concentrations in the cuticular wax of pasture plants. *Australian Journal of Agricultural Research* 47, 1333–1347.

Doyle, P.T., Casson, T., Cransberg, L. and Rowe, J.B. (1994) Faecal output of grazing sheep measured by total collection or using chromium sesquioxide. *Small Ruminant Research* 13, 231–236.

Dufty, J.H. (1972) Clinical studies on bovine parturition. *Australian Veterinary Journal* 48, 1–6.

Edwards, G.R., Parsons, A.J., Penning, P.D. and Newman, J.A. (1996) Relationship between vegetation state and bite dimensions of sheep grazing contrasting plant species and its implication for intake rate and diet selection. *Grass and Forage Science* 50, 378–388.

Engles, E.A.N. and Hugo, J.M. (1969) A technique for the collection of urine of grazing Merino wethers. *Proceedings of the South African Society of Animal Production* 8, 209.

Entwistle, K.W. (1986) Measurement of progesterone levels in the cow and their diagnostic significance. In: Burgess, G.W. (ed.) *Elisa Technology in Diagnosis and Research.* James Cook University, Queensland, pp. 309–312.

Fisher, A.V. (1997) A review of the technique of estimating the composition of livestock using the velocity of ultrasound. *Computers and Electronics in Agriculture* 17, 217–231.

Fitzpatrick, L.A. and Finlay, P.J. (1993) Fixed-time insemination for controlled breeding of *Bos indicus* heifers under extensive management conditions in north Queensland. *Australian Veterinary Journal* 70, 77–78.

Forbes, J.M. (1986) *The Voluntary Food Intake of Farm Animals.* Butterworth, Leeds, UK.

Frisch, J.E. and O'Neill, C. (1996) Calving rates in a tropical beef herd after treatment with a synthetic progestogen, norgestomel or a prostaglandin analogue, cloprostenol. *Australian Veterinary Journal* 73, 98–102.

Furnival, E.P., Corbett, J.L. and Inskip, M.W. (1990a) Evaluation of controlled release devices for administration of chromium sesquioxide using fistulated grazing sheep. 1. Variation in marker concentration in faeces. *Australian Journal of Agricultural Research* 41, 969–975.

Furnival, E.P., Ellis, K.J. and Pickering, F.S. (1990b) Evaluation of controlled release devices for administration of chromium sesquioxide using fistulated grazing sheep. 2. Variation in rate of release from the device. *Australian Journal of Agricultural Research* 41, 977–986.

Gibb, M.J. (1998) Animal grazing/intake terminology and definitions. In: Keane, M.G. and O'Riordan, E.G. (eds) *Potential for and Consequences of Extensification of Beef and Sheep Production on the Grasslands of the EC. Proceedings of a Workshop held in Dublin, Sept 1996.* EU Concerted Action AIR3-CT93-0947, Occasional Publication no. 3, pp. 21–37.

Gibb, M.J. and Treacher, T.T. (1980) The effect of ewe body condition at lambing on the performance of ewes and their lambs at pasture. *Journal of Agricultural Science, Cambridge* 95, 631–640.

Gibb, M.J., Rook, A.J., Huckle, C.A. and Nuthall, R. (1995) Estimation of grazing behaviour by dairy cows from measurements of grazing behaviour and weight change. In: *Proceedings of the 29th International Congress of the International Society for Applied Ethology, August 1995*, pp. 71–72.

Gibb, M.J., Huckle, C.A., Nuthall, R. and Rook, A.J. (1997) Effect of sward surface height on intake and grazing behaviour by lactating Holstein Friesian cows. *Grass and Forage Science* 52, 309–321.

Goering, H.K. and Van Soest, P.J. (1970) *Forage Fiber Analyses (Apparatus, Reagents, Procedures and some Applications).* USDA-ARS Agricultural Handbook 379. US Government Printing Office, Washington, DC.

Gordon, I.J. (1995) Animal-based techniques for grazing ecology research. *Small Ruminant Research* 16, 203–214.

Hamilton, B.A. and Hall, D.G. (1975) Estimation of the botanical composition of oesophageal extrusa samples. 1. A modified microscope point technique. *Journal of the British Grassland Society* 30, 229–235.

Hart, R.H., Hepworth, K.W., Smith, M.A. and Waggoner, J.W. Jr (1991) Cattle grazing behaviour on a foothill elk winter range in southeastern Wyoming. *Journal of Range Management* 44, 262–266.

Hatfield, P.G., Clanton, D.C., Sanson, D.W. and Eskridge, K.M. (1990) Methods of administering ytterbium for estimation of fecal output. *Journal of Range Management* 43, 316–320.

Hodgson, J. (1979) Nomenclature and definitions in grazing studies. *Grass and Forage Science* 34, 11–18.

Hodgson, J. (1982) Ingestive behaviour. In: Leaver, J.D. (ed.) *Herbage Intake Handbook.* British Grassland Society, Hurley, UK, pp. 113–138.

Hoehne, O.E., Clanton, D.C. and Streeter, C.L. (1967) Chemical changes in esophageal fistula samples caused by salivary contamination and sample preparation. *Journal of Animal Science* 26, 628–631.

Holechek, J.L., Vavra, M. and Pieper, R.D. (1982) Botanical composition determination of range herbivore diets: a review. *Journal of Range Management* 35, 309–315.

Hollingsworth, K.J., Adams, D.C., Klopfenstein, T.J., Lamb, J.B. and Villalobos, G. (1995) Supplement and forage effects on fecal output estimates from an intra-ruminal marker device. *Journal of Range Management* 48, 137–140.

Hughes, J.G. (1976) Short-term variation in animal live weight and reduction of its effect on weighing. *Animal Breeding Abstracts* 44, 111–118.

Johnson, E.R. and Charles, D.D. (1976) An evaluation of the Australian beef carcase appraisal system. *Australian Veterinary Journal* 52, 149–154.

Johnson, K., Huyler, M., Westberg, H., Lamb, B. and Zimmerman, P. (1994) Measurement of methane emissions from ruminant livestock using an SF_6 tracer technique. *Environmental Science Technology* 28, 359–367.

Jones, R.J. (1981) The use of natural carbon isotope ratios in studies with grazing animals. In: Wheeler, J.L. and Mochrie, R.D. (eds) *Forage Evaluation: Concepts and Techniques.* CSIRO Australia and the American Forage and Grassland Council, Melbourne, pp. 277–286.

Jones, R.J. and Lascano, C.E. (1992) Oesophageal fistulated cattle can give unreliable estimates of the proportion of legume in the diets of resident animals grazing tropical pastures. *Grass and Forage Science* 47, 128–132.

Jones, R.J., Ludlow, M.M., Throughton, J.H. and Blunt, C.G. (1979) Estimation of the proportion of C_3 and C_4 plant species in the diet of animals from the ratio of natural ^{12}C and ^{13}C isotopes in the faeces. *Journal of Agricultural Science, Cambridge* 92, 91–100.

Kennedy, P.M. (1995) Intake and digestion in swamp buffaloes and cattle. 3. Comparisons with four forage diets, and with rice straw supplemented with energy and protein. *Journal of Agricultural Science, Cambridge* 124, 265–275.

Keyserlingk, M.A.G. von and Mathison, G.W. (1989) Ruminant Feed Evaluation Unit: nylon bag digestibility and rates of passage. *Agriculture and Forestry Bulletin* 68, 18–20.

Killedar, N.S., Maheshkumar, Naikare, B.D. and Jagtap, D.Z. (1987) Factors influencing lamb growth rate in Deccani and its halfbreds with Merino and Dorset. *Indian Veterinary Journal* 64, 1039–1042.

Kimmich, H.P. (1980) Artifact free measurement of biological parameters: biotelemetry, a historical review and layout of modern development. In: Amlaner, C.J. and MacDonald, D.W. (eds) *A Handbook on Biotelemetry.* Pergamon Press, Oxford, pp. 3–20.

Kock, S.W. and Preston, R.L. (1979) Estimation of bovine carcase composition by the urea dilution technique. *Journal of Animal Science* 48, 319–327.

Kotb, A.R. and Luckey, T.D. (1972) Markers in nutrition. *Nutrition Abstracts and Reviews* 42, 813–845.

Kowalczyk, J., Skiba, B., Buczkowski, Z. and Kowalik, B. (1996) A device for quantitative urine collection from male sheep in balance trials. *Journal of Animal and Feed Sciences* 5, 297–301.

Krueger, W.C. (1972) Evaluating animal forage preference. *Journal of Range Management* 25, 471–475.

Krysl, L.J., Galyean, M.L., Estell, R.E. and Sowell, B.F. (1988) Estimating digestibility and faecal output in lambs using internal and external markers. *Journal of Agricultural Science, Cambridge* 111, 19–25.

Kuchida, K., Yamagishi, T., Takeda, H. and Yamaki, K. (1995) Live body volume and density measuring method for estimation of carcase traits in Japanese Black steers by computer image analysis. *Animal Science and Technology* 66, 1–6.

Laby, R.H., Graham, C.A., Edwards, S.R. and Kautzner, B. (1984) A controlled release intraruminal device for the administration of faecal dry-matter markers to the grazing ruminant. *Canadian Journal of Animal Science* (Supplement) 64, 337–338.

Laca, E.A., Ungar, E.D., Seligman, N. and Demment, M.W. (1992) Effect of sward height and bulk density on bite dimensions of cattle grazing homogeneous swards. *Grass and Forage Science* 47, 91–102.

Lang, D.R., Hight, G.K., Ulgee, A.E. and Young, J. (1968) A marking device for detecting oestrus activity in cattle. *New Zealand Journal of Agricultural Research* 11, 955–958.

Langlands, J.P. (1966a) Studies on the nutritive value of the diet selected by grazing sheep. I. Differences in composition between herbage consumed and material collected from oesophageal fistulae. *Animal Production* 9, 253–259.

Langlands, J.P. (1966b) Creatinine as an index substance for estimating the urinary excretion of nitrogen and potassium by grazing sheep. *Australian Journal of Agricultural Research* 17, 757–763.

Le Du, Y.L.P., Baker, R.D. and Barker, J.M. (1978) The use of short-term secretion rate measurements for estimating the milk production of suckler cows. *Journal of Dairy Research* 45, 1–4.

Le Du, Y.L.P., MacDonald, A.J. and Peart J.N. (1979) Comparison of two techniques for estimating the milk production of suckler cows. *Livestock Production Science* 6, 277–281.

Le Feuvre, R. and Jones, R.J. (1988) The static combustion of biological samples sealed in glass tubes as a preparation for $\delta^{13}C$ determination. *The Analyst* 13, 817–823.

Ledger, H.P., Gulliver, B. and Rob, J.M. (1973) An examination of sample joint dissection and specific gravity techniques for assessing the carcase composition of steers slaughtered in commercial abattoirs. *Journal of Agricultural Science, Cambridge* 80, 381–392.

Leite, E.R. and Stuth, J.W. (1995) Fecal NIRS equations to assess diet quality of free-ranging goats. *Small Ruminant Research* 15, 223–230.

Little, D.A. (1972) Studies on cattle with oesophageal fistulae. The relation of the chemical composition of feed to that of the extruded bolus. *Australian Journal of Experimental Agriculture and Animal Husbandry* 12, 126–130.

Little, D.A. (1975) Studies on cattle with oesophageal fistulae: comparison of concentrations of mineral nutrients in feeds and associated boluses. *Australian Journal of Experimental Agriculture and Animal Husbandry* 15, 437–439.

Little, D.A., McLean, R.W. and Winter, W.H. (1977) Prediction of the phosphorus content of herbage consumed by grazing cattle. *Journal of Agricultural Science, Cambridge* 88, 533–538.

Lockyer, D.L. (1997) Methane emissions from grazing sheep and calves. *Agriculture, Ecosystems and Environment* 66, 11–18.

Low, W.A., Dudzinski, M.L. and Muller, W.J. (1981) The influence of forage and climatic conditions on range community preference of Shorthorn cattle in central Australia. *Journal of Applied Ecology* 18, 11–26.

Lunt, D.K., Smith, G.C., McKeith, F.K., Savell, J.W., Riewe, M.E., Horn, F.P. and Coleman, S.W. (1985) Techniques for predicting beef carcase composition. *Journal of Animal Science* 60, 1201–1207.

Lupton, C.J. (1996) Prospects for expanded mohair and cashmere production and processing in the United States of America. *Journal of Animal Science* 74, 1164–1172.

Lynch, J.J., Hinch, G.N. and Adams, D.B. (1992) *The Behaviour of Sheep: Biological Principles and Implications for Production.* CAB International, Wallingford, UK and CSIRO, East Melbourne, Australia.

Lyons, R.K. and Stuth, J.W. (1992) Fecal NIRS equations for predicting diet quality of free-ranging cattle. *Journal of Range Management* 45, 238–244.

Magner, T., Sim, W.D. and Bardsley, D.H. (1988) Apparatus for urine collection from female cattle in metabolism crates. *Australian Journal of Experimental Agriculture* 28, 725–727.

Mayes, R.W., Dove, H., Chen, X.B. and Guada, D.A. (1995) Advances in the use of faecal and urinary markers for measuring diet composition, herbage intake and nutrient utilisation in herbivores. In: Journet, M., Grentt, E., Farce, M.-H. and Thericz, C. (eds) *Recent Developments in the Nutrition of Herbivores. Proceedings of the IVth International Symposium on the Nutrition of Herbivores*. INRA Editions, Paris, pp. 381–406.

McCloghry, C.E. (1997) Alternative dye banding method for measuring the length growth rate of wool in sheep. *New Zealand Journal of Agricultural Research* 40, 569–571.

McCloghry, C.E., Brown, G.H. and Uphill, G.C. (1997) Computer-assisted image analysis for the measurement of wool follicle density and fibre diameter in skin sections. *New Zealand Journal of Agricultural Research* 40, 239–244.

McLean, R.W., McCown, R.L., Little, D.A., Winter, W.H. and Dance, R.A. (1983) An analysis of cattle live-weight changes on tropical grass pasture during the dry and early wet seasons in northern Australia. *Journal of Agricultural Science, Cambridge* 101, 17–24.

McLeod, M.N. and Minson, D.J. (1978) The accuracy of the pepsin–cellulase technique for estimating the dry matter digestibility *in vivo* of grasses and legumes. *Animal Feed Science and Technology* 3, 277–287.

McManus, W.R. (1980) Oesophageal fistulation technique as an aid to diet evaluation of the grazing ruminant. In: Wheeler, J.L. and Mochrie, R.D. (eds) *Forage Evaluation: Concepts and Techniques*. CSIRO Australia and the American Forage and Grassland Council, Melbourne, pp. 249–260.

Menke, K.H., Raab, L., Salewski, A., Steingass, H., Fritz, D. and Schneider, W. (1979) The estimation of the digestibility and metabolizable energy content of ruminant feedingstuffs from the gas production when they are incubated with rumen liquor *in vitro*. *Journal of Agricultural Science, Cambridge* 93, 217–222.

Minson, D.J. (1990) *Forage in Ruminant Nutrition*. Academic Press, New York.

Minson, D.J. and McDonald, C.K. (1987) Estimating forage intake from the growth of beef cattle. *Tropical Grasslands* 21, 116–122.

Minson, D.J. and Whiteman, P.C. (1989) A standard livestock unit (SLU) for defining stocking rate in grazing studies. In: *Proceedings of the XVI International Grassland Congress, 4–11 October 1989*. Nice, France, pp. 1117–1118.

Minson, D.J., Taylor, J.C., Alder, F.E., Raymond, W.F., Rudman, J.E., Line, C. and Head, M.J. (1960) A method for identifying the faeces produced by individual cattle or groups of cattle grazing together. *Journal of the British Grasslands Society* 15, 86–88.

Moore, R.W. (1985) A comparison of electro-ejaculation with the artificial vagina for ram semen collection. In: *Annual Report 1983/84*. New Zealand Ministry of Agriculture and Fisheries, Agriculture Research Division, Wellington, New Zealand, p. 134.

Morgan, P.J.K., Pienaar, J.P. and Clark, R.A. (1976) Animal based methods of determining herbage intake and quality under grazing conditions. *Proceedings of the Grassland Society of Southern Africa* 11, 73–78.

Moule, G.R. (1965) *Field Investigation with Sheep: a Manual of Techniques*. CSIRO, Melbourne.

Nagorcka, B.N., Dollin, A.E., Hollis, D.E. and Beaton, C.D. (1995) A technique to quantify and characterize the density of fibres and follicles in the skin of sheep. *Australian Journal of Agricultural Research* 46, 1525–1534.

Neville, W.E. (1962) Influence of dam's milk production and other factors on 120 and 240-day weight of Hereford calves. *Journal of Animal Science* 21, 315–320.

Newman, J.A., Penning, P.D., Parsons, A.J., Harvey, A. and Orr, R.J. (1994a) Fasting affects intake behaviour and diet preference of grazing sheep. *Animal Behaviour* 47, 185–193.

Newman, J.A., Parsons, A.J. and Penning, P.D. (1994b) A note on the behavioural strategies used by grazing animals to alter their intake rates. *Grass and Forage Science* 49, 502–505.

Newman, J.A., Thompson, W.A., Penning, P.D. and Mayes, R.W. (1995) Least-squares estimation of diet composition from n-alkanes in herbage and faeces using matrix mathematics. *Australian Journal of Agricultural Research* 46, 793–805.

Orr, R.J., Penning, P.D., Parsons, A.J. and Champion, R.A. (1995) Herbage intake and N excretion by sheep grazing monocultures or a mixture of grass and white clover. *Grass and Forage Science* 50, 31–40.

Orr, R.J., Harvey, A., Kelly, C.L. and Penning, P.D. (1997a) Bite dimensions and grazing severity for cattle and sheep. In: *Proceedings of the Vth British Grassland Society Research Meeting, September 1997.* Seal Hayne, UK, pp. 185–186.

Orr, R.J., Penning, P.D., Harvey, A. and Champion, R.A. (1997b) Diurnal patterns of intake rate by sheep grazing monocultures of grass or white clover. *Applied Animal Behaviour Science* 52, 65–77.

Owen, J.B. (1957) A study of the lactation and growth of hill sheep in their native environment and under lowland conditions. *Journal of Agricultural Science, Cambridge* 48, 387–412.

Parsons, A.J., Newman, J.A., Penning, P.D., Harvey, A. and Orr, R.J. (1994a) Diet preference of sheep: effects of recent diet, physiological state and species abundance. *Journal of Animal Ecology* 63, 465–478.

Parsons, A.J., Thornley, J.H.M., Newman, J.A. and Penning, P.D. (1994b) A mechanistic model of some physical determinants of intake rate and diet selection in a two-species temperate grassland sward. *Functional Ecology* 8, 187–204.

Peart, J.N. (1982) Lactation of suckling ewes and does. In: Coop, I.E. (ed.) *Sheep and Goat Production.* World Animal Science Series C, Elsevier, Amsterdam and New York, pp. 119–134.

Pell, A.N. and Schofield, P. (1993) Computerised monitoring of gas production to measure forage digestion *in vitro. Journal of Dairy Science* 76, 1063–1073.

Penning, P.D. (1983) A technique to record automatically some aspects of grazing and ruminating behaviour in sheep. *Grass and Forage Science* 38, 89–96.

Penning, P.D. and Gibb, M.J. (1979) The effect of milk intake on the intake of cut and grazed herbage by lambs. *Animal Production* 29, 53–67.

Penning, P.D. and Hooper, G.E. (1985) An evaluation of the use of short-term weight changes in grazing sheep for estimating herbage intake. *Grass and Forage Science* 40, 79–84.

Penning, P.D., Steel, G.L. and Johnson, R.H. (1984) Further development and use of an automatic recording system in sheep grazing studies. *Grass and Forage Science* 39, 345–351.

Penning, P.D., Orr, R.J., Parsons, A.J. and Rutter, S.M. (1993a) Factors controlling meal length and herbage intake rate by grazing sheep. In: *Proceedings of the International Congress on Applied Ethology.* Berlin, pp. 498–500.

Penning, P.D., Parsons, A.J., Newman, A.J., Orr, R.J. and Harvey, A. (1993b) The effects of group size on grazing time in sheep. *Applied Animal Behaviour Science* 37, 101–109.

Penning, P.D., Parsons, A.J., Hooper, G.E. and Orr, R.J. (1994) Intake and behaviour responses by sheep to changes in sward characteristics under rotational grazing. *Grass and Forage Science* 49, 476–486.

Penning, P.D., Johnson, R.H. and Orr, R.J. (1996) Effects of continuous stocking with sheep or goats on sward composition and animal production from grass and white clover pasture. *Small Ruminant Research* 21, 19–29.

Penning, P.D., Newman, J.A., Parsons, A.J., Harvey, A. and Orr, R.J. (1997) Diet preferences of adult sheep and goats grazing ryegrass and white clover. *Small Ruminant Research* 24, 175–184.

Phillips, C.J.C. (1993) *Cattle Behaviour.* Farming Press Books. Ipswich, UK.

Pickup, G. and Bastin, G.N. (1997) Spatial distribution of cattle in arid rangelands as detected by patterns of change in vegetation cover. *Journal of Applied Ecology* 34, 657–667.

Pickup, G. and Chewings, V.H. (1988) Estimating the distribution of grazing and patterns of cattle movement in a large arid zone paddock: an approach using animal distribution models and Landsat imagery. *International Journal of Remote Sensing* 9, 1469–1490.

Pinchak, W.E., Smith, M.A., Hart, R.H. and Waggoner, J.W. Jr (1991) Beef cattle distributions patterns on a foothill range. *Journal of Range Management* 44, 267–275.

Provenza, F.D. (1995) Postingestive feedback as an elementary determinant of food preference and intake in ruminants. *Journal of Range Management* 48, 2–17.

Provenza, F.D., Pfister, J.A. and Cheney, C.D. (1992) Mechanisms of learning in diet selection with reference to phytotoxicocis in herbivores. *Journal of Range Management* 45, 36–45.

Qi, K., Lupton, C.J., Pfeiffer, F.A. and Minikheim, D.L. (1994) Evaluation of the Optical Fibre Diameter Analyser (OFDA) for measuring fiber diameter parameters of sheep and goats. *Journal of Animal Science* 72, 1675–1679.

Qi, K., Lupton, C.J., Pfeiffer, F.A., Minikhiem, D.L., Kumar, N.S. and Whittaker, A.D. (1995) Automatic image analysis system for objective measurement of animal fibres. *Sheep and Goat Research Journal* 11, 71–77.

Raats, J.G., Webber, L., Tainton, N.M. and Pepe, D. (1996) An evaluation of the equipment for the oesophageal fistula valve technique. *Small Ruminant Research* 21, 213–216.

Radford, H.M., Watson, R.H. and Wood, G.F. (1960) A crayon and associated harness for the detection of mating under field conditions. *Australian Veterinary Journal* 36, 57–66.

Reis, P.J. and Sahlu, T. (1994) The nutritional control of the growth and properties of mohair and wool fibers – a comparative review. *Journal of Animal Science* 72, 1899–1907.

Ridout, M.S. and Robson, M.J. (1991) Diet composition of sheep grazing grass/white clover swards: a re-evaluation. *New Zealand Journal of Agricultural Research* 34, 89–93.

Roberts, C.R. (1980) Effect of stocking rate on tropical pastures. *Tropical Grasslands* 14, 225–231.

Roberts, G., Williams, A., Last, J.D., Penning, P.D. and Rutter, S.M. (1993) A low-powered portable post-processed DGPS package for precise position logging of sheep on hill pasture. *Proceedings Institute of Navigation, September 1993.* Salt Lake City, Utah, p. 9.

Romney, D.L., Sendalo, D.S.C., Owen, E., Mtenga, L.A., Penning, P.D., Mayes, R.W. and Hendy, C.R.C. (1996) Effects of tethering management on feed intake and behaviour of Tanzanian goats. *Small Ruminant Research* 19, 113–120.

Rule, D.C., Arnold, R.N., Hentges, E.J. and Beitz, D.C. (1986) Evaluation of urea dilution as a technique for estimating body composition of beef steers *in vivo*: validation of published equations and comparison with chemical composition. *Journal of Animal Science* 63, 1935–1948.

Russel, A.J.F. (1994) Fibre production from South American camelids. *Journal of Arid Environments* 26, 33–37.

Rutter, S.M., Champion, R.A. and Penning, P.D. (1997) An automatic system to record foraging behaviour in free-ranging ruminants. *Applied Animal Behaviour Science* 54, 185–195.

Rutter, S.M., Orr, R.J., Penning, P.D., Yarrow, N.H., Champion, R.A. and Atkinson, L.D. (1998) Dietary preference of dairy cows grazing grass and clover. *Proceedings Winter Meeting British Society of Animal Science*, Scarborough, UK, pp. 51.

Sasser, R.G. and Ruder, C.A. (1987) Detection of early pregnancy in domestic ruminants. *Journal of Reproduction and Fertility* (Supplement) 34, 261–271.

Scheibe, K.M., Schleusner, Th., Berger, A., Eichhorn, K., Langbein, J., Dal Zotto, L. and Streich, W.J. (1998) ETHOSYS® – new system for recording and analysis of behaviour of free-ranging domestic animals and wildlife. *Applied Animal Behaviour Science* 55, 195–211

Schofield, P., Pitt, R.E. and Pell, A.N. (1994) Kinetics of fiber digestion from *in vitro* gas production. *Journal of Animal Science* 72, 2980–2991.

Scott, R.F. and Roberts, E.M. (1978) Objective measurement of clean fleece weight by infrared reflectance spectroscopy. *Wool Technology and Sheep Breeding* 26, 27–30.

Sehested, E. (1984) Computerized tomography in sheep. In: In Vivo *Measurement of Body Composition in Meat Animals.* Elsevier Applied Science Publishers, London, pp. 67–74.

Sibly, R.M., Nott, H.M.R. and Fletcher, D.J. (1990) Splitting behaviour into bouts. *Animal Behaviour* 39, 63–69.

Silvey, M.W. (1977) Problems associated with the use of beef cows and calves in evaluating pastures. *Journal of the Australian Institute of Agricultural Science* 43, 31–37.

Silvey, M.W. and Haydock, K.P. (1978) A note on live-weight adjustment for pregnancy in cows. *Animal Production* 27, 113–116.

Slater, J. and Jones, R.J. (1971) Estimation of the diets selected by grazing animals from microscopic analysis of the faeces – a warning. *Journal of the Australian Institute of Agricultural Science* 37, 238–239.

Snowder, G.D. and Glimp, H.A. (1991) Influence of breed, number of suckling lambs, and stage of lactation on ewe milk production and lamb growth under range conditions. *Journal of Animal Science* 69, 923–930.

Spurling, D. (1974) A note on the use of a weighband in estimating the liveweight of pure and crossbred zebu cattle. In: *Annual Report of the Department of Agriculture (Animal Husbandry Research) 1970–71.* Government Printer, Zomba, Malawi, pp. 48–52.

Stobbs, T.H. and Cowper, L.J. (1972) Automatic measurement of the jaw movements of dairy cows during grazing and rumination. *Tropical Grasslands* 6, 107–112.

Susmel, P., Stefanon, B., Spanghero, M. and Mills, C.R. (1996) Ability of mathematical models to predict faecal output with a pulse dose indigestible marker. *British Journal of Nutrition* 75, 521–532.

Ternouth, J.H., Poppi, D.P. and Minson, D.J. (1979) The voluntary food intake, ruminal retention time and digestibility of two tropical grasses fed to cattle and sheep. *Proceedings of the Nutrition Society of Australia* 4, 152.

Tilley, J.M.A. and Terry, R.A. (1963) A two-stage technique for the *in vitro* digestion of forage crops. *Journal of the British Grassland Society* 18, 104–111.

Van Dyne, G.M. and Torell, D.T. (1964) Development and use of the oesophageal fistula: a review. *Journal of Range Management* 17, 7–19.

Van Soest, P.J. (1994) *Nutritional Ecology of the Ruminant*, 2nd edn. Cornell University Press, Ithaca, New York, and London, 476 pp.

Volesky, J.D. and Coleman, S.W. (1996) Estimation of botanical composition of oesophageal extrusa samples using near infrared reflectance spectroscopy. *Journal of Range Management* 49, 163–166.

Wade, M.H., Peyraud, J.-L., Lemaire, G. and Comeron, E.A. (1989) The dynamics of daily area and depth of grazing and herbage intake of cows in a five-day paddock system. *Proceedings of the 16th International Grassland Congress.* Nice, France, pp. 1111–1112.

Warriss, P.D. and Edwards, J.E. (1995) Estimating the liveweight of sheep from chest girth measurements. *Veterinary Record* 137, 123–124.

Weiss, W.P. (1994) Estimation of digestibility of forages by laboratory methods. In: Fahey, G.C. Jr, Collins, M., Mertens, D.R. and Moser, L.E. (eds) *Forage Quality, Evaluation, and Utilization.* American Society of Agronomy/Crop Science Society of America/Soil Science Society of America, Madison, Wisconsin, pp. 644–681.

White, I.R. and Russel, A.J.F. (1987) Pregnancy diagnosis and fetal number determination. In: *New Techniques in Sheep Production.* Butterworths, London, pp. 207–220.

White, P.F., Treacher, T.T., Termanini, A. and Rihawi, S. (1997) The accuracy of using the ratio of nitrogen to acid detergent fibre in faeces to partition nitrogen between faeces and urine in total excreta collections from ewes. *Grass and Forage Science* 52, 122–124.

Wilson, J.W., English, P.R., Macdonald, D.C., Bampton, P.R., Warren, M., Birnie, M. and Macpherson, O. (1985) Factors affecting lamb growth rate in an upland flock of Blackface ewes producing Greyface lambs. *British Society of Animal Production* 153, 2.

Winks, L., O'Rourke, P.K., Venamore, P.C. and Tyler, R. (1978) Factors affecting birth weight and performance to weaning of beef calves in the dry tropics of north Queensland. *Australian Journal of Experimental Agriculture and Animal Husbandry* 18, 494–499.

Winter, W.H. (1988) Supplementation of steers grazing *Stylosanthes hamata* pastures at Katherine, Northern Territory. *Australian Journal of Experimental Agriculture* 28, 669–682.

Wolff, J.E., Mitra, S., Garrett, R. and Webb, P.A. (1996) Measuring body composition by fast neutron activation analysis. *Proceedings of the New Zealand Society of Animal Production* 56, 212–215.

Woodward, S.J.R. (1997) Formulae for predicting animal's daily intake of pasture and grazing time from bite weight and composition. *Livestock Production Science* 52, 1–10.

Wright, D.E. and Wolff, J.E. (1976) Measuring milk intake of lambs suckling grazing ewes by a double isotope method. *Proceedings New Zealand Society of Animal Production* 36, 99–102.

Wright, D.E., Jones, B.A. and Geenty, K.G. (1974) Measurement of milk consumption in young ruminants using tritiated water. *Proceedings New Zealand Society of Animal Production* 34, 145–150.

Young, D.L. (1972) The estimation of liveweight from heartgirth within specified age/sex groups of Kenya range cattle. *East African Agricultural and Forestry Journal* 38, 193–200.

Development-oriented Socioeconomic Methods in Grassland and Animal Production Research

16

A. Waters-Bayer and W. Bayer

Rohnsweg 56, Göttingen, Germany

Introduction

Applied grassland research should contribute to developing more profitable systems of grassland use and better management of natural resources. It must therefore deal not only with plants and animals, but also with people and their perceptions, aims, problems and needs.

The classical approach was to regard farmers as the 'end-users' of research findings. Scientists took the end-users' problems and needs into account by collecting and analysing socioeconomic data; they then decided on research priorities and the required characteristics of new technologies, and developed what they thought was needed. Extension services were supposed to disseminate the new technologies to farmers for adoption. Analyses of the linkages between research and practice have revealed that this 'transfer of technology' model has not worked well (Russell and Ison, 1991; Scoones, 1997).

In the final analysis, the decision as to the appropriateness of grassland research will depend on the land-users' interpretation of their own situations and how they think the research results can help them. This may differ from what is seen as the 'truth' from the scientific point of view. The possibility that scientists and land-users have different perceptions may be more self-evident in countries where the two groups are of different cultural backgrounds and do not speak the same language. However, problems of communication resulting from different perceptions also occur in industrialized countries (Russell and Ison, 1991).

©CAB *International* 2000. *Field and Laboratory Methods for Grassland and Animal Production Research* (eds L. 't Mannetje and R.M. Jones)

In this chapter we discuss approaches and methods of people-centred and development-oriented grassland research that try to bridge these communication gaps. We argue that the application of socioeconomic research methods should not be viewed primarily as a support to biophysical research, but as an integral part of an interactive research process that brings the different worlds of experience of producers and biophysical and social scientists into dialogue and mutual enrichment.

Forms of Interaction between Scientists and Producers

The percentage of people who derive their living from agriculture (including livestock keeping) is very small in industrialized countries, but as high as 90% in some developing countries. Property sizes and animal holdings vary greatly. The relationship between scientists and producers will be quite different if a producer owns several thousand cattle and can hire an adviser, who may have attended the same college, than if a producer has four goats and is illiterate. In Australia, New Zealand, North America or Europe, research and extension staff may be working with a small number of large-scale private properties, whereas among smallholders in Africa or Asia they may be working with groups of numerous people using the same village resources.

Also, within an industrialized or a developing country, grasslands are managed in many different socioeconomic, cultural and institutional settings. The recognition that grassland research must be placed in these different contexts gave rise to Livestock Systems Research (LSR). The on-farm or 'in-herd' component of LSR was intended primarily to adapt scientist-developed technologies to existing systems of livestock husbandry. Studies by social scientists were meant to help biotechnical scientists to explain farmer behaviour, especially the social and cultural constraints to adoption of the new technologies. Experience in LSR soon revealed that interactions between researchers and farmers can take different forms, and scientists can play different roles.

Biggs (1989) has classified scientist–farmer interactions as follows:

- *Contractual*: scientists contract with farmers to provide land, animals or services; experiments are planned and evaluated by scientists.
- *Consultative*: scientists consult farmers about their problems, interpret the responses and then try to develop appropriate solutions.
- *Collaborative*: scientists and farmers collaborate as research partners in identifying research questions, planning experiments, and collecting and interpreting data jointly.
- *Collegial*: scientists work to strengthen farmers' informal research and development systems.

Farmers can also contract scientists to carry out research on topics identified by farmers.

After briefly describing consultative socioeconomic research, this chapter will focus on the collaborative form, in which socioeconomic and cultural factors become most evident. What will be referred to as 'collaborative' research aims at improving grassland systems through increasing the capacity of grassland users to improve their systems. It therefore includes Biggs's 'collegial research' and represents a unity of research and development.

Consultative Socioeconomic Research

Particularly in situations where the researchers have little knowledge of existing farming and livelihood systems, consultative socioeconomic research is necessary in order to gain an initial understanding of the situation. At later stages of research, formalized quantitative methods can be applied to monitor socioeconomic change, to test hypotheses about human behaviour related to grassland and livestock husbandry, and to check wider validity of research findings. Consultative socioeconomic research includes formal surveys, structured interviews, farm record keeping and case studies. In recent years, some of these methods have been complemented or even replaced by more rapid, informal survey methods.

Formal surveys

In formal surveys, questionnaires are used to gather information from a deliberately selected sample of respondents. In countries with high levels of literacy and good communication services, surveys can be done by post, telephone or electronic mail. However, returns tend to be biased, as only a certain type of producer (those who are able and willing) responds. In countries with low levels of literacy and poor communication services, questionnaires are usually administered by enumerators, who must be trained and closely supervised. This makes formal surveys costly and time consuming, and justifiable only when the outcome of an informal survey (p. 409) indicates a need for good quantification and rigorous sampling (Roeleveld and Van den Broek, 1996).

Researchers should be clear about the purpose of the survey, the type and minimum amount of data required, and the way in which the data will be analysed. No more data should be collected than necessary, and researchers should avoid the pitfall of collecting data to an exaggerated degree of accuracy. Detailed questionnaires that take several hours to complete strain the relationship between interviewers and respondents, and jeopardize the quality of the responses. A long period of data analysis away from the field will reduce producers' interest in future collaboration. Points of attention in designing, administering and analysing formal surveys in livestock systems were described by ILCA (1990) and in farming systems more generally by Moser and Kalton (1971) and Mettrick (1993).

Structured interviews

In structured interviews, individuals or groups are questioned according to an interview schedule. If exploratory studies are being made, open-ended questions are suitable, as these allow respondents a wide variety of reactions. However, the researcher must then spend much time on content analysis. Closed or fixed-alternative questions give respondents a set of categories from which to choose. These are easier to code and analyse, but may overlook important issues. They should therefore be used only after a small number of key questions and relevant alternative responses have been identified during informal surveys or case studies. Structured interviews are useful for obtaining comparable information from different categories of livestock keepers identified by means of an exploratory study.

Keeping farm records

In early LSR work, multiple-visit surveys were made over 1 year or more in order to collect household-economic and production data. It is now more common to make a rapid survey to obtain approximate information sufficient for situation analysis, and to collect quantifiable socioeconomic and production data alongside on-farm research with producers. The measurements and record keeping can be done by the producers, freely if they are keen on obtaining these data themselves, or paid for by the researchers (Fig. 16.1). People without formal education can record quantitative data (cf. Waters-Bayer, 1988).

Case studies

Case studies are suitable for gaining insight into socioeconomic processes in production systems or for identifying key factors that influence application of an innovation. They can be intensive studies of selected communities or households during initial situation analysis, or can involve repeated visits to the same communities or households over several months or years during collaborative research. The researchers make observations, conduct semi-structured interviews and keep written records, both descriptive and quantitative. Hypotheses based on case-study findings can be investigated subsequently in a well-focused formal survey covering a larger sample.

A form of case study that helps to put the situation analysis into a socio-political and historical context is the life history. For example, the life history of a pastoral woman can give a vivid picture of the sociocultural and economic role of livestock through the household cycle: as a girl in her father's household, as a young bride, as a mother, and as a grandmother. This will point to aspects that deserve attention during design of collaborative research to ensure that gender-differentiated roles and needs are taken into account.

During producers' experimentation with a new technology, case studies allow intensive observation of household and community decision making and the technology's socioeconomic impact. Cases are selected deliberately according to characteristics of interest for the technology being tested – for example, producers with small, medium and large herds using a communal pasture where improvements are being tested. The cases must also be selected according to the willingness of the households or communities to cooperate.

Case studies can provide useful insight into socioeconomic and political–institutional aspects of land husbandry on levels above the farm,

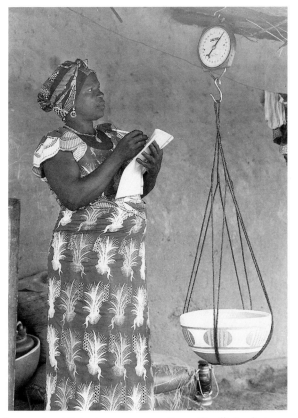

Fig. 16.1. Agropastoral Fulani woman recording milk offtake during participatory 'in-herd' research. (Source: A. Waters-Bayer, central Nigeria.)

in areas used by several individuals or groups (e.g. pastoralists, tourists, hunters). In studies of such land use units, e.g. a watershed, many of the tools described later in the section on visualization can help to elicit the viewpoints of different user groups and encourage debate. Involvement of policy makers from national or regional levels increases the likelihood that the findings of the case studies become more widely known at these levels.

Rapid informal methods

The detailed systems studies conducted in early LSR proved to be very labour and data intensive. It often took years before the analysis was completed and suggestions for improving the production system were made. The producers and funders became impatient for constructive action. In recent years, there has been a trend to more rapid methods of enquiry and analysis. Particularly in grassland systems where different social groups have interests in the resources, rapid methods of stakeholder analysis are proving valuable. Informal survey techniques are being applied with the aim of gaining sufficient initial understanding of production systems and producers' needs to be able to commence on-farm research sooner.

Stakeholder analysis
Grassland resources are often used by different groups for different purposes, not only as pasture for domestic ruminants. Also, among livestock keepers there may be distinct groups, e.g. sedentary farmers and mobile pastoralists. The various interest groups can be identified by means of a stakeholder analysis. This is an approach to understanding a system by identifying key actors, assessing their respective interests in the system, and probing into the various uses of the resources, differences in access rights, and stakeholders' perspectives and aims in natural resource management.

Examples of local stakeholders in grassland systems are households with livestock and those without, those who own land and those who do not but use the resources, indigenes, immigrants, hunters and city-based environmental groups. There will often be a need to build or strengthen institutions for facilitating negotiation of resource use, including joint experimentation, monitoring and evaluation to improve local management of the resources. Involving stakeholders in the analysis of their own differences and common interests can be a first step towards this process of building local capacities.

Stakeholder analysis can be done in a workshop or 'round-table' setting, but this may be inappropriate in cases of serious conflict of interest, particularly where certain groups have weak bargaining positions. In such cases, the analyses should be done with different subgroups. Approaches to stakeholder analysis have been discussed by Grimble and Wellard (1997).

A particular form of stakeholder analysis is gender analysis. This involves comparing profiles of men's and women's activities, access to and control over resources in the household and community, use of benefits, areas of decision making, and needs. Innovation development can then be based on awareness of these differences. Methods of gender analysis in agricultural research have been described by Lightfoot *et al.* (1991a) and Feldstein *et al.* (1993).

Informal surveys

A team of researchers, ideally including both technical and social scientists, spends several days or weeks making field observations and conducting semi-structured interviews and group discussions with stakeholders in the study area. An initial checklist serves as a guide, but further issues that emerge as important during the survey are also explored. Suggested economic and sociocultural questions for teams surveying livestock systems are outlined in Table 16.1. Visualization tools such as those described later

Table 16.1. Sample checklist for initial economic and sociocultural analysis of livestock systems.

Economic considerations:
- What types of animals are kept and for what reasons?
- How large are the animal and land holdings of the richest, poorest and majority of households?
- What labour resources are available within these household categories?
- Who (gender, age, ethnic group) is concerned with livestock grazing and/or feeding?
- What proportion of their time do they devote to this?
- What other activities demand their time, and how important are these for the livestock keepers?
- What grassland and feed resources are used, and when?
- What livestock products are sold, when and where?
- What is the price ratio between livestock products and production inputs?
- What other uses are made of potential forages, and by whom?
- What are the economic alternatives to livestock keeping?

Socio-cultural factors, including innovation behaviour:
- How do men and women, rich and poor, indigenes and immigrants, etc. differ in their rights to use potential forages?
- What institutions, formal and informal, influence access to resources, inputs and information?
- What types of information are livestock keepers seeking?
- What constraints and risks do they perceive in their livestock keeping?
- What informal experiments do they conduct on their own?
- What changes have they seen in their use of forages and livestock, and why have these changes occurred?
- How have livestock keepers adapted past innovations in forage husbandry suggested by outsiders?

(pp. 423–431) give some structure to the interviews and help to stimulate and focus the discussions.

Semi-structured interviews require good listening and communication skills. The interviewer must keep the discussion on the research topic yet be open to unexpected aspects, and must recognize when it is appropriate to pose focused questions such as 'What do you think about this plant here?' yet avoid leading questions such as: 'Do you think that growing stylo improves soil properties?' The individuals involved in the interviews may be encountered by chance or selected on the basis of certain characteristics such as gender, age, relative wealth, ethnic background, or specialist knowledge. In group discussions, issues confronted jointly by several individuals, such as multiple users of a water source, or by certain categories of people, such as women-headed households, can be explored.

Quantitative data can also be collected. For example, recall methods can be applied to record costs and benefits of production: the interviewee is asked to recall expenditures, sales, consumption, labour inputs for activities, etc. over a specific period of time. ILCA (1990) described how single-visit surveys using recall methods can be used as a relatively fast and low-cost tool for collecting data. Examples of successful recall approaches have been reported by Gbégo and Van den Broek (1996) and Wella *et al.* (1996).

A review of efforts to focus LSR (Roeleveld and Van den Broek, 1996) came to the conclusion that rapid informal surveys: (i) improve understanding of the overall resource-use system, its dynamics and variability; (ii) reduce the time span between situation analysis and the first on-farm trials; and (iii) make more efficient use of scarce resources such as funds and staff time. Moreover, the collaboration of different specialists in the surveys improves the integration of technical and socioeconomic disciplines in the subsequent research.

After the researchers have gathered information from resource users and have made their own interpretation of research needs, subsequent research is likely to be more relevant if this interpretation is returned to the resource users for validation. This can be done through research committees including producer representatives, or through debriefing sessions in the communities where the information was gathered. During these sessions, information gaps can be filled and misunderstandings corrected; proposals for research can be discussed and joint activities decided upon. In the case of research that will be conducted subsequently by scientists on-station, such meetings are likely to increase producers' interest in the research and encourage use of the findings.

Collaborative Action Research and Innovation Development

Interview-based methods, whether formal or not, harbour the danger that the information collected reflects what respondents would like to do or what they think they should respond, rather than what they actually do. People's perceptions and reactions to change are best observed deliberately in the process of change. If local people are involved in assessing their situation and reactions, they can give their own interpretations of why they acted as they did. Also the scientists learn more through this process than if they made only their own interpretations.

It is in the collaborative (including collegial) form of scientist–farmer interaction that learning processes among the producers are most stimulated. It is also in this form of interaction that the social, economic, cultural and institutional aspects of farming systems become most apparent. In grassland-based farming systems, these aspects play an extremely important role. The decisions of grassland users depend on a multitude of factors, such as rights of access to the vegetation and water, functions and values of the animals and their products, differing rights within households or communities to the animals and their products, local perceptions of risks and constraints, and visions of families and communities for their future.

In many parts of the world, the natural resources being used for livestock production also serve other functions in the society and local economy. Where grassland management is communal, many decisions are made at community level. Socioeconomic aspects of such complex systems are best studied in the course of collaborative action research.

The complexities of livestock systems in many parts of the world offer little scope for researchers to conduct their own trials in producers' herds. Pastoralists, by definition, depend on their herds for survival. In on-farm (in-herd) trials, they will ultimately want to decide how the animals and vegetation are used, and their decisions will be based on much more than just biological aspects of the system. Experimental control cannot lie in the hands of the scientists, who are obliged to enter a collaborative form of research that combines scientific and local knowledge in developing, testing and adapting a new technology, as in the example below.

Combining scientific and local pastoral knowledge

In central Nigeria, lack of dry-season feed was identified by scientists and Fulani pastoralists as a major problem. The scientists suggested intercropping stylosanthes in sorghum to improve stubble grazing, but the stylo depressed cereal yields when sown with the cereal and yielded poorly when sown later. One Fulani involved in these trials relocated his sorghum field, let the stylo come back as a sole crop and used it as a small pasture reserve for his herd. Thus the idea of the 'fodderbank' was born.

The scientists developed a basic model for establishing a fodderbank: fence in 4 ha for a herd of 50 cattle; prepare the land by animal trampling; broadcast stylo; and graze the pasture early to reduce competition for the stylo, which cattle do not like when they can eat tender grass. The stylo could then be used in the dry season to supplement the diet of pregnant and lactating cows.

A dozen trial fodderbanks were established. Not one Fulani followed the scientists' suggestions exactly. The most significant adaptations were: (i) using the fodderbank only in the late dry season, because crop residues offered good feed during the first half; (ii) supplementing only weak animals, thus halving calf mortality rates and eliminating emergency slaughter of adult animals; (iii) using live fence-posts from selected indigenous woody species that resisted termites; and (iv) growing cereals in parts of the fodderbank, to take advantage of the nitrogen fixed by the stylo – the seed reserves in the soil ensured spontaneous stylo regeneration after 1–2 years of cropping.

The scientists monitored these adaptations, discovered the reasons for them through discussion with the Fulani and helped to disseminate the improvements on the original fodderbank model to other pastoralists and scientists. What is important in this example is not the technical result, which is site specific, but the process: the way scientists interacted with livestock keepers to develop the technology (Taylor-Powell and Von Kaufmann, 1986).

A new input, such as a forage species, becomes a technology only when it is applied. In the above case, development of the technology involved developing ways to manage the new forage species within the existing livestock system. Incorporation of producers' criteria and management ideas is best achieved through trials managed by them. Technical and social scientists support the producers in conducting their trials and evaluating the outcome. Socioeconomic factors that influence grassland and livestock systems, such as land tenure, grazing control, risk-avoidance behaviour, inter- and intra-household decision making, or labour availability at critical periods, will emerge during the process of experimentation.

Particularly in natural resource management on a scale larger than individual enterprises, the innovations that will have the greatest impact on livestock production are likely to be of an organizational nature, such as conflict resolution and regulating access to water and forage, rather than new forage species or production techniques. Organizational innovation can be tested only through action research, as in the example below.

Action research in grassland management

Having experienced severe drought, pastoralists in northern Mali were open to new ideas as to how to manage the natural vegetation on which their herds depended. They entered into discussions with government livestock services and external consultants to identify possible improvements in resource management. They jointly observed current range conditions and analysed how these had changed. Some older pastoralists recalled that, in the past, certain pastures were not grazed during the rains and were then available in the dry season. They also noted that fonio or hungry rice (*Panicum laetum*), which the pastoralists collected to eat in times of need, had become scarce.

They started experimenting on a small scale with the reservation of fonio areas from grazing. The experiments soon expanded to include areas reserved for deferred grazing. In a meeting at the end of the rains, the pastoralists assessed vegetation needs and availability and decided whether and when to open up the protected areas. At subsequent twice-yearly meetings, they drew lessons from experience and adjusted the management regime, e.g. by changing the size of the reserved areas, the period of reservation or the way in which fines were imposed on herders who did not comply. The pastoralists took the lead in this action research in local-level natural resource management, with government agents and consultants providing support where needed (Marty, 1985; A. Marty, 1994, personal communication).

Iterative cycles of analysis, planning, implementation and evaluation allow the various factors interacting in the grassland system to be experienced by the research collaborators in the process of experimenting with change. Facilitation of the social process and organizational capacity to make desired changes is part of action research (Jiggins, 1993). The distinction between research and development is erased.

Methods that can be used in the major phases of collaborative research will now be described.

Situation analysis and needs assessment

Good analysis of the existing situation, trends and needs is the key to making research relevant. This allows identification of questions that can be addressed by research, both in direct interaction with producers and on-station, and prioritization of these questions from the producers' viewpoint.

The livestock system must be understood within the broader farming and livelihood systems of the family and community. Also non-farming activities must be taken into account, since these may have a bearing on labour availability and other important factors determining grassland and livestock husbandry.

Initial orientation about the socioeconomic situation can be gained by consulting secondary sources of information: reports from regional and local institutions, previous research and development projects, anthropological studies, economic data, census data, market surveys, and historical studies related to livestock keeping. The reliability of the data must be critically assessed. The review of secondary sources will yield a picture of the existing production systems and their dynamics, and should identify key questions to explore or verify during subsequent investigations in the field.

In consultative research, scientists collect information and then interpret it. In collaborative research, local people are involved in collecting the data on their own behalf and in analysing the results. In this way, their local knowledge is integrated into the analysis and their capacities to analyse their own situation are strengthened. Identification of needs is the result of negotiation between local and external interests and views of the situation, achieved through shared analysis and debate (Clark, 1993; Campbell, 1994).

Several tools have been developed to visualize the points of discussion so that all participants can see, comprehend and contribute their viewpoints. These tools include transects, maps, time charts, matrices, institutional (Venn) diagrams (Fig. 16.2) and flow charts (Davis, 1990; Pretty *et al.*, 1995; Narayan, 1996). Some tools that are particularly valuable for grassland and livestock research are described on pp. 423–431.

In a system of natural resource management larger than a farm, visualization tools help the stakeholders to see how events and processes in their own enterprises are affected by, and contribute to, the larger-scale system dynamics (Jiggins, 1993). Making diagrams helps them to think through the situation they are trying to visualize, and stimulates discussion between

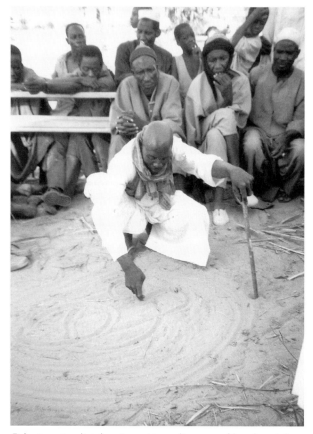

Fig. 16.2. Fulani pastoralist drawing a Venn diagram of local social organization in land use matters. (Source: A. Waters-Bayer, northern Burkina Faso.)

all concerned. Organizing separate meetings or splitting a meeting into sub-groups allows different groups using the resources to make an assessment from their viewpoint, before presenting it to others. This process brings out differences in interests and priorities. It can also initiate negotiation of new positions and so stimulate socioeconomic change. Researchers and extensionists facilitating the process must ensure that less eloquent and less powerful local groups have a chance to express their interests. Needs assessment must be recognized as a political process; only then can questions of power in identifying needs be adequately addressed (cf. Scoones, 1997).

In a few days or weeks of situation analysis, it is not possible to gain deep insight into the political and cultural aspects that determine what is voiced by local groups or 'the community'. In order to reduce bias, the same issue should be studied from different angles (triangulation), using a variety of information-gathering techniques (e.g. case studies, observations, key-informant interviews, focus-group discussions, topical quantitative surveys), a variety of units of observation (individuals, households, communities) and a variety of disciplines in the research team. The initial analysis will need critical review from time to time. Focused studies, such as on the relationship between wealth distribution and local experimenters, will have to be carried out at a later stage in the research process.

In the initial situation analysis prior to on-farm experimentation, the scientists do not need to gain an exhaustive understanding of all aspects of the livelihood system(s). The main aims are to reach agreement with producers about priority topics for development-oriented research, and to identify communities, groups or individuals with whom the collaborative research will be carried out. During the course of the on-farm trials, a deeper understanding will be gained of the socioeconomic conditions and producers' decision making. Situation analysis is an iterative process of approaching a moving target.

Identification and prioritization of research topics

The methods used in situation analysis as described above should give enough insight into key constraints and relevant innovations to be able to plan joint action. A large amount of exact quantitative data is not needed; estimates based on existing data from secondary sources and informal surveys usually suffice. During analytical workshops with producers, research topics can be prioritized using cause-and-effect diagrams and possibly modelling of land management units, and potential solutions for producers' trials can be identified.

Analytical workshops
During analytical workshops, issues are explored through open debate and a consensus is sought on priorities for collaborative research. When large

numbers of producers are involved, especially if they represent different resource-user groups, it is advisable to form smaller discussion groups who later report to the plenum for a broader discussion. A common sequence in such workshops is: (i) comparison of past and present situations; (ii) discussion of visions of the future; (iii) analysis of present problems, possibly based on preliminary results of rapid surveys, or through an analysis of Strengths, Weaknesses, Opportunities and Threats (SWOT); (iv) consideration of potential solutions; and (v) planning of experiments and possible other types of action.

It is important that the scientists and producers discuss frankly whether research can help to find solutions for the perceived problems. It must then be clarified what questions can be investigated by whom, and which questions should be tackled first.

A cause-and-effect diagram is a useful tool for stimulating analysis and pinpointing researchable and priority questions. This can be depicted, for example, as a tree drawn on the ground, on paper or on a board. A problem important to the producers forms the trunk, their ideas about causes are written or drawn in the roots, and the effects are shown in the branches. The diagram is then used as a focus for probing the causes of the problem. The analysis will normally reveal linkages between biophysical, socioeconomic, cultural and political/institutional aspects. Not all cause–effect relationships will be clear-cut and some will merit further investigation, but potential solutions can be sought for those problems for which the probable causes are understood. These may be selected for testing either on-farm or on-station (Roeleveld and Van den Broek, 1996).

Farm and land management modelling

Models are useful for depicting the use of resources and interactions between different components of a system, as well as for analysing the likely effects and implications of introducing innovations. For livestock keepers producing for a market, modelling also helps in calculating budgets, an important basis for their decision making. The models need to be built so that they can be comprehended and discussed by researchers and land users together (Dorward *et al.*, 1997). They can be physical models, conceptual models drawn on paper or mathematical ones compiled on a computer (Chapter 3).

In simple bioeconomic models (e.g. Lightfoot *et al.*, 1991b), the use of resources can be quantified to a sufficient degree to assist producers and scientists to identify researchable constraints and opportunities. Bioeconomic modelling can be done at farm level, as well as on a larger scale – for example, for modelling change in community-managed grazing land or a watershed including several communities. Farm management modelling can be conducted with individuals, selected by researchers and/or by the community as representative of different socioeconomic classes. Land management modelling is best done with groups of persons who know the area well or represent different user groups, and can be conducted in the framework of analytical workshops.

Particularly when working with groups having low levels of literacy, bioeconomic modelling using visualization tools such as flow charts (p. 429) provides good support for participatory budgeting, in which the estimates of costs and benefits and the construction of the actual budget are done jointly by producers and scientists. Depending on the degree of system complexity and the extent of the changes being considered, participatory budgeting may involve various types of economic evaluation, including the following examples:

- *Enterprise budgets* link production and financial aspects. Production levels, costs involved in meeting these levels, and returns from production are evaluated for a particular enterprise. Such budgets are useful for judging whether a proposed innovation will be of economic interest to the producers, and for comparing different enterprises – for example, whether it is worth investing research money and time in forage improvement for the one or the other enterprise. Attention needs to be given to gross margins per unit of scarce resource for the category of livestock keepers concerned. In many livestock-keeping systems, labour is scarce. Here, gross margin per person or labour-day will be of greatest interest. Attention must also be given to division of labour and, therefore, returns to the labour time of this category of person from one enterprise compared with another.

  Calculation of enterprise budgets will not be meaningful in livestock-keeping systems where inputs are bought and income is earned by different individuals in the household. For example, in the Fulani cattle-keeping system in central Nigeria, costs of most herd inputs are paid by men, while other costs (e.g. dairy equipment) are paid by women. Income from milk is controlled by the women, while most of the income from animal sales is controlled by the men. Gender analysis of enterprises will reveal where cases such as these exist. Here, enterprise budgets could still be useful if applied as a tool to encourage the women and men to discuss their inputs and outputs and how the partners can adjust responsibilities and benefits so that both can gain from an innovation.

- *Partial budgets* can be drawn up when small changes in a production practice are being considered that do not involve complex interactions with other inputs and outputs in the enterprise. They allow comparison of any added costs and returns, and any reduced costs and returns of the change. Partial budgeting can be done with individual producers or with groups of producers with the same type of enterprise. A process diagram (p. 430) can aid in identifying the points of costs and returns. The merit of the partial budget lies more in tabulating the factors affected by the innovation than in the prices attached to these factors.

Its major weakness is that the focus on one component to be changed may obscure the secondary character of that component in the entire production system. More details about economic analyses in livestock systems can be found in Amir and Knipscheer (1989) and Jansen *et al.* (1997).

- *Land-unit budgets.* In managing grassland and selecting potential improvements to be researched, bioeconomic flows have to be considered at farm and community level, for the local perspective, and at the level of the watershed or agroclimatic zone for the perspective of regional or national policy makers (Breman and De Ridder, 1991). At levels above the livestock enterprise, land-unit budgets are needed to clarify who is likely to benefit to what extent from a proposed innovation, who should carry the major costs, and who should be involved in monitoring and evaluating the results.

Identifying research priorities

Scientists' criteria for ranking problems to address will depend partly on government policy (e.g. self-sufficiency in animal products, equity). However, to the extent that collaboration with producers and their acceptance of innovations are sought, the criteria of different categories of resource users will play an important role. These can be elicited through semi-structured interviews and discussions conducted with individuals representative of the different categories, and with focus groups having common interests (Krueger, 1994). Ranking and matrix-scoring techniques (p. 427–428) can be used as aids in prioritizing research questions.

Grasslands subject to communal or open-access use may be governed by both customary and government regulations. Even where land is privately owned, other persons, civil groups or government levels hold interests and rights (tourism, watershed management, mining, environmental protection, etc.). The stakeholders will differ in their perception of the major problems. In a workshop setting, each interest group can make its own problem analysis, but a process of reaching consensus is still needed if concrete research is to be planned. Priority setting is not a one-off exercise. Priorities must be reviewed, when the actions of groups concerned do not correspond with their stated priorities.

Identifying potential solutions

When groups of producers with common interests or resources have agreed on priorities, they can start to identify specific issues that need further investigation or innovations that merit testing. Brainstorming techniques encourage wide participation. All participants are asked to express any ideas on a given topic. Individuals may write these on cards, or 'buzz groups' of two or three people may discuss quietly for a few minutes before suggesting an idea to the larger group. The workshop facilitator lists all contributions on a board or sheet of paper on the wall, and helps the participants to organize the ideas by grouping similar ones and finding consensus about what they have in common.

The main sources of ideas for potential solutions to explore will be: (i) best practices and innovations of producers in the area or elsewhere with similar conditions (Clark, 1997; McCartney *et al.*, 1997); and (ii) new technologies developed by scientists during previous research in the area or during research conducted elsewhere and reported in the literature. In discussing these options for on-farm testing, the producers can provide essential elements of local knowledge regarding the feasibility of the proposed solutions for their particular situation, just as scientists can give their judgement of feasibility from their knowledge. Options or questions to be investigated using more formal scientific methods can also be identified.

Ashby (1990) described three ways to make explicit the producers' criteria in choosing among options for testing:

- *Absolute evaluation*: each option is judged on its own merits (e.g. 'What do you like or dislike about this technique?').
- *Pair-wise comparison*: each option is compared successively with all others and/or with actual practice ('If you had to choose between these two alternatives, which one would you select and why?').
- *Ranking*: options are ranked from most to least preferred (e.g. by giving points), and participants discuss reasons for the ranking that emerges.

Once a particular option has been chosen for testing, this is expressed as a hypothesis. This step helps the participants to define more exactly what they want to find out and why, and enables them to analyse more clearly the results of the trial.

Technology development and evaluation with producers

Identifying appropriate management of trials

It is important to clarify what research topics are best addressed in scientist-managed trials and what topics in producer-managed trials. The socio-economic aspects of a technology can best be explored in the latter – for example, to discover how biologically promising forage plants can fit into existing production systems and how producers can best manage the plants. The main aim of producer-managed trials is not to make precise measurements, such as of differences in plant yield from different species, but to see how producers can adapt new ideas to suit specific purposes. This gives all participants a better understanding of the range of possible options offered by a new technology.

Scientist-managed trials, in which more precise measurements are made to support analysis of producers' trials, may be conducted on-station or on land borrowed from the community or private landowners. Particularly in production systems primarily oriented to subsistence, it may not be possible to conduct scientist-managed trials with animals borrowed from livestock owners. In such cases, animals have to be bought and kept locally under conditions similar to those on-farm.

If producers are interested in new pasture plants, it may be necessary to screen numerous accessions to identify 'best bets'. When such screening is done on-station, producers should be invited to join the scientists in evaluating the results. For multi-site evaluation of new plants under different agrobiological conditions, on-farm trials have become common. Discussions between scientists and producers about species evaluation can bring out important socioeconomic criteria to feed back into the search for suitable cultivars.

Designing producer-managed trials

Basically, the designs of scientists' and producers' trials differ little. However, complex designs that can show differences between treatments only after detailed statistical analysis should be avoided in producer-managed trials (Van Veldhuizen *et al.*, 1997).

The producers in a given area need to agree who should carry out the on-farm trials (everybody in the group, or a few on behalf of the others) and how the results should be recorded, assessed and communicated. In areas where the daily work of livestock care is done by women, older children or elderly people, not just the male household heads should be involved in the planning, monitoring and evaluation.

In participatory design workshops, the interested producers can plan how components of the livestock system will be tested. Several of the visualization tools described later can help in this planning – for example, cause-and-effect diagrams to formulate hypotheses to test, or process charts to help to design implementation procedures that fit into the producers' work pattern.

The scientists and the producers must agree on qualitative and quantitative criteria for assessing the innovations being tested. The criteria elicited as described on p. 428 will form the basis for monitoring and evaluation. Other criteria are likely to emerge during joint analysis of the trials in progress. It cannot be assumed that increased animal production will always be a top priority for livestock keepers; other factors, such as accumulating capital or saving labour, may prove to be more important (cf. Laurent and Centres, 1990).

Implementing, monitoring and evaluating producer-managed trials

The partners in collaborative research will have initially agreed on their roles and time plan, but during the research process unexpected events, such as a fire, pest or disease outbreak, may occur, new insights may be gained or new opportunities may arise. These oblige or invite changes in the producers' experiments. The changes need to be recorded so that the reasons for them can be discussed and their effects on the outcome of the experiments can be better understood.

An integral part of collaborative research is joint monitoring and evaluation (M&E) of the process and results. This is the key to a shared understanding, particularly of the socioeconomic factors involved in the enterprise(s) or communities concerned. When the M&E procedures are designed and implemented jointly with the producers, the M&E system will be relevant for their conditions and they will be more likely to use the output from the system. Many of the tools used in situation analysis and prioritization of research topics (e.g. ranking exercises) can be used for M&E of the socioeconomic impacts of technical innovation. Formal surveys and/or structured interviews, using short and focused questionnaires and drawing on farmer recall, can be applied periodically over several years in order to monitor socioeconomic changes in comparison with the initial baseline.

Where livestock research involves changes in the use of land with multiple values to multiple stakeholders, it will not be sufficient to involve only the livestock keepers in the M&E. Land used for grazing may also be used for ecotourism, aboriginal livelihoods, 'alternative' lifestyles, horticulture, conservation, wood harvesting and mining (Pringle and Burnside, 1996). Monitoring systems must include data that allow these stakeholders to interpret the findings using their own value systems. Focus-group discussions and semi-structured interviews, possibly using visualization tools, will be needed to elicit their particular interests.

To gain a picture of longer-term impacts of present practices and innovations on the condition of grassland resources (vegetation, water, wildlife), participatory monitoring methods promise to be more effective than monitoring carried out by external observers only. Indicators meaningful to local people and easily observed and recorded must be identified together with those people. Monitoring can also be a learning tool for local action, if it is combined with reflection by the resource users on the causes of observed changes and on what must be done to support favourable changes and to correct emerging problems.

Local resource monitoring can be combined with geographic information system (GIS) data for a region, derived partly from land users' own soil, vegetation and topological classifications, and – in places where properties are large – with satellite images. This combination proved important for visualizing the nature, incidence and scale of resource problems experienced by Australian Landcare groups. 'Making things visible' is important not only for systematizing information and experience, but also for stimulating participation in the higher levels of organization needed to manage large-scale natural resource systems (Jiggins, 1993). Also the example from New Zealand given by Bosch et al. (1996), where local and scientific knowledge were combined in a system of community-based monitoring and adaptive management of rangeland, shows that participatory research and local monitoring are closely intertwined.

Collaborative research supported by monitoring and reflection on the results of joint experiments (or the results of ongoing land management decisions and actions) is a process of experiential learning. It leads into renewed cycles of producer-led experimentation or action research. It also raises questions of high practical relevance that require more conventional research under controlled conditions. The learning process can continue in small groups of research-minded producers with common interests, along the lines of the farmer study groups in The Netherlands, who are supported by agricultural advisors (Oerlemans *et al.*, 1997).

Dissemination

In collaborative research for developing grassland and livestock systems, the boundary to 'extension' is less clearly defined than in the conventional transfer-of-technology model. Field agents in agricultural services or development projects are in a good position to facilitate interaction between scientists and producers in the type of research described above, and the 'extension' of the new ideas to land users in other areas is rarely possible without local experimentation and adaptation. As grassland and livestock scientists do not have the time and resources to work directly with all producers, the majority of these must depend on their own ingenuity and the support of other producers and agricultural services in pursing their informal research and development activities.

Joint analysis, experimentation and evaluation by scientists and producers is already an important step toward disseminating the results. Those producers and communities directly involved in the research will understand and value the results, and will be the best promoters of successful innovations. It is through personal communication with their peers that producers gain much of the new information they use in their informal experimentation, innovation and development activities. Field days, agricultural fairs or open-door events provide opportunities to invite a wider group, including producers from neighbouring areas, agricultural advisors and local administrators, to see and discuss the results of on-farm and on-station research.

Scientists' experiences with collaborative research and the results of this research are shared within the scientific community by fairly conventional means: publication in scientific journals, newsletters and books, and papers and presentations at conferences and workshops. As interest in collaborative research and participatory methods of technology development is quite recent, so-called 'grey' literature is an important source of information.

The recent rise in popularity of participatory methods harbours the danger of their misuse. Many agencies apply rapid informal surveys, which they refer to as 'participatory', in order to identify problems. But then they proceed to business as usual, either trying to transfer technologies developed under other conditions, or retreating to their stations and offices to produce publishable but not applicable results. Often, a conflict of interests arises for scientists employed by research organizations or universities, who are judged primarily on their performance in terms of publications in recognized scientific journals. Participatory research and development requires a commitment to serve the producers.

Particularly in the case of the so-called Participatory Rural Appraisal (PRA) tools, there is a danger of ritualism, when they are applied without clarity about the reasons for choosing a particular tool or about the purpose for which the results will be used. This can discredit participatory approaches to research and development. Collaboration between people depends more on attitude and behaviour than on methods. Therefore, the methods of collaboration cannot be so strictly codified as can statistical methods or chemical analyses. Scientists are more likely to learn how to engage in collaborative research with producers by being exposed to this type of interaction and by reflecting on their own research practices and agendas than through training in particular techniques.

Some Visualization Tools for Socioeconomic Research in Grassland Systems

Visualization tools that are particularly useful in guiding discussions with resource users, analysing how grassland and livestock systems function and focusing the related negotiation processes, are described briefly here. These descriptions are based primarily on experiences with smallholder farming and pastoral communities in developing countries, in cases where grazing land is communal and animals are controlled by herding or tethering. However, more recent experience in grassland research in production systems with private ownership and control of a discrete property and lower intensity of labour inputs, e.g. in Australia (Ison and Ampt, 1992), has shown the value of this approach to research in these settings as well. The tools have also been applied in more intensive systems in Europe, e.g. in the UK (Anderson *et al.*, 1999) and Switzerland (Scheuermeier and Ison, 1992), where mixed forms of private and communal grazing occur.

In many cases, a given tool can be applied at various stages and for various purposes during the research process. Table 16.2 gives an overview of how some of the tools mentioned below, as well as others described in Kirsopp-Reed and Hinchcliffe (1994) and Waters-Bayer and Bayer (1994), can be used. The appropriateness of a research tool depends on factors such as the cultural distance between researchers, extension agents and producers; the detail and reliability of available secondary information; population density; and farm size.

Table 16.2. Methods for selected purposes in collaborative livestock research (semi-structured interviews can be used in all stages and to explore all types of information mentioned below).

Phase of interaction	
Type of information or purpose	Methods and tools suggested

Establishing rapport

History of area (past trends, accomplishments, livestock-related events, e.g. re/destocking, introduction of plough)	Timelines Oral history Life histories
Overview of farming systems, natural resources and production conditions	Transect walks Participating in daily tasks
General information on people and relationships	Taking photographs/films and discussing them together

Analysing the situation

Relative importance of livestock in livelihood system	Livelihood analysis Proportional piling
Resources available to livestock	Seasonal resource mapping
Natural resource use (and changes/trends)	Bioresource flow diagram Mapping Proportional piling Matrix
Nutrient flows	Bioresource flow diagram
Grazing pattern/forage resource availability and use	Forage calendar Resource-use mapping
Fodder preferences	Ranking
Animal husbandry practices	Seasonal calendars Mobility maps Flow charts
Frequency and purpose of travel by household members for livestock-related activities	Mobility maps
History of livestock diseases	Timelines
Preferred traits of livestock breeds	Matrix scoring
Livestock productivity parameters	Progeny histories Herder recall
Livestock linkages with other sectors	Flow diagram Systems analysis diagram

Continued

Table 16.2. *Continued.*

Phase of interaction	
Type of information or purpose	Methods and tools suggested

Seasonal differences in, e.g.
    livestock sales and prices,
    prices of inputs and products,
    milk yield, home consumption and sales
	Calendars
	Proportional piling

Proportional income from livestock products	Proportional piling Diagramming
Labour requirements	Activity calendar Daily timelines Learning local tasks
Stock loaning and sharing relationships	Social mapping
Social organization	Venn diagram Social mapping
Location of households with certain characteristics (e.g. owning livestock)	Social mapping Wealth mapping
Institutional links	Venn diagram
Wealth differences	Wealth ranking
Marketing structure	Flow diagram
Conflict analysis	Venn diagram Flow diagram Critical incident
Innovation history	Pathway diagram charts
Services available	Venn diagram Services and opportunity map

Identifying innovations

Analysing and prioritizing problems	Brainstorming/Ranking Calendars Flow diagrams Problem tree
Identifying potential solutions	Visits to other farmers Visits to research stations Seeking local best practices Seeking local innovators

Continued

Table 16.2. *Continued.*

Phase of interaction	
Type of information or purpose	Methods and tools suggested
Prioritizing solutions	Brainstorming/Ranking
	Problem and solution game
	Proportional piling
Planning experiments	
Designing experiments	Participatory design workshop
Allocating tasks/time planning	Process diagram
	Matrix
Assessing results	
Monitoring	Herder recall
	Calendars
	Series of calendars or maps
	Series of photographs
	Meetings with experimenting farmers
Evaluation	Cross-visits
	Impact diagram
	Proportional piling
	Ranking/scoring
	Farmers' evaluation workshops

The appropriateness of research tools and the choice of groups with whom they are applied will vary according to land use system. For example, participatory mapping to clarify multiple use of natural resources around a village will not be suitable in extensive range systems in Australia. Here, the actors would have to include the widely dispersed property operators as well as representatives of regional or national groups such as environmentalists and national tour operators. The way in which the tools are applied will depend on local availability of materials and equipment. Maps may be drawn with a stick in the sand or by digitalized GIS. Creativity is demanded of researchers to choose and adapt tools to suit the local situation.

Transects

Transects made together with local people help to systematize direct observations in the field. The scientists travel (usually on foot but over longer distances by horse or vehicle) with a few local people through the area they use, characterize it jointly and record their observations in a cross-sectional sketch (Fig. 16.3). Particularly important are the informal discussions among the mixed team making the transect, and between them and people met along the way, about what is observed, e.g. herd composition, animal condition, people working with livestock, grazing areas, watering techniques, and differences in ways of doing things.

Ranking

Various ranking tools allow people to compare items and show their preferences, e.g. among forage species. They are means of discovering local people's categories, differences in priorities of different social groups, and local criteria for evaluating innovations. The aim is to obtain values that are not absolute and exact, but approximate and relative. Certain information, such as family income, may be sensitive, i.e. people are reluctant to reveal it,

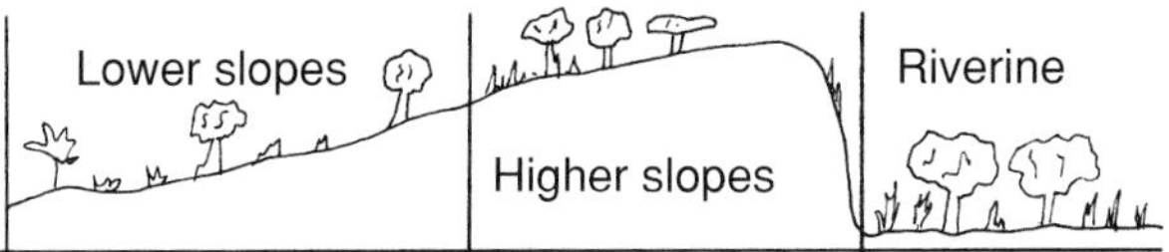

Sererit area	Lower slopes	Higher slopes	Riverine
Trees/ shrubs	*itepes* *laturdai* *lgirigiri* *lororoi*	*itepes* *siteti* *laishimi*	*lkidash* *laminira* *lmomoi* *iti*
Grasses	*loturei* *maititai* *ntalakwen*	*ntorees* *etekeek*	*loobene* *seketet* *lararas* *seiyai*
Livestock	cattle goats	cattle goats	–
People	few *manyattas*	few *manyattas*	–
Wildlife	kudu baboons	birds	warthog many birds
Water	–	–	river
Problems	wild animals	gully erosion	–
Opportunities	medicinal plants food plants	fruits fencing materials	beehives permanent water

Fig. 16.3.   Transect of a pastoral area in Kenya. (Source: Birch, 1994, simplified.)

or it may be difficult for informants to give exact figures. Relative rankings are easier to obtain, less threatening (and so more likely to lead to honest responses) and often just as useful as exact figures.

A very simple form of ranking is *proportional piling*. Producers show their perceptions of relative proportions by placing counters (e.g. beans) in different piles or rows for each item. Pie or bar charts can be drawn from these piles. Depending on how well acquainted the participants are with such diagrams, they may draw them directly, without forming piles. Discussion is then generated around reasons for differences and, if done for different periods, reasons for variations in proportions over time. This tool can be used to obtain rough quantitative figures, in relative terms.

A more complex form of ranking is *matrix scoring*. Local criteria for assessing comparable items, such as fodder trees, are identified through pair-wise comparison or by asking what is good or bad about each. A table is drawn in which the column headings are the items and the rows consist of the criteria (e.g. palatability, feeding value, availability). This tool encourages debate on a theme, helps producers to decide what they would like to test, and identifies criteria for evaluating the results.

A useful tool for identifying socioeconomic classes in a community is *wealth ranking*. After a discussion with local people about their understanding of wealth and poverty, the name of each household head is written on a separate card and the cards are sorted by key informants from the community. This gives insights into local perceptions of well-being and permits targeting of research activities to particular groups. Grandin (1988) provided details of how the cards from several informants can be tabulated to produce a list of all households in a community ranked according to wealth. However, it is much easier to use the above-mentioned tool of proportional piling to discover the characteristics of different wealth classes and the proportion of households in each category, without identifying specific households.

Venn diagram

Individuals or groups are asked to identify key institutions, groups or individuals that are important in a specific connection, such as resource use in a watershed. Different-sized circles represent the relative importance of each institution, group and individual. They can be placed to show their contact or overlap in activities or responsibilities, or lines can be drawn to show the relative strength of links between the circles. The diagram serves as a basis for discussing the functions and interrelationships of the circles. It can reveal the interdependency of various organizations, or points where linkages need to be established or improved, or possibilities of alliances or conflicts. If drawn by an individual or members of a household, a Venn diagram can indicate social links such as animal-sharing relationships.

Maps

Maps are especially important for studying the use of grassland resources, as it is necessary to look beyond the farm to community and watershed levels. Local people can be asked to draw maps on paper or on the ground; also existing maps can be used as a base for marking features important to them. Either the knowledge of large mixed groups can be combined in one map, or small groups subdivided according to age, gender, ethnic group, etc. can make separate maps and compare them to see differences in perceptions. For planning purposes, maps offer an impersonal focus of attention, which can help in working toward a consensus on activities to be undertaken, e.g. the siting of pasture trials. Two types of map are particularly useful in analysing grassland and livestock systems:

- Resource maps, showing natural resources according to local classifications, which may include different types of grazing and browsing areas and water points. In areas with strong seasonal differences, resource maps can be made for each main season. Resource mapping is a useful vehicle for discussing differences between individuals and groups in terms of access to the resources.
- Mobility maps, showing the seasonal and annual movements of herds. Comparing maps representing different years provides insight into strategies in normal and adverse years, changes in mobility over time (e.g. 10 years ago and now) or responses of resource users to interventions such as dam construction.

Comparison of maps depicting the present situation and different periods in the past can reveal evolution in land use. Also time-series photographs (either aerial or fixed ground views of the landscape) are valuable for examining vegetation trends and discussing reasons for them. Such discussions often reveal socioeconomic changes in the grassland system.

Flow charts

Flow charts depict the flow of events in a resource use system. Of particular interest for livestock systems are *bioresource flow diagrams*. The producers draw the flows of nutrients and other inputs into a farm and between components of it. The diagram provides an inventory of available resources and a basis for discussing alternative ways of using the resources. Lightfoot *et al.* (1991b) have produced a guide for participatory modelling of bioresource flows. The diagrams can also depict flows in areas larger than farms, showing the linkages between cropping, livestock keeping, wood cutting, gathering and other uses of natural resources, and how actions of different users influence the well-being of others. On this basis, experiments in forms of shared use of these resources can be negotiated.

Another form of flow chart is the *process diagram* for analysing selected economic activities of a household or community. Key informants or a discussion group list the steps in the production process and the inputs and outputs at each step, and show how different people are involved. The information is noted in words or symbols on the chart. This gives a focus for discussing costs and returns, who incurs or gains them, and the likely impact of proposed changes in the enterprise. A process diagram of dairy production (Fig. 16.4) revealed that the people (men) paying for improved

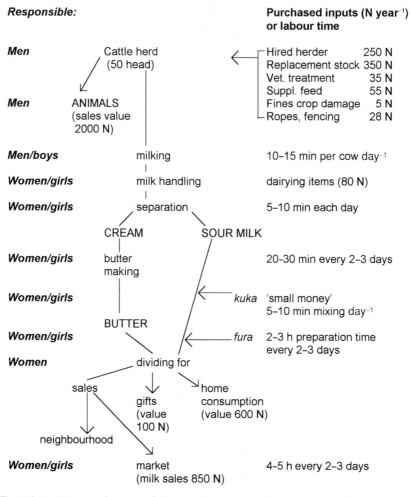

Fig. 16.4. Process diagram of dairy production. Products are in capital letters; N = naira year^{-1} (naira = local currency); *kuka* = pith from baobab pods; *fura* = millet dumplings. (Source: Waters-Bayer, 1988, based on measurements by Fulani women plus observations and interviews by FSR team in central Nigeria.)

pasture were not the people (women) who would benefit from the expected increase in milk sales. Particularly in enterprises with a marked division of labour and benefits according to gender, joint analysis of such charts makes it clearer to researchers and producer families whether innovations are likely to lead to the desired results.

Time charts

Various tools have been developed to visualize sequence of events, seasonality of activities and use of time. *Historical matrices* can show how resource use has changed over decades, and the causes and effects of these changes on relative availability of resources. Elderly men and women, either together or separately, distinguish the time periods to compare; divisions can be marked by major events, such as droughts or wars. These form the horizontal axis of the matrix. Components of the issues being studied (e.g. resource abundance) are listed vertically. The relative importance of each activity or resource in each historical period is then shown. Open-ended questions stimulate discussion about reasons for differences between the periods. Good examples of the use of this tool are given from Senegal and The Gambia by Schoonmaker Freudenberger and Schoonmaker Freudenberger (1994) and from Mongolia by Cooper and Gelezhamtsin (1994).

Seasonal analysis diagrams or *calendars* are made by asking local people to distinguish divisions of the year (months, seasons) in their own terms, and to mark these with symbols or local names. Counters are then placed, or marks made, to show the relative importance of the different periods. One example is a forage calendar showing the importance of different forages in different seasons (Bayer and Waters-Bayer, 1998). This helps to pinpoint major problems in forage supply or accessibility. When considering innovations that could solve problems identified by means of a forage calendar, it should be compared with a calendar of household labour inputs, differentiated according to gender and age. This will help to assess the feasibility of allocating labour at a particular time of year to developing a new forage resource.

Intra-household division of labour and time spent on livestock keeping and other activities throughout a day can be visualized in *daily timelines*. These are made like a calendar, but using time divisions of the day rather than year. Separate time charts can be made by men and women to depict their own activities and their perceptions of the other gender's activities. Availability and management of time for new activities can then be discussed. This and other tools for participatory situation analysis and planning from a gender perspective are described by Westphal *et al.* (1994) and Narayan (1996).

Conclusions

The emphasis in this chapter has been on research methods that integrate different perceptions and forms of knowledge held by producers and scientists of different disciplines. Experience with people-centred research in grassland and livestock systems that has been gained in recent years reveals that it is just as applicable and necessary in industrialized countries as in the 'Third World' (Pearson and Ison, 1997).

In collaborative research, the land users play a major role in deciding on research questions and how to address them, manage the experiments themselves and interpret the results with scientists' support. In addition to revealing the socioeconomic factors that drive grassland systems, this type of research serves several purposes:

- It incorporates local knowledge and insights into the design and analysis of the research.
- It helps to develop the land users' own knowledge systems.
- It supports local efforts to plan and implement change.
- It strengthens local capacities to innovate and to adjust the production systems to changing conditions, and to demand relevant support from agricultural services, including influence on the formal research agenda.
- It increases the likelihood that the research results will be relevant for and applied by the land users.

During the research process, the land users and scientists will identify questions that require study under controlled conditions, either to validate results or to investigate elements needed in developing new technologies. Collaborative research can give the ownership of innovation development to local people and, through its linkage with formal research, can make this more responsive to stakeholders' needs.

References

Amir, P. and Knipscheer, H.C. (1989) *Conducting On-farm Animal Research: Procedure and Economic Analysis.* Winrock International Institute for Agricultural Development, Morrilton/International Development Research Centre (IDRC), Ottawa, 244 pp.

Anderson, S., Gündel, S., Marais, M. and Wondewossen, T. (1999) Consultative appraisal: linking farmers' and researchers' perspectives for a mediation of a more sustainable agriculture. In: Doppler, W. and Calatrava, J. (eds) *Technical and Social Systems Approaches for Sustainable Rural Development: Proceedings of the Second European Symposium of the Association of Farming Systems Research and Extension in Granada, Spain.* Margraf Verlag, Weikershem, pp. 100–112.

Ashby, J.A. (1990) *Evaluating Technology with Farmers: a Handbook.* International Centre for Tropical Agriculture (CIAT), Cali, Colombia, 95 pp.

Bayer, W. and Waters-Bayer, A. (1998) *Forage Husbandry*. Macmillan, London, 192 pp.

Biggs, S.D. (1989) *Resource-poor Farmer Participation in Research: a Synthesis of Experiences from Nine National Agricultural Research Systems*. International Service for National Agriculture Research, The Hague, 37 pp.

Birch, I. (1994) 'The whole big world is here': PRA training workshop, Baragoi, 2–10 February 1994. Oxfam, Nairobi, 60 pp.

Bosch, O.J.H., Williams, J.W., Allen, W.J. and Ensor, A.H. (1996) Integrating community-based monitoring into the adaptive management process: the New Zealand experience. In: West, N.E. (ed.) *Proceedings Fifth International Rangeland Congress 1995*, Vol. II. Society for Range Management, Denver, Colorado, pp. 105–106.

Breman, H. and De Ridder, N. (eds) (1991) *Manuel sur les pâturages des pays sahéliens*. Karthala, Paris, 485 pp.

Campbell, A. (1994) *Community First: Landcare in Australia*. Gatekeeper Series No. 42, International Institute for Environment and Development (IIED), London, 19 pp.

Clark, R. (1993) Local consensus data, grazing management practices needed and constraints to be overcome. In: *Will Cells Sell? Proceedings of a Grazing Systems Seminar, Rockhampton, 26 October 1993*. Soil and Water Conservation Association of Australia, Queensland Branch, Brisbane, pp. 34–46.

Clark, R. (1997) Starting with a vision or the mess: a new technique to enable people to identify opportunities to change their practices. In: *2nd Australasia Pacific Extension Network Conference, 18-21 November 1997*. Albury, New South Wales, 8 pp.

Cooper, L. and Gelezhamtsin, N. (1994) Historical matrices: a method for monitoring changes in seasonal consumption patterns in Mongolia. In: Kirsopp-Reed, K. and Hinchcliffe, F. (eds) *RRA Notes 20: Special Issue on Livestock*. International Institute for Environment and Development (IIED), London, pp. 124–126.

Davis, C.D. (1990) *The Community's Toolbox: the Idea, Methods and Tools for Participatory Assessment, Monitoring and Evaluation in Community Forestry*. FAO, Rome, 146 pp.

Dorward, P.T., Shepherd, D.D. and Wolmer, W.L. (1997) Developing farm management type methodologies for participatory needs assessment. *Agricultural Systems* 55(2), 239–256.

Feldstein, H.S., Butler Flora, C. and Poats, S.V. (1993) *The Gender Variable in Agricultural Research*. International Development Research Centre, Ottawa, 58 pp.

Gbégo, I.T. and Van den Broek, A. (1996) Rapid appraisal and in-depth topical surveys in participatory diagnostic research on small ruminant production systems: Southern Benin. In: Roeleveld, A.C.W. and Van den Broek, A. (eds) *Focusing Livestock Systems Research*. Royal Tropical Institute, Amsterdam, pp. 119–132.

Grandin, B.E. (1988) *Wealth Ranking in Smallholder Communities: a Field Manual*. Intermediate Technology Publications (ITP), London, 49 pp.

Grimble, R. and Wellard, K. (1997) Stakeholder methodologies in natural resource management: a review of principles, contexts, experiences and opportunities. *Agricultural Systems* 55(2), 173–193.

ILCA. (1990) *Livestock Systems Research Manual*, 2 vols. International Livestock Centre for Africa, Addis Ababa, 412 + 130 pp.

Ison, R.L. and Ampt, P.R. (1992) Rapid rural appraisal: a participatory problem formulation method relevant to Australian agriculture. *Agricultural Systems* 38, 363–386.

Jansen, H.G.P., Ibrahim, M.A., Nieuwenhuyse, A., Mannetje, L. 't, Joenje, M. and Abarca, S. (1997) The economics of improved pasture and silvipastoral technologies in the Atlantic Zone of Costa Rica. *Tropical Grasslands* 31, 588–598.

Jiggins, J. (1993) From technology transfer to resource management. In: Baker, M.J. (ed.) *Grasslands for Our World*. SIR Publishing, Wellington, New Zealand, pp. 184–191.

Kirsopp-Reed, K. and Hinchcliffe, F. (eds) (1994) *RRA Notes 20: Special Issue on Livestock*. International Institute for Environment and Development (IIED), London, 172 pp.

Krueger, R.A. (1994) *Focus Groups: a Practical Guide for Applied Research* 2nd edn. Sage Publications, London, 255 pp.

Laurent, C. and Centres, J.M. (1990) *Dairy Husbandry in Tanzania: a Development Programme for Smallholders in Kilimanjaro and Arusha Regions*. Document de travail de l'Unité de Recherche sur les Systèmes Agraire et le Développement, Versailles–Dijon–Mirecourt, 112 pp.

Lightfoot, C., Feldman, S. and Abedin, M.Z. (1991a) *Households, Agroecosystems and Rural Resources Management: a Guidebook for Broadening the Concepts of Gender and Farming Systems*. Bangladesh Agricultural Research Institute, Joydebpur/ International Center for Living Aquatic Resources Management (ICLARM), Manila, Philippines, 86 pp.

Lightfoot, C., Noble, R. and Morales, R. (1991b) *Training Resource Book on a Participatory Method for Modelling Bioresource Flows*. International Center for Living Aquatic Resources Management (ICLARM), Manila, Philippines, 29 pp.

Marty, A. (1985) La gestion des pâturages en zone pastorale (Région de Gao, Mali). *Cahiers de la Recherche-Développement* 6, 22–24.

McCartney, A., Rea, E., Clark, R. and Robinson, E. (1997) Best practices: extension that makes a difference to practices and performance. 2nd Australasia Pacific Extension Network Conference, 18-21 November 1997, Albury, New South Wales, 7 pp.

Mettrick, H. (1993) *Development Oriented Research in Agriculture: an ICRA Textbook*. International Centre for Development Oriented Research in Agriculture (ICRA), Wageningen, The Netherlands, 291 pp.

Moser, C.A. and Kalton, G. (1971) *Survey Methods in Social Investigation*, 2nd edn. Heinemann, London, 352 pp.

Narayan, D. (1996) *Toward Participatory Research*. Technical Paper No. 307, World Bank, Washington DC, 265 pp.

Oerlemans, N., Proost, J. and Rauwhorst, J. (1997) Farmers' study groups in the Netherlands. In: Van Veldhuizen, L., Waters-Bayer, A., Ramírez, R., Johnson, D.A. and Thompson, J. (eds) *Farmers' Research in Practice: Lessons from the Field*. Intermediate Technology Publications (ITP), London, pp. 263–277.

Pearson, C.J. and Ison, R.L. (1997) *Agronomy of Grassland Systems*, 2nd edn. Cambridge University Press, Cambridge, 222 pp.

Pretty, J.N., Guijt, I., Thompson, J. and Scoones, I. (1995) *Participatory Learning and Action: a Trainer's Guide*. International Institute for Environment and Development (IIED), London, 267 pp.

Pringle, H. and Burnside, D. (1996) Range condition assessment in a multi-value world. In: West, N.E. (ed.) *Proceedings Fifth International Rangeland Congress 1995* Vol. I, Society for Range Management, Denver, Colorado, pp. 456–457.

Roeleveld, A.C.W. and Van den Broek, A. (eds) (1996) *Focusing Livestock Systems Research.* KIT, Amsterdam, 151 pp.

Russell, D.B. and Ison, R.L. (1991) The research–development relationship in rangelands: an opportunity for contextual science. In: *Proceedings of Fourth International Rangeland Congress.* Montpellier, Vol. 3, pp. 1047–1054.

Scheuermeier, U. and Ison, R.L. (1992) Together get a grip on the future: an RRA in the Emmental of Switzerland. *RRA Notes 15.* International Institute for Environment and Development (IIED), London, pp. 56-64.

Schoonmaker Freudenberger, M. and Schoonmaker Freudenberger, K. (1994) Livelihoods, livestock and change: the versatility and richness of historical matrices. In: Kirsopp-Reed, K. and Hinchcliffe, F. (eds) *RRA Notes 20: Special Issue on Livestock.* International Institue for Environment and Development (IIED), London, pp. 144–148.

Scoones, I. (1997) Knowledge, power and grazing management: new challenges for research and extension systems. In: *Proceedings of XVII International Grassland Conference, 8–17 June 1997, Winnipeg and Saskatoon, Canada,* CD ROM, Vol. III.

Taylor-Powell, E. and Von Kaufmann, R. (1986) Producer participation in livestock systems research: experience with on-farm research among settled Fulani agropastoralists in central Nigeria. In: Flora, C.B. and Tomacek, M. (eds) *Selected Proceedings of Kansas State University's 1986 Farming Systems Research Symposium.* Kansas State University, Kansas City, pp. 257-276.

Van Veldhuizen, L., Waters-Bayer, A. and De Zeeuw, H. (1997) *Developing Technology with Farmers: a Trainer's Guide for Participatory Learning.* ZED Books, London, 230 pp.

Waters-Bayer, A. (1988) *Dairying by Settled Fulani Agropastoralists in Central Nigeria: The Role of Women and Implications for Dairy Development.* Wissenschaftsverlag Vauk, Kiel, Germany, 328 pp.

Waters-Bayer, A. and Bayer, W. (1994) *Planning with Pastoralists: PRA and More – a Review of Methods Focused on Africa.* GTZ Division 422 Livestock Farming, Veterinary Services and Fisheries, Eschborn, Germany, 173 pp.

Wella, E.B., Roeleveld, A.C.W., Ngendello, A.M. and Bunyecha, K.F.N. (1996) Setting livestock research priorities through a participatory rapid appraisal: Northwestern Tanzania. In: Roeleveld, A.C.W. and Van den Broek, A. (eds) *Focusing Livestock Systems Research.* KIT, Amsterdam, pp. 91–107.

Westphal, U., Bogmeier, U., van Gemmigen, G., Hanke, M., Hinrichs, A., Holthusen, B., Schneider, M. and Schwanz, V. (1994) *Participatory Methods for Situation Analysis and Planning of Project Activities: Experiences with Women and Youth in the Communal Areas of Namibia.* Humboldt University, Berlin, 186 pp.

Index

Page numbers in *italics* refer to figures.